Chimeric Antigen Receptor T-Cell Therapies for Cancer

A Practical Guide

Chimeric Antigen Receptor T-Cell Therapies for Cancer

A Practical Guide

Edited by

DANIEL W. LEE, MD
Assistant Professor
Department of Pediatrics
University of Virginia School of Medicine
Charlottesville, Virginia
United States

NIRALI N. SHAH, MD, MHSc
Lasker Clinical Research Scholar
Pediatric Oncology Branch
National Cancer Institute
Bethesda, Maryland
United States

ELSEVIER

Elsevier
Radarweg 29, PO Box 211, 1000 AE Amsterdam, Netherlands
The Boulevard, Langford Lane, Kidlington, Oxford OX5 1GB, United Kingdom
50 Hampshire Street, 5th Floor, Cambridge, MA 02139, United States

Notices
Knowledge and best practice in this field are constantly changing. As new research and experience broaden our
understanding, changes in research methods, professional practices, or medical treatment may become
necessary.

Practitioners and researchers must always rely on their own experience and knowledge in evaluating and using
any information, methods, compounds, or experiments described herein. In using such information or methods
they should be mindful of their own safety and the safety of others, including parties for whom they have a
professional responsibility.

To the fullest extent of the law, neither the Publisher nor the authors, contributors, or editors, assume any
liability for any injury and/or damage to persons or property as a matter of products liability, negligence or
otherwise, or from any use or operation of any methods, products, instructions, or ideas contained in the
material herein.

This research was supported in part by the Intramural Research Program of the NIH, National Cancer Institute,
Pediatric Oncology Branch

The content of this publication does not necessarily reflect the views of policies of the Department of Health and
Human Services, nor does mention of trade names, commercial products, or organizations imply endorsement
by the U.S. Government.

Library of Congress Cataloging-in-Publication Data
A catalog record for this book is available from the Library of Congress

British Library Cataloguing-in-Publication Data
A catalogue record for this book is available from the British Library

ISBN: 978-0-323-66181-2

For information on all Elsevier publications visit our website at
https://www.elsevier.com/books-and-journals

Publisher: Dolores Meloni
Acquisition Editor: Robin R Carter
Editorial Project Manager: Anna Dubnow
Production Project Manager: Kiruthika Govindaraju
Cover Designer: Alan Studholme

Typeset by TNQ Technologies

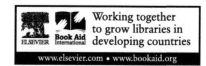

Dr. Lee would like to dedicate this book to his son, wife, and all his patients who, through their trust and generosity, have taught the CAR T-cell field so much.

Dr. Shah would like to dedicate this book to her family and friends, colleagues and mentors, but most importantly to the patients who have served as brave pioneers in advancing this new field of immunotherapy. The advances made in CAR T-cell therapy would not be possible without you.

List of Contributors

Nabil Ahmed, MD, MPH
Associate Professor, Pediatrics
Baylor College of Medicine
Houston, TX, United States

Jacob S. Appelbaum, MD, PhD
Fred Hutchinson Cancer Research Center
Seattle, WA, United States

Division of Hematology/Oncology
University of Washington School of Medicine
Seattle, WA, United States

Ben Towne Center for Childhood Cancer Research
Seattle Children's Research Institute
Seattle, WA, United States

Karen Ballen, MD
Professor of Medicine
Department of Medicine/Division of Hematology and
    Oncology
University of Virginia
Charlottesville, VA, United States

Cathy Conry Cantilena, MD
Department of Transfusion Medicine
National Institutes of Health Clinical Center
Bethesda, MD, United States

Francesco Ceppi, MD
Mother Women Child
Pediatric Oncology Unit
CHUV
Lausanne, VD, Switzerland

Kenneth Cornetta, MD
Professor of Clinical Medical and Molecular Genetics
Indiana University School of Medicine
Indianapolis, IN, United States

Kevin J. Curran, MD
Department of Pediatrics
Memorial Sloan Kettering Cancer Center
New York, NY, United States

Department of Pediatrics
Weill Cornell Medical College
New York, NY, United States

Center for Cell Engineering
Department of Medicine
Memorial Sloan Kettering Cancer Center
New York, NY, United States

Terry J. Fry, MD
Professor, Pediatrics and Hematology
University of Colorado Anschutz Medical Campus
Denver, CO, United States

Robert and Kathleen Clark Endowed Chair in Pediatric
    Cancer Therapeutics
Center for Cancer and Blood Disorders
Children's Hospital Colorado
Denver, CO, United States

Co-Director
Human Immunology and Immunotherapy Initiative
University of Colorado Anschutz Medical Campus
Denver, CO, United States

Rebecca A. Gardner, MD
Associate Professor Pediatrics
University of Washington
Seattle, WA, United States

Juliane Gust, MD, PhD
Center for Integrative Brain Research
Seattle Children's Research Institute
Seattle, WA, United States

Acting Instructor
Department of Neurology
Division of Pediatric Neurology
University of Washington
Seattle, WA, United States

Cristina Gutierrez, MD
Assistant Professor
Critical Care and Respiratory Care
University of Texas at MD Anderson Cancer Center
Houston, TX, United States

Steven L. Highfill, PhD
Center for Cellular Engineering
Department of Transfusion Medicine
Clinical Center
Bethesda, MD, United States

Assistant Director
Center for Cellular Engineering
NIH
Bethesda, MD, United States

Elad Jacoby, MD
Head, Pediatric Cancer Immunotherapy
Division of Pediatric Hematology, Oncology and BMT
The Edmond and Lily Safra Children's Hospital
Sheba Medical Center
Tel Hashomer, Ramat Gan, Israel

Sackler Faculty of Medicine
Tel Aviv University
Tel Aviv, Israel

Ping Jin, PhD
Center for Cellular Engineering
Department of Transfusion Medicine
Clinical Center
Bethesda, MD, United States

Sujith K. Joseph, PhD
Senior Staff Scientist
Pediatrics, Hematology/Oncology
Baylor College of Medicine
Houston, TX, United States

Senior Staff Scientist
Cancer and Hematology Centers
Texas Children's Hospital
Houston, TX, United States

Tamila L. Kindwall-Keller, DO
Associate Professor
Division of Hematology/Oncology
Department of Medicine
University of Virginia School of Medicine
Charlottesville, VA, United States

Krishna V. Komanduri, MD
Division of Transplantation and Cellular Therapy
Departments of Medicine, Microbiology and Immunology
Sylvester Comprehensive Cancer Center
University of Miami, Miller School of Medicine
Miami, FL, United States

Daniel W. Lee, MD
Assistant Professor
Director Pediatric Hematopoietic Stem Cell Transplantation and Immunotherapy

Division of Pediatric Hematology/Oncology
Departments of Pediatrics and Internal Medicine
University of Virginia School of Medicine
Charlottesville, VA, United States

Kris M. Mahadeo, MD, MPH
Doctor, Pediatric Stem Cell Transplantation and Cellular Therapy
CARTOX Program
University of Texas at MD Anderson Cancer Center
Houston, TX, United States

Eoghan Molloy, MB BCh, MRCPI, FRCPath
Department of Transfusion Medicine
National Institutes of Health Clinical Center
Bethesda, MD, United States

Victor M. Orellana-Noia, MD
Fellow Division of Hematology and Oncology
Department of Medicine
University of Virginia School of Medicine
Charlottesville, VA, United States

Rimas J. Orentas, PhD
Ben Towne Center for Childhood Cancer Research
Seattle Children's Research Institute
Seattle, WA, United States

Department of Pediatrics
University of Washington School of Medicine
Seattle, WA, United States

Sandhya Ramanathan Panch, MD, MPH
Center for Cellular Engineering
Department of Transfusion Medicine
Clinical Center
Bethesda, MD, United States

Staff Clinician, Hematology/Transfusion Medicine
Clinical Center
National Institutes of Health
Bethesda, MD, United States

Jae H. Park, MD
Center for Cell Engineering
Department of Medicine
Memorial Sloan Kettering Cancer Center
New York, NY, United States

Karlo Perica, MD, PhD
Center for Cell Engineering
Department of Medicine
Memorial Sloan Kettering Cancer Center
New York, NY, United States

Navin Pinto, MD
Ben Towne Center for Childhood Cancer Research
Seattle Children's Research Institute
Seattle, WA, United States

Department of Pediatrics
University of Washington School of Medicine
Seattle, WA, United States

Craig A. Portell, MD
Associate Professor of Medicine
Division of Hematology/Oncology
Department of Medicine
University of Virginia School of Medicine
Charlottesville, VA, United States

Michael A. Pulsipher, MD
Section Head, Transplantation and Cellular Therapy
Cancer and Blood Disease Institute
Children's Hospital Los Angeles
USC Keck School of Medicine
Los Angeles, CA, United States

Khaled Sanber, MD, PhD
MeRIT Resident
Department of Medicine
Center for Cell and Gene Therapy
Baylor College of Medicine
Houston, TX, United States

Nirali N. Shah, MD, MHSc
Associate Research Physician
Pediatric Oncology Branch
National Cancer Institute
National Institutes of Health
Bethesda, MD, United States

Haneen Shalabi, DO
Assistant Research Physician
Pediatric Oncology Branch
National Cancer Institute
National Institutes of Health
Bethesda, MD, United States

David Stroncek, MD
Center for Cellular Engineering
Department of Transfusion Medicine
Clinical Center
Bethesda, MD, United States

Chief, Cell Processing Section
Department of Transfusion Medicine
NIH Clinical Center
Bethesda, MD, United States

Corinne Summers, MD
Assistant Member Clinical Research Division Fred
 Hutchinson Cancer Research Center
Seattle, WA, United States

Assistant Professor Department of Pediatrics
University of Washington
Seattle Children's Hospital
Seattle, WA, United States

Francesco Paolo Tambaro, MD, PhD
Doctor
Bone Marrow Transplant Unit
AORN Santobono-Pausilipon
Naples, Italy

Agne Taraseviciute, MD, PhD
Assistant Professor of Clinical Pediatrics
Cancer and Blood Disease Institute
Children's Hospital Los Angeles
USC Keck School of Medicine
Los Angeles, CA, United States

Cameron J. Turtle, MBBS, PhD, FRACP, FRCPA
Associate Member
Clinical Research Division and Integrated Immuno-
 therapy Research Center
Fred Hutchinson Cancer Research Center
Seattle, WA, United States

Associate Professor
Department of Medicine
University of Washington
Seattle, WA, United States

Indumathy Varadarajan, MBBS
Assistant Professor
Division of Hematology/Oncology
Department of Medicine
University of Virginia School of Medicine
Charlottesville, VA, United States

Alan S. Wayne, MD
Professor of Pediatrics and Medicine
Director, Cancer and Blood Disease Institute
Head, Division of Hematology-Oncology
Vice Chair, Department of Pediatrics
Children's Hospital Los Angeles

Associate Director
USC Norris Comprehensive Cancer Center
USC Keck School of Medicine
Los Angeles, CA, United States

Kamille A. West, MD
Chief, Blood Services Section
Department of Transfusion Medicine
National Institutes of Health Clinical Center
Bethesda, MD, United States

Introduction

Never has a treatment paradigm evolved as rapidly, or in as short a period of time, as has the field of chimeric antigen receptor (CAR) T-cell therapy. From the initial work of Zelig Eshhar who provided the foundation for the earliest version of T-bodies that would evolve into current CAR T-cell constructs, to the FDA approval in 2017 of the first CAR T-cell therapy for children and young adults with acute lymphoblastic leukemia, the promise of CAR T-cell therapy has revolutionized the field of cancer immunotherapy.

Along with the success of this therapy, however, has come the realization of all the many components that are required to lead to a successful outcome and where obstacles may lie. From the very basic elements of when to refer a patient and optimizing the apheresis product to the intricacies of CAR T-cell manufacturing, simply getting to the infusion requires a significant amount of planning and careful considerations. Following infusion comes the difficult task of managing acute toxicities associated with cytokine release syndrome, neurotoxicity, and beyond, and then monitoring for response, relapse, and other more delayed complications. Future directions will require development of novel constructs which can overcome issues of relapse and optimize responses in cancers that extend beyond B-cell targeting. The development and implementation of such strategies also requires a deep understanding of the current regulatory guidance providing oversight of these genetically modified T-cells.

While there have been many recent reviews and single-center reports on CAR T-cell therapy, never has there been one comprehensive work devoted to providing a complete summary of the experiences to date. Accordingly, *Chimeric Antigen Receptor T-Cell Therapies for Cancer*, is the first such complete book to take on the daunting task of summarizing exactly this. We are deeply indebted to the many experts in the field who contributed to this work and to the brave patients, young and old, who embarked with us on a new frontier where very little was known. Indeed, this first book dedicated solely to CAR T-cell therapy is intended to provide a guide toward the practical considerations of the many multifaceted aspects of CAR T-cell therapy.

Sincerely,
Daniel W. Lee
Nirali N. Shah

Contents

CHAPTER 1

When to Refer a Patient for CAR T-Cell Therapy

VICTOR M. ORELLANA-NOIA, MD • CRAIG A. PORTELL, MD • KAREN BALLEN, MD

INTRODUCTION

Chimeric antigen receptor (CAR) T-cell immunotherapy is a rapidly emerging and highly publicized new treatment modality, which has gained significant attention for its effectiveness, side effects, and costs. Early-phase clinical trials have shown dramatic results in patients with often heavily pretreated disease, including those with relapsed/refractory childhood acute lymphoblastic leukemia (ALL)[1,2] and adult diffuse large B-cell lymphomas (DLBCL).[3–5] With recent US Food and Drug Administration (FDA) approval of two CAR T-cell products in these disease groups and ongoing clinical trials in many other clinical contexts, the number of patients who will receive CAR-based adoptive immunotherapy is expected to grow substantially in the coming years. The criteria by which providers will decide who and when to refer for CAR T-cell therapy will continue to evolve considerably as the field matures, and considerations of referral timing, therapeutic target, and treatment-related toxicity will remain important factors going forward.

In this chapter, we propose a series of questions which the referring provider should consider in deciding when to refer a patient for CAR T-cell therapy. These aim to address key factors in this process including which diseases are appropriate for CAR T therapy, what the expected timelines are for treatment, and what organ function criteria are needed to tolerate therapy. Finally, we will review the use of CAR T-cells in special populations, including elderly and human immunodeficiency virus (HIV)–positive patients, for whom the use of CAR T therapy is less established and will warrant further study as the field continues to grow.

CAN MY PATIENT WAIT FOR CHIMERIC ANTIGEN RECEPTOR T-CELL THERAPY?

One of the most significant limitations in access to CAR T-cell therapy is the waiting period needed for product manufacturing. From apheresis to infusion, most CAR T-cell products studied to date have required at least two if not several weeks to complete the necessary procedural steps.[1,2,6,7] For some centers with extensive experience and on-site manufacturing, the process and time requirements may be significantly reduced. However, most institutions considering CAR T-cell therapy for a patient now are either referring a patient to one of these established centers or relying on commercial products that are manufactured at a separate facility and shipped back for the patient's infusion when a sufficient cellular dose has been produced. Numerous attempts have been made to shorten this highly complex and heavily regulated process, including novel cellular processing methods and ongoing efforts to create "off-the-shelf" CAR T-cell products. For now, CAR T-cells remain a therapy requiring significant time investment, which by necessity dictates that only those who are able to wait for treatment are able to receive it.

Knowing that these and other delays may affect the timing of an eventual CAR T-cell infusion, early consideration of potential rate-limiting steps is an important part of a successful referral for CAR T-cell therapy. A few such possibilities include timing of apheresis, additional screening procedures for patients enrolling onto clinical trials, insurance approvals, and coordination of travel to a specialized center.

For some patients, rapidly progressive or CNS-penetrant disease (see below) may require more expedited therapy, either as a temporizing maneuver or instead of CAR T-cells depending on the clinical scenario. Bulky disease has also been postulated as a reason to consider alternative therapies, given that patients with higher disease burden appear to have more pronounced cytokine release following CAR T-cell infusion and may derive less benefit from therapy.[1,2,8,9] Debulking therapy prior to CAR T-cell administration, either in the form of alternative preparative course or via one or more cycles of chemotherapy prior to beginning a dedicated lymphodepletion regimen, may be appropriate on a case-by-case basis. However, this remains an area of active investigation, where no particular strategy in a given context can necessarily be considered standard of care. For patients potentially enrolling onto clinical trials, this is especially important, as different protocols may have varying limitations on prior therapies including bridging or debulking regimens. For now, deciding when to refer patients who may benefit from CAR T-cell therapy but have pressing treatment needs remains a challenge, and providers should weigh the risks of delaying referral carefully against those of earlier intervention with more conventional therapies.

CAN MY PATIENT TOLERATE THE TOXICITIES FROM CHIMERIC ANTIGEN RECEPTOR T-CELL THERAPY?

Deciding whether a patient can withstand the unique toxicities of CAR T-cell therapy is another important early consideration in deciding when to refer a patient. These toxicities, which can range from mild to life-threatening, are described in greater detail elsewhere (see Chapters 5–8). It is worth noting that while many efforts are being made to better describe these toxicities and how to manage them when they occur, our ability to accurately predict who will develop life-threatening or fatal CAR-related toxicity remains limited. As such, one general principle when considering any patient for CAR T-cell therapy is whether they could potentially endure the physiologic stress of severe cytokine release syndrome (CRS) or neurotoxicity.

At present, there are no uniformly applied screening criteria for those set to receive CAR T-cell therapy, as compared with allogeneic stem cell transplantation, which requires rigorous screening and published comorbidity assessment scores prior to deciding a patient's candidacy for treatment.[10] Likewise the FDA labels for both tisagenlecleucel and axicabtagene ciloleucel, the two commercially available CAR T-cell products, do not list any absolute contraindications to therapy.[11,12] However, there are some populations where risk of CRS is thought to be significantly increased. As mentioned, bulky disease appears to correlate with severe CRS and decreased therapeutic efficacy, though CAR T-cells can still be effective in a number of patients with high disease burden. Otherwise eligible patients with poor performance status may be unable to withstand severe CRS and should be

considered for other therapies. Patients with an active infection should have their infection adequately treated prior to CAR T-cell infusion. Furthermore, patients who require an external drain for an organ (nephrostomy tube, pleural drain, peritoneal drain, cholecystostomy, etc.) are at high risk of infection and subsequent CRS. Central venous catheters, however, are not considered high risk and are often required for the CAR T-cell infusion.

Most CAR T-cell products are currently prescribed within the context of a clinical trial requiring patients to satisfy screening criteria necessary for trial enrollment. There is currently a gap between this and the necessary screening for patients receiving commercial products. Most clinical trials to date have employed similar restrictions in terms of performance status (usually ECOG 0–1) and cardiopulmonary function. Patients with evidence of heart failure clinically or by cardiac imaging have typically been excluded from trials, as have those requiring supplemental oxygen for any reason. However, other impairments in pulmonary function such as COPD are less consistent, and pulmonary function testing, which is a prerequisite for stem cell transplantation, is not necessarily a requirement at this time.

Further study is still needed in several key groups (see Table 1.1), primarily those excluded from the cadre of early-phase clinical trials currently published. Notably the FDA labels for both tisagenlecleucel and axicabtagene ciloleucel caution against use in patients above the age of 65 years; though as mentioned, none of these factors (including age) are currently listed as an absolute contraindication.[11,12]

When considering patients in one of these categories for CAR T-cell therapy, limiting such referrals to those

TABLE 1.1 **High-Risk or Unstudied Populations for CAR T-Cell Therapy.**
Elderly (age >65)
HIV-positive
Hepatitis B/C
CNS disease
Organ dysfunction[a]
Bulky nodal disease burden
Rapidly progressive disease

[a] Cardiac, pulmonary, renal, hematologic (i.e., prior thrombotic or bleeding diathesis).

who are otherwise in good health and ensuring careful communication may help ensure an overall safer outcome in these understudied populations.

CAN MY PATIENT RECEIVE THEIR CARE AT A SPECIALIZED CENTER?

Though many institutions without prior CAR T-cell clinical trial experience are now treating their first patients with commercially available products, this is for now limited to selected institutions with appropriate training, resources, and monitoring in place. Many of these steps, and much of the posttreatment monitoring that is performed, fall under the Risk Evaluation and Mitigation Strategies (REMS), which are part of the conditional approvals by the FDA for each of the commercial CAR T-cell products.[13,14]

The goals of these, as listed by the FDA, are the same for each product:

1. Ensuring that hospitals and their associated clinics that dispense (the CAR T-cell product) are specially certified and have on-site, immediate access to tocilizumab
2. Ensuring those who prescribe, dispense, or administer (the CAR T-cell product) are aware of how to manage the risks of CRS and neurological toxicities

Similar REMS programs are anticipated for any future CAR T-cell product brought to market, though the exact nature and requirements of such a program may evolve as the field continues to gain experience with CAR T-cell therapy and its complications. It should also be expected that, like other cellular therapies, CAR-T-cell administration will remain restricted to specialized centers for the foreseeable future and that patients will need to remain in close proximity to these centers for at least some prespecified period of time following their initial therapy. Whether a uniform accreditation process for CAR T therapy emerges, through the Foundation for the Accreditation of Cellular Therapy (FACT) or some other organization, remains to be determined. For now, eligibility to administer each commercial product is granted through the pharmaceutical company responsible for the individual product, although FACT accreditation for autologous stem cell transplantation is frequently part of the criteria used in selecting CAR T-cell centers.

IS THERE A CHIMERIC ANTIGEN RECEPTOR FOR MY PATIENT?

As with any targeted therapy, CAR products are limited by whether a patient's disease bears the requisite therapeutic target. For example, T-cell lymphomas do not typically express B-cell markers such as CD19 and would not be expected to respond to therapy with a CD19 CAR. However, multiple CAR products are currently in use or under investigation, each at different stages of therapeutic development based on target and indication. These have primarily shown efficacy in hematologic malignancies, beginning with anti-CD19 CARs in relapsed/refractory CLL.[15] CARs against CD20, CD22, CD30, and BCMA are all in various stages of development, as are combination CARs with bi- and trispecific constructs. Many other targets and diseases have been studied, with varying results in terms of efficacy and toxicity. While many of the specific details for CAR development and disease-specific considerations will be discussed in later chapters, we will briefly explore a few key concepts as they pertain to deciding which patients can and should be referred for CAR T-cell therapy.

First, the use of CAR T-cell therapy remains largely experimental, with the exception of the two FDA approved products for use under specific indications (see Table 1.2). Most CAR products continue to be given within the context of a clinical trial, meaning the decision of when to refer a patient will depend in part on a working familiarity with which centers and

TABLE 1.2			
FDA-Approved Chimeric Antigen Receptor T-Cell Products.			
Product Name	**Generic Name**	**Target**	**Indication**
Kymriah (Novartis)	Tisagenlecleucel	CD19	Pediatric ALL (up to age 25), r/r after 2+ lines of therapy Adult DLBCL, including transformed FL and HGBL (age 18+), r/r after 2+ lines of therapy
Yescarta (Kite)	Axicabtagene ciloleucel	CD19	Adult DLBCL, including transformed FL and HGBL (age 18+), r/r after 2+ lines of therapy

trials are available as well as a consideration of the specific trial's entry criteria. Second, most CAR T-cell products have been studied in the setting of multiply relapsed disease, typically after at least two lines of previous therapy. Moving CAR T-cell therapy earlier in the treatment course for a given disease may provide better outcomes but will need to be weighed carefully against the efficacy and risks of current regimens. Third, what therapy should follow CAR T-cell treatment, including possible autologous or allogeneic stem cell transplantation depending on the underlying disease, remains an open question in many of these settings and will be discussed later in Chapter 10.

B-Cell Acute Lymphoblastic Leukemia

Relapsed/refractory pediatric B-cell ALL remains one of the strongest indications for CAR T-cell therapy, particularly using CD19 CAR products. The first approved indication for CAR T-cell therapy was in this population with tisagenlecleucel, and other products are currently under investigation. Likewise, expanding the use of CAR T-cell therapy to young and older adults remains an active area of study, though its use in these contexts remains limited to clinical trials and referrals for older patients should be carefully selected for those who could withstand potential treatment-related toxicities. Incorporating disease risk profile for individual patients may help guide the decision of who to refer for CAR T-cell therapy and when in the course of their disease. This is especially being explored in patients with MRD-positive disease after induction or consolidation therapy, given the clear efficacy of CD19 CAR T-cell therapy in this disease, low tumor burden in this particular context, and the steep decline in treatment outcomes when failing frontline therapy. CAR T-cell therapy in standard or low-risk B-cell ALL may not be worth the toxicity risk given that these patients are often cured of their disease with standard treatments. However, should the therapy be seen as safer than a prolonged chemotherapy course needed to treat this population, it may prove to be beneficial.

Diffuse Large B-Cell Lymphoma

Similar to B-cell ALL, CD19 CAR T-cells are now available as standard of care in the relapsed/refractory setting after two lines of prior therapy and have shown significant promise even for heavily pretreated patients. These therapies are being tested earlier in the conventional treatment paradigm, most notably with the ongoing clinical study evaluating axicabtagene ciloleucel against salvage chemotherapy and autologous stem cell rescue in first relapse (ZUMA-7; NCT03391466).

This important study may change how we treat patients failing anthracycline-based chemotherapy regimens. However, as noted previously the decision of when to refer patients with rapidly progressive disease should balance the need for definitive therapy with ensuring adequate disease control during the CAR T-cell manufacturing period.

We do not anticipate that CAR T-cell therapy will replace anthracycline-based chemoimmunotherapy as the front line choice for the majority of patients, given the favorable outcomes and minimal toxicity with regimens such as R—CHOP. Challenging these regimens with earlier use of CAR T-cell therapy should therefore be undertaken carefully and likely limited to those with higher risk features (double- or triple-hit, transformed disease, etc.) who historically have shown less favorable outcomes with conventional therapies. Meanwhile, our practice in referring patients with DLBCL continues to be in the second relapse with standard-of-care commercial CAR T-cell products or by enrolling patients in clinical trials in either the first or second relapse depending on patient, disease, and clinical trial specifics.

Follicular Lymphoma

While the majority of follicular lymphoma is very indolent and therefore unlikely to derive significant benefit from CAR T-cell therapy compared with its inherent risks, there are some follicular lymphomas that behave very aggressively, despite having a low-grade histology. Unfortunately, we cannot reliably identify these patients with standard methods. Many of them will demonstrate evidence of transformed disease and thus would be eligible for the commercial CD19-directed CAR T-cell therapies. For those with multiply refractory low-grade disease, several studies are currently underway to examine who among these may benefit from CAR T-cell therapy.

Chronic Lymphocytic Leukemia

Similar to follicular lymphoma, CLL presents heterogeneously and will remain indolent for the majority of patients. However, for a subset of patients with aggressive disease or certain high-risk features (i.e., del 17p or TP53 mutant), treatment of CLL often warrants an aggressive approach. With many new targeted therapies available to patients with this disease, such as ibrutinib or venetoclax, CAR T-cell therapy remains a consideration that is relegated to the multiply relapsed setting and strictly within the contexts of a clinical trial. Of note, none of these targeted agents are curative, whereas the goal for CAR T-cell therapy in this context would likely be to establish long-term remissions either with CAR T-cells alone or as a bridge to allogeneic stem cell transplantation. With the first published reports of successful CAR T-cell therapy being in patients with heavily pretreated CLL,[15] there is likely to be a role for CAR T-cell therapy in young, otherwise healthy patients with CLL, and multiple studies are currently ongoing to better clarify its use in this setting.

Additional Diseases

The role for CAR T-cell therapy in other hematologic malignancies and solid tumors remains experimental, though progress is being made in several diseases with novel antigen targets. These include CD30 in Hodgkin's disease and T-cell lymphomas[16,17] as well as BCMA in multiple myeloma.[18,19] As these therapies are still earlier in development compared with other CAR products, referring patients with these diseases is necessarily limited to clinical trials that typically restrict enrollment to those with multiply relapsed disease and otherwise fit enough to withstand potential toxicities. Deciding who and when to refer for non–CD19-directed CAR T-cell therapy remains an open question for further study. It remains to be seen whether similar toxicities will be seen as CAR T-cell therapy is expanded to additional targets or whether new antigen-specific toxicities will emerge.

IS CAR T-CELL THERAPY WORTH THE RISK FOR MY PATIENT?

Perhaps the most challenging question in referring patients for CAR T-cell therapy is assessing what their individual risk will be compared with that of pursuing alternative treatment options. This is especially true for populations where CAR T-cells have been less well studied (see Table 1.1) and for those with poor performance status, where the therapeutic potential may be eclipsed by toxicity risk. As mentioned previously, there is no standardized approach to quantifying risk of CAR-T-cell therapy. This is in large part due to the significant heterogeneity of CAR products, each of which acts differently based on the underlying disease state, numerous patient factors, and the CAR construct itself. Individual toxicities will be addressed in later chapters but should be considered early on when determining if CAR T-cell therapy can be given safely.

Other factors to consider may not fall under physiologic complications of therapy but can pose significant challenges to patients. The cost of commercial CAR products gained attention early on, ranging from $373,000 to $475,000 based on product and indication, with the full cost of therapy, including hospitalizations and supportive care, significantly higher than this.[20,21] Patients should have medical insurance coverage to consider these therapies; however, those insurance companies and governmental agencies have not yet come to consensus on how to cover the cost of the CAR T-cell product and expenses around it. At the time of writing this chapter, the Centers for Medicare and Medicaid Services (CMS) have not given guidelines on their coverage though ruling is expected soon. Private insurers are approving each patient on a case by case basis, and thus, these prior authorizations will extend the time required prior to getting the CAR T-cell product. Prior authorizations are likely to be needed before the apheresis procedure.

Similar to stem cell transplantation, patients will be required to remain within close proximity of their treatment center for a prespecified period of time. This is set at 4 weeks within 2 hours travel distance for the current FDA-approved products but may be different if treatment is through a clinical trial. For those living further away, time from home should be discussed early on with a focus on maintaining good psychosocial support during their treatment.

CONCLUSIONS

Cited as the most important oncologic advance in 2018, more than 300 clinical trials exploring the use of CAR T-cell therapy across a multitude of solid tumors and hematologic malignancies are currently underway. To date, there are no standardized eligibility criteria or comorbidity scores to predict success or toxicities with CAR T-cell therapy, meaning that the decision of who and when to refer for this modality of treatment remains highly individualized and variable. We have outlined several key questions to ask when considering referring a patient for CAR T-cell therapy, noting that much of this is based on experience rather than standardized practice. As one example of addressing this unmet need, many transplant centers currently use a pretransplant comorbidity score to select patients and predict outcomes for allogeneic stem cell transplantation.[10] This score incorporates organ, body mass index, history of infections, and psychiatric disease, with higher scores being associated with poorer survival. We propose a similar scoring system with CAR T-cell therapy and believe a pre-CAR T-cell comorbidity score will aid in helping to decide when to refer a patient.

REFERENCES

1. Lee DW, Kochenderfer JN, Stetler-Stevenson M, et al. T cells expressing CD19 chimeric antigen receptors for acute lymphoblastic leukaemia in children and young adults: a phase 1 dose-escalation trial. *Lancet.* 2015; 385(9967):517–528. https://doi.org/10.1016/S0140-6736(14)61403-3.

2. Maude SL, Frey N, Shaw PA, et al. Chimeric antigen receptor T cells for sustained remissions in leukemia. *N Engl J Med.* 2014. https://doi.org/10.1056/NEJMoa1407222.

3. Kochenderfer JN, Dudley ME, Kassim SH, et al. Chemotherapy-refractory diffuse large B-cell lymphoma and indolent B-cell malignancies can be effectively treated with autologous T cells expressing an anti-CD19 chimeric antigen receptor. *J Clin Oncol.* 2015;33(6):540–549. https://doi.org/10.1200/JCO.2014.56.2025.

4. Locke FL, Neelapu SS, Bartlett NL, et al. Phase 1 results of ZUMA-1: a multicenter study of KTE-C19 anti-CD19 CAR T cell therapy in refractory aggressive lymphoma. *Mol Ther.* 2017;25(1):285–295. https://doi.org/10.1016/j.ymthe.2016.10.020.

5. Neelapu SS, Locke FL, Bartlett NL, et al. Axicabtagene ciloleucel CAR T-cell therapy in refractory large B-cell lymphoma. *N Engl J Med.* December 2017. https://doi.org/10.1056/NEJMoa1707447. NEJMoa1707447.

6. Turtle CJ, Hanafi L-A, Berger C, et al. Immunotherapy of non-Hodgkins lymphoma with a defined ratio of CD8+ and CD4+ CD19-specific chimeric antigen receptor-modified T cells. *Sci Transl Med.* 2016;8(355). https://doi.org/10.1126/scitranslmed.aaf8621, 355ra116-355ra116.

7. Davila ML, Riviere I, Wang X, et al. Efficacy and toxicity management of 19-28z CAR T cell therapy in B cell acute lymphoblastic leukemia. *Sci Transl Med.* 2014;6(224). https://doi.org/10.1126/scitranslmed.3008226, 224ra25.

8. Park JH, Rivière I, Gonen M, et al. Long-term follow-up of CD19 CAR therapy in acute lymphoblastic leukemia. *N Engl J Med.* 2018;378(5):449–459. https://doi.org/10.1056/NEJMoa1709919.

9. Hay KA, Hanafi L-A, Li D, et al. Kinetics and biomarkers of severe cytokine release syndrome after CD19 chimeric antigen receptor-modified T cell therapy. *Blood.* September 2017. https://doi.org/10.1182/blood-2017-06-793141. blood-2017-06-793141.

10. Sorror ML. How I assess comorbidities before hematopoietic cell transplantation. *Blood.* 2013;121(15):2854–2863. https://doi.org/10.1182/blood-2012-09-455063.

11. FDA – U.S. Food & Drug Administration Approved Products – KYMRIAH (tisagenlecleucel). https://www.fda.gov/biologicsbloodvaccines/cellulargenetherapyproducts/approvedproducts/ucm573706.htm. Accessed July 6, 2018.

12. FDA - U.S. Food & Drug Administration Approved Products - YESCARTA (axicabtagene ciloleucel). https://www.fda.gov/biologicsbloodvaccines/cellulargenetherapyproducts/approvedproducts/ucm581222.htm. Accessed July 6, 2018.

13. FDA. Approved Risk Evaluation and Mitigation Strategies (REMS) – Kymriah. https://www.accessdata.fda.gov/scripts/cder/rems/index.cfm?event=IndvRemsDetails.page&REMS=368. Accessed June 9, 2018.

14. FDA. Approved Risk Evaluation and Mitigation Strategies (REMS) – Yescarta. https://www.accessdata.fda.gov/scripts/cder/rems/index.cfm?event=IndvRemsDetails.page&REMS=375. Accessed June 9, 2018.

15. Porter DL, Levine BL, Kalos M, Bagg A, June CH. Chimeric antigen receptor–modified T cells in chronic lymphoid leukemia. *N Engl J Med.* 2011;365(8):725–733. https://doi.org/10.1056/NEJMoa1103849.

16. Ramos CA, Ballard B, Zhang H, et al. Clinical and immunological responses after CD30-specific chimeric antigen receptor–redirected lymphocytes. *J Clin Invest.* 2017; 127(9):3462–3471. https://doi.org/10.1172/JCI94306.

17. Wang C-M, Wu Z-Q, Wang Y, et al. Autologous T cells expressing CD30 chimeric antigen receptors for relapsed or refractory Hodgkin lymphoma: an open-label phase I trial. *Clin Cancer Res.* 2017;23(5):1156–1166. https://doi.org/10.1158/1078-0432.CCR-16-1365.

18. Ali SA, Shi V, Maric I, et al. T cells expressing an anti-B-cell maturation antigen chimeric antigen receptor cause remissions of multiple myeloma. *Blood.* 2016;128(13):1688–1700. https://doi.org/10.1182/blood-2016-04-711903.

19. Brudno JN, Maric I, Hartman SD, et al. T cells genetically modified to express an anti–B-cell maturation antigen chimeric antigen receptor cause remissions of poor-prognosis relapsed multiple myeloma. *J Clin Oncol.* 2018;36(22):2267–2280. https://doi.org/10.1200/JCO.2018.77.8084.

20. Hagen T. *Novartis Sets a Price of $475,000 for CAR T-Cell Therapy;* 2017. Published http://www.onclive.com/web-exclusives/novartis-sets-a-price-of-475000-for-car-tcell-therapy.

21. Clarke T, Berkrot B. *FDA Approves Gilead Cancer Gene Therapy; Price Set at $373,000.* Reuters; 2017. Published https://www.reuters.com/article/us-gilead-sciences-fda/fda-approves-gilead-cancer-gene-therapy-price-set-at-373000-idUSKBN1CN35H.

CHAPTER 2

Optimizing the Apheresis Product*

EOGHAN MOLLOY, MB BCH, MRCPI, FRCPATH • CATHY CONRY CANTILENA, MD • KAMILLE A. WEST, MD

INTRODUCTION

Definition and Early Beginnings of Apheresis

Apheresis, named after the ancient Greek word meaning "taking away," is a medical procedure in which blood is drawn from a donor or patient and separated into its component parts outside of the body, allowing selective retention of a particular component and return of the remainder by reinfusion. The most common modern application of apheresis is the collection of specific blood components for transfusion from allogeneic donors, such as platelets, plasma, red cells, and granulocytes. Apheresis may also be employed in a therapeutic context to treat disease by removing pathologic cells or plasma-bound substances. Leukapheresis is the general term for white blood cell (WBC) collection by apheresis.

The history of modern leukapheresis had its beginnings in the National Cancer Institute at the National Institutes of Health. In the 1960s, George Judson, an IBM engineer whose son had chronic myelogenous leukemia, worked with Dr. Emil Freireich to develop an instrument comprising a reusable centrifugal bowl connected to the patient, to separate and deplete excess leukocytes from venous whole blood (WB) in a continuous manner, reinfusing the remaining red cells, platelets, and plasma.[1] Subsequently, leukapheresis was optimized for granulocyte collections, hematopoietic progenitor cell (HPC) and lymphocyte collection from healthy donors. Over 50 years later, collection of autologous lymphocytes from patients has been increasing with the development of novel cellular therapies such as CAR T-cells. Compared with healthy donors, patients undergoing CAR T-cell treatment have a number of characteristics that may impact the collection procedure, the quality of the apheresis material, and downstream processing in the cell manufacturing facility.

Managing each unique apheresis procedure ultimately affects the successful manufacture of the CAR T-cell product and is therefore of the utmost importance.

APHERESIS BASICS

Principles and Technical Considerations in Apheresis

Modern apheresis devices for cellular collections work on the principle of centrifugal separation of blood components based on their density or specific gravity (see Fig. 2.1). Mononuclear cell (MNC) apheresis targets the layer comprising mostly lymphocytes (60%) and monocytes (20%), as well as granulocytes (15%), red blood cells (RBCs; 3%–5%) and platelets; however, absolute demarcation of specific cell populations (e.g., T-lymphocytes) is not possible. Further processing or purification of the apheresis product by elutriation, or antibody-bound magnetic beads, is required to select for the targeted cell type.

The apheresis procedure begins with the removal of WB from the patient via an IV catheter or central line. The apheresis machine is generally prepared before the patient arrives and contains a sterile, single-use, functionally closed disposable tubing set or kit that has been primed with normal saline. The extracorporeal circuit must be anticoagulated to prevent blood clotting in the tubing and kit during the procedure. Citrate-based anticoagulant (AC) is routinely used, generally AC citrate dextrose solution A (ACD-A), which is added to tubing sets during apheresis procedures and returns to the patient with the reinfusion of blood from the circuit. It exerts its AC effect by chelating ionized calcium (iCa), a necessary cofactor in the clotting cascade, as well as other divalent cations such as magnesium (iMg). Citrate AC may cause symptoms due to hypocalcemia and/or hypomagnesemia during the apheresis procedure; however, these are generally mild, and due to its rapid metabolism, with a short half-life of 36 minutes, residual effects are not prolonged. Because citrate is quickly

---

*Contributed by Eoghan Molloy, Cathy Conry Cantilena & Kamille West is under Public Domain, as they are US Government employee.

Separation by centrifugation

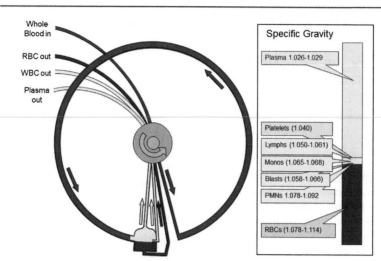

FIG. 2.1 **Schematic diagram depicting separation of whole blood components in the centrifugal apheresis circuit.** (Adapted with permission from David M. Ward, MD, FRCP, HP (ASCP), Emeritus Professor, Division of Nephrology and Hypertension, Department of Medicine, University of California San Diego.)

metabolized, it is not a systemic AC and therefore will not cause sustained bleeding risk in patients postprocedure. Supplemental heparin anticoagulation may be used routinely in some centers according to institutional practice or limited to select cases at the discretion of the Apheresis Medical Director to minimize the risk of bleeding or heparin-induced thrombocytopenia (HIT).

Citrate delivery rates generally range from 1.0 to 1.8 mg/kg/minute. The ratio of WB to AC in the circuit (WB:AC) is typically 12:1 but can be changed depending on the instrumentation and procedure involved. The rate of citrate infusion is coupled to the WB flow rate and therefore to the length of the procedure. The faster the AC infusion rate, the greater the decline in iCa and iMg, with proportionally increased risk of symptoms and complications. When citrate accumulation outpaces metabolism, toxicity occurs. Citrate is metabolized by the Krebs (citric acid) cycle, mainly in the liver, but also in muscles and kidneys. Thus, patients predisposed to citrate toxicity include those with renal and hepatic insufficiency, low body mass, female gender, small children, and those undergoing longer procedures. An example worksheet used to calculate the ACD-A infusion rates, inlet flow rate, and prophylactic calcium and magnesium replacement in a pediatric patient is shown in Table 2.1.

During the procedure, a portion of the patient's blood volume, termed the extracorporeal volume (ECV), will be outside the body within the apheresis apparatus. The ECV

is dependent on the specific device and type of kit used. For a given patient, the ECV should not exceed 15% of the patient's total blood volume (TBV), as this will result in unsafe volume and RBC loss. In patients for whom the ECV slightly exceeds 15% of their TBV, the apheresis device may be primed with colloid (albumin) to limit the effects of the volume shift. Small children under 25 kg generally require a prime with an RBC unit to prevent severe intraprocedural anemia. Due to infusion of crystalloids and AC solution, the patient is often fluid positive after leukapheresis and may even have peripheral edema, with adequate renal function, this excess fluid is eliminated shortly after the procedure.

The patient's blood passes through the extracorporeal circuit in a continuous fashion; hence, apheresis procedures are described in terms of liters processed or blood volumes processed. To collect sufficient numbers of lymphocytes ($\approx 60-600 \times 10^6$/kg body weight) for CAR T-cell manufacture, processing at least two to four times the patient's TBV, termed large-volume leukapheresis (LVL), is required. Occasionally, up to six times the patient's TBV may be processed in pediatric cases to collect sufficient cells, provided that patient is tolerating the procedure well. Typical flow rates range from 50 to 90 mL/minute in adult patients and 30–50 mL/minute in children; thus, the procedure takes several hours to complete. The number of targeted cells to be collected and the peripheral blood counts determine the duration of the procedure. Therefore,

---

TABLE 2.1
Example of Infusion Calculation Worksheet for Pediatric Apheresis.

For Patient of Weight 19.8 kg

ACD-A:

- **Citrate infusion rate (CIR):** Default is 3.0 mg/kg/minute (acceptable range 2.5–3.5 mg/kg/minute)
- **ACD-A rate** = weight (kg) × CIR/21.4 = **19.8 × 3.0/21.4 = 2.8 mL/minute**
- **WB:AC ratio:** Default is 12:1, may change to 13:1 after first liter processed
- **Inlet flow rate** = ACD-A rate × AC ratio
  - 34 mL/minute when AC ratio 12:1
  - 36 mL/minute when AC ratio 13:1

IV CALCIUM AND MAGNESIUM PROPHYLAXIS:

- **CaCl rate: 20 × 2.8** mL/minute ACD-A = **56 mL/hour** (corresponds to 0.66 mg Ca/mL ACD-A)[a]
- **MgSO$_4$ admin rate:** 25% of Ca infusion rate → 56 mL/hour Ca × 0.25 = **14 mL/hour**

[a] Calcium Chloride 10% Injection 20 mL (2 g) in 0.45% Sodium Chloride, total volume 270 mL; final concentration of Elemental Ca = 2 mg/mL.
Magnesium Sulfate 50% Injection 7.5 mL (3.75 g) in 0.45% Sodium Chloride, total volume 125 mL; final concentration of Elemental Mg = 3 mg/mL.

---

patients with reduced absolute lymphocyte count (ALC) require a longer procedure to collect sufficient lymphocytes for CAR T-cell manufacture.

Investigators at the National Institutes of Health demonstrated that the CD3$^+$ count preapheresis correlates to the yield of CD3$^+$ cells in the collected product.[2] The use of preapheresis CD3$^+$ count as a prediction tool builds on the long established experience in apheresis clinics using preapheresis peripheral blood CD34$^+$ count to extrapolate collection yield during HPC harvest.[3] To utilize this approach, the apheresis clinic must have access to a flow cytometry laboratory during the collection procedure.

ORGANIZATION OF THE APHERESIS CLINIC

Apheresis clinics may be located within a hospital, blood collection facility or in stand-alone units. When the apheresis clinic is involved in provision of services to patients, in addition to healthy donors, it is most practical for them to be located at the hospital or site of primary patient medical care. Apheresis clinics must be appropriately staffed and equipped, have access to resources to care for sick patients, and comply with standards and guidelines for cell therapy collections.

Accrediting bodies provide guidance on the fundamental operations of the clinic and an outline of the personnel required to operate an apheresis service. Highly trained and competent apheresis operators, usually registered nurses, are essential to operate procedures. Necessary skills for personnel working in an apheresis clinic include assessment of donor/patient suitability/eligibility for apheresis, handling vascular access, operation of the apheresis device(s), management

of adverse clinical events, safe handling and labeling of collected products, and quality control of supplies and equipment. The apheresis clinic is operated under the supervision of an experienced medical director who is a licensed physician trained in transfusion medicine and/or hematology, with sufficient experience in apheresis, and knowledge of the federal regulations, and accreditation standards.[4] Standard operating procedures are mandatory for every type of apheresis procedure and should be readily available to performing staff.

Adequate storage space in the apheresis center is needed for apheresis disposable tubing, IV sets, saline, AC solutions, and other supplies. Since patients must sometimes tolerate several hours in the clinic, they and their family members must be made comfortable in hospital beds and nearby waiting areas. For small children, enough room must be available at the bedside for their parent(s) or caretaker(s) to stay with them. Nurses must have access to computers and printers at a station with view of the patient.

Helpful adjunctive services for the clinic include proximity to interventional radiology for central venous catheter (CVC) insertion; pharmacy support to provide intravenous calcium and magnesium solutions to mitigate citrate toxicity; and a nearby blood bank to issue RBC units when needed to prime the extracorporeal circuit. Ideally, a high complexity laboratory would also be on-site to provide cell counts and flow cytometry in real time; immediate access to stat laboratory results is mandatory for the workup and management of unexpected, urgent, or emergent adverse events. The shipping process requires coordination between the apheresis clinic and the manufacturing laboratory, which will often be at different sites, as the shipping and handling procedures must be congruent and timely.

REGULATORY CONSIDERATIONS

Emerging cellular therapies such as CAR T-cells provide promising therapeutic options for life-threatening diseases; however, these are not without risks of adverse outcomes. Regulations governing CAR T-cell manufacture are designed to ensure the safety and efficacy of biological products for human use and aid in the transition from translational research to clinical practice. In the United States, CAR T-cell manufacture, starting with the apheresis product, is regulated by the Food and Drug Administration (FDA). The FDA has issued guidelines concerning human cells, tissues, and cellular and tissue-based products (HCT/Ps). International organizations such as the Foundation for the Accreditation of Cellular Therapy (FACT) and AABB (formerly the American Association of Blood Banks) have also developed community-based standards with requirements for accredited cellular therapy programs.

Current good manufacturing practice (cGMP) for CAR T-cells starts at the apheresis facility, with stipulations for the environment (cleanliness, temperature, humidity) of the collection facility, and qualification of critical supplies such as IV fluids. The collection center must demonstrate evidence of appropriate training and competence of the apheresis operators, standard operating procedures,

good documentation practices, and appropriate retention of procedure records. Evaluation of the donor prior to collection is also a regulated step. The FDA does not mandate history screening and infectious disease testing tor autologous donors; however, if testing is performed for biohazard handling purposes, this must be done within ±7 days of MNC collection. Currently, many CAR T-cell therapies are still at the investigational stage, conducted under investigational new drug application in clinical trials; apheresis procedures must comply with applicable institutional review board requirements.

Quality assurance personnel within each facility verify compliance with requirements by conducting internal audits and facilitating external inspections from regulatory or accrediting bodies. If collections are to be shipped to another facility for manufacture, the apheresis clinic must be qualified by the cell manufacturing facility. This is generally conducted by a review of relevant records or an on-site audit of the apheresis center.

PATIENT/DONOR EVALUATION

At this stage, most CAR T-cell apheresis collections are collected from autologous donors; for the remainder of this chapter, we will discuss the process as it pertains to these patients/donors. Evaluation of the patient prior to autologous collection is primarily aimed at assessing and optimizing modifiable patient or disease

TABLE 2.2
Preparing for Autologous MNC Apheresis for CAR T-Cell Manufacture.

Preassessment	Parameter	Action Points
History	Age, weight, history of liver, renal, cardiopulmonary disease	If custom prime required, perform type and screen, order RBC unit, and ensure blood transfusion consent in chart Pediatric patients: Calculate TBV, SEV, WB flow rate, citrate, calcium ± magnesium infusion rate, heparin infusion if appropriate
Physical assessment	Arm veins, performance status	Recommend CVC if peripheral veins inadequate for LVL
Laboratory results	CBC, WBC, ALC $CD3^+$, peripheral blast %	Determine target lymphocyte/$CD3^+$ yield for manufacture, make preparation for repeat procedure if goal not met
Vascular access	Preexistent CVC	Confirm appropriateness of catheter for apheresis

ALC, absolute lymphocyte count; *CAR*, chimeric antigen receptor; *CBC*, complete blood count; *CVC*, central venous catheter; *LVL*, large-volume leukapheresis; *MNC*, mononuclear cell; *RBC*, red blood cell; *SEV*, safe extracorporeal volume; *TBV*, total blood volume; *WB*, whole blood; *WBC*, white blood cell.

factors that could affect the safety and success of the collection. A summary of the factors considered in patient evaluation in preparation for apheresis is shown in Table 2.2.

Physical Assessment

Prior to apheresis collection, physical assessment of the patient includes the patient age, height and weight, vital signs, vascular access, and performance status. Given that fluid shifts inherently occur during the procedure, evaluation of underlying cardiac, pulmonary, or renal disease is pertinent. Depending on the patient's baseline lymphocyte count, the procedure may take up to 6 hours and may require more than one procedure to collect the apheresis target. The ability of the patient to tolerate lying in bed attached to the apheresis machine for a prolonged period should be taken into account with any underling physical impairments. During preassessment, apheresis nurses examine peripheral veins to determine if they are acceptable for apheresis; patients should be well hydrated prior to examination.

Laboratory Assessment

Baseline laboratory data at preassessment should include at a minimum a complete blood count (CBC), renal function, baseline electrolytes, and mineral panel (calcium and magnesium), with other testing as indicated by the clinical history. Due to their primary treatment or underlying disease, patients who are candidates for CAR T-cell therapy may have a significant degree of anemia and thrombocytopenia. Standard operating procedures should include a minimum hemoglobin and platelet threshold prior to apheresis, for example, Hb $\geq$ 8 g/dL and platelet count $\geq$50,000/μL. If necessary, arrangements can be made for RBC or platelet transfusions prior to the procedure. Lymphopenia secondary to disease or prior treatment, or specifically a low CD3$^+$ count, portends a longer apheresis collection, and a second day of collection may be required to meet the target. Coagulopathy identified prior to the procedure should be corrected to reduce the risk of bleeding associated with vascular access insertion or as a consequence of platelet depletion during apheresis.[5] If a patient is known to be calcium or magnesium deficient prior to the procedure, these can be corrected preemptively; additional replacement calcium or magnesium can be administered during the procedure.

Disease Assessment

The current disease status of a patient planned for leukapheresis provides vital information that may affect the success of the collection procedure, as well as the purity and manufacture of the CAR T-cell product. CAR T-cell therapies are, at the time of writing, most commonly used to treat hematologic malignancies, primarily B-cell acute lymphoblastic leukemia (ALL) or lymphoma; other indications include multiple myeloma and prostate cancer. For patients with leukemia, lymphocyte apheresis yields may differ in patients in remission, or in a state of controlled disease, versus a patient with very active disease who requires bridging chemotherapy during the apheresis window.[2]

Patients who are heavily pretreated prior to leukapheresis, or those who have previously undergone stem cell transplantation or received lymphodepleting chemotherapy, may have significantly reduced total white cell count and lymphocyte counts. This poses both a technical challenge to the apheresis procedure in terms of establishing a stable buffy coat interface in the centrifuge and a numerical challenge in collecting sufficient T-cells to allow for CAR T-cell manufacture. In such cases, it is useful to measure the CD3$^+$ count during a patient preassessment to inform the anticipated success of the leukapheresis.

Pharmaceutical companies manufacturing CAR T-cells have recommended minimum peripheral blood lymphocyte counts prior to MNC collection, such as an ALC > 500/μL or CD3$^+$ >150/μL for the manufacture of tisagenlecleucel.[6] Collection of sufficient CD3$^+$ cells for CAR T-cell manufacture can be very challenging in patients with very low ALC; it can be helpful to obtain a CD3 count by flow cytometry prior to apheresis, to extrapolate the number of cells that will be collected per liter of blood processed.[2] Additionally, a sample can be drawn from the apheresis product midway through the procedure to assess whether the number of cells collected is in keeping with projected yields; the apheresis procedure may be extended to collect more cells as needed. However, flow cytometry is not readily available during apheresis in all centers; therefore, the alternative approach is to determine a set number of blood volumes to be processed and plan for a second day of collection if the cell yield was inadequate for CAR T-cell manufacture. Despite the challenges of collection in such patients, adequate collection in one MNC apheresis procedure has been reported in some patients with CD3$^+$ counts <150/μL.[7] Circulating blasts or tumor cells may contaminate the collected product and be deleterious to the successful manufacturing process and efficacy of the CAR T-cell product. In cases where this potential contamination may be suspected, the manufacturing laboratory should be informed prior to receipt of the apheresis product so that appropriate manufacturing steps can be taken to optimize the product (see Chapter 4, Role of the Local Cytotherapy Lab).

Timing of Apheresis

Planning the optimal timing for the apheresis collection is vital and requires multidisciplinary communication between the primary clinical team, the apheresis clinic, vascular access service, and the cell manufacturing facility, so that each step from the collection of CD3$^+$ cells onward to CAR T-cell manufacturing and ultimately infusion is coordinated successfully. If malignant disease is rapidly progressive, there may be a limited window of opportunity when apheresis can be safely undertaken. In such cases, bridging chemotherapy prior to apheresis may be performed to achieve disease stability, followed by a period of time for hematological recovery of sufficient lymphocyte counts to allow the patient to undergo leukapheresis.

Patients may undergo leukapheresis and have their cells immediately put into culture and manufacture, followed by fresh infusion. However, it has also been demonstrated successfully that the cells collected at apheresis can be cryopreserved prior to culture and manufacture or be cryopreserved postmanufacture for infusion to the patient at later date.[8] If a patient is anticipated to undergo CAR T-cell therapy at a future date not yet specified, apheresis can be performed when the patient is in remission or stable disease, with cryopreservation of the cells, which would then be thawed in the future for manufacture of the CAR T-cell product. Indeed, with the high success rates seen in CAR T-cell trials targeting B-cell malignancies, many providers are referring patients with high-risk disease for an apheresis much earlier in their treatment course to ensure a successful collection. This is somewhat similar to the collection and storage of autologous HPCs from patients with multiple myeloma to allow for future high-dose chemotherapy and autologous stem cell transplantation.

VASCULAR ACCESS FOR APHERESIS

Where possible, peripheral veins should be used in preference to inserting a CVC for vascular access; however, pediatric autologous CAR T-cell patients rarely have suitable peripheral veins to accommodate LVL. Some patients may already have a vascular access device in place to facilitate chemotherapy or other treatment; this device should be assessed for suitability for MNC apheresis. If a new CVC must be inserted for the procedure, either a temporary device solely for the cellular collection or long-term vascular access device may be selected as needed. Placement of an adequate CVC is particularly challenging in

children, requiring coordination with interventional radiology, sedation, analgesia, and postanesthesia recovery.

Peripheral Venous Access

Large-bore peripheral venous catheters are required to achieve flow rates needed for LVL. The draw site needle is typically a straight 16-gauge apheresis needle in the antecubital fossa, and the return site needle on the contralateral arm may be identical; alternatively, a 16–18 gauge peripheral IV catheter in the return antecubital fossa or forearm veins may be suitable. Veins may be dilated using warm packs or warming blankets. Ultrasound-guided peripheral venous access can also be considered in challenging cases to avoid the insertion of a CVC where possible.

Central Venous Access

Double-lumen catheters are required for LVL apheresis, to allow separate channels for WB draw and return. Temporary nontunneled central apheresis catheters are most commonly inserted into the internal jugular, subclavian, or femoral veins. To achieve satisfactory flow rates, a sufficiently large catheter should be inserted, considering patient size. Adult patients should have 10–13.5 French catheters inserted, and pediatric collections in patients weighing <25 kg may require 7 to 8-French catheters.[9] For examples of CVCs suitable for MNC apheresis, see Table 2.3. Catheter placement must be performed by experienced operators, using image guidance where applicable to minimize risk of complications and malposition.[10] Risks associated with CVC insertion include complications of anesthesia, infection, pneumothorax, bleeding, line thrombosis, cardiac arrhythmia, and vessel puncture; in one study, children under 4 years of age were at higher risk.[11,12] The apheresis clinic staff should examine the CVC for bleeding, discharge, or signs of infection prior to each use. Hospital policies vary, but routinely CVCs are flushed with saline and may be capped with heparin after use to avoid line thrombosis. Tissue plasminogen activator installation can be used to clear catheter occlusion by clots.

Long-term access CVCs may be inserted for patients undergoing autologous MNC collection, as they may facilitate both cellular collection and subsequent medication administration (e.g., chemotherapy) and infusion of the CAR T-cell product. Some patients will already have had a long-term CVC inserted prior to the date of MNC collection. These devices must be assessed by the apheresis clinic for suitability, as not all long-term CVCs are suitable for apheresis due to insufficient flow rates, due to their collapsible nature.

TABLE 2.3
Examples of Central Venous Catheters Suitable for Mononuclear Cell Apheresis.

Type	Name	Manufacturer	Gauge (Fr)	Comments
Nontunneled (Temporary)	Arrow	Arrow	12	Excellent flow rates up to 120 mL/minute. Polyurethane, easy to insert. Comfortable for patients in femoral location.
Tunneled	MedComp	MedComp	8–9, 7 for patients <15 kg	Excellent flow rates up to 60 mL/minute. Preferred pediatric catheter. Pliable silicon. More difficult to insert, but comfortable in jugular or femoral location.
	Quinton Mahurkar	Covidien	11.5	Excellent flow rates. Polyurethane, easy to insert. Preferred for jugular site due to curved externalized tubing; preferred catheter for course of plasma exchange.
Tunneled	Hemodialysis/ apheresis CVC	Hickman/Bard	13.5	Larger diameter may cause greater patient discomfort.
	Quinton PermCath	Covidien	11.5	Excellent flow rates. Preferred for plasma exchange. Easy to insert though slightly more stiff-walled and uncomfortable.

Manufacturers provide information on each of their CVC devices, with specifications. The options for long-term CVCs include tunneled CVCs and tunneled CVC ports. Tunneled CVCs are inserted through a subcutaneous "tunnel" on the anterior chest wall, prior to entry into a large central vein such as the subclavian vein, under image guidance. There is a cuff on the catheter, which induces granulation within the tunnel, serving as an anchor ensuring the line remains securely in place. Tunneled CVCs have a lower infection risk compared with temporary CVCs.

Tunneled CVC ports are another option for long-term access but are not often used for apheresis. A subcutaneous port is placed anterior chest wall, and this port is connected to the catheter, which is inserted into a large central vein. Ports may either be dual lumen or single lumen. Dual lumen ports available include the Vortex port (AngioDynamics, Inc., NY, United States), with reported flow rates of 40–50 mL/minute. Single lumen ports can used as the draw site for apheresis, and a return site such as peripheral venous catheter must be inserted. One such single lumen port is the Powerflow port (Bard, Inc., NJ, USA), with reported flow rates of up to 150 mL/minute in simulated testing. Both single and dual lumen ports have been used for apheresis procedures, including red cell exchange and extracorporeal photopheresis. The data on their use in cellular collection are more limited but expected to increase.

APHERESIS DEVICES FOR MONONUCLEAR CELL COLLECTION

There are multiple commercially available apheresis devices, which work by similar principles with slight technical differences. In 2019, the Spectra Optia (Terumo BCT Inc.; CO, USA) and the Amicus Cell Separator (Fenwal Inc., Fresenius Kabi AG; IL, USA) are FDA cleared for MNC collection. In other countries, other devices such as the COM.TEC (Fresenius Kabi AG, Germany) are also used. Performance characteristics of apheresis collections include (1) total yield of desired cells, (2) minimizing collection of off-target cells (RBCs, platelets), and (3) collection efficiency (CE), the proportion of circulating cells of interest that are harvested by the apheresis procedure.

Since the 1980s, MNC apheresis has primarily been optimized in two clinical settings: first in mobilized donors for HPC collection[13] and then for allogeneic donor lymphocyte infusions for HPC transplant recipients.[14] In both these settings, abundant or adequate numbers of leukocytes are available for collection. In contrast, CAR T-cell candidates are often lymphopenic; thus, targeting this narrow MNC layer for collection can be technically difficult. Published comparisons of mobilized HPC collections on different instruments generally show that CE and yields are relatively similar, with lower red cell contamination using the (now defunct) COBE Spectra and COM.TEC, and lower platelet

TABLE 2.4
Autologous MNC Collections for CAR T-Cell Manufacture on Different Apheresis Devices.

References	Patient Diagnosis	Target	Device	N	Volume Processed (L)	CE (%)
Allen et al.[2]	ALL, solid tumors	CD3$^+$	COBE	71	8.4 (4.0–18.0)	(CE1) 58.97[a], 67.97[b]
Even-Or et al.[20]	Precursor B-ALL	MNC	COBE	11	10.0 ± 1.2	40.3 ± 6.2%
			Optia	15	10.0 ± 1.4	57.9 ± 4.6%
Ceppi et al.[6]	ALL, neuroblastoma	Lymph	COBE	102	8.0 (2.8–13.3)	83.4 (13.7–6103.2)%
Tuazon et al.[21]	B-cell malignancies	Lymph	COBE	71	11.6 (11.1–17.4)[c]	32 < 40%, 39 > 40%
			Optia	21		9 < 40%, 12 > 40%

N = number of procedures. Volumes processed reported as mean ± SD, or median (range). CE = CE2 unless otherwise specified. *ALL*, acute lymphoblastic leukemia; *CAR*, chimeric antigen receptor; *CE*, collection efficiency; *MNC*, mononuclear cell.
[a] Collection below target.
[b] Collections above target yield of >2 × 10^9 CD3$^+$ cells.
[c] Volume of blood processed not specified per device.

contamination with Amicus.[15] In a prospective randomized multicenter study, the Spectra Optia showed superior CE for CD34$^+$ cells compared with the COBE, with reduced granulocyte and platelet contamination.[16] However, the optimal parameters for HPC collection may not be applicable to collection of mature T-cells for CAR T-cell manufacture for several reasons. First, nonmobilized CAR T-cell patients often have low total WBC counts, making identification and continued isolation of the WBC interface challenging. Second, mature lymphocytes are smaller and denser than immature HPCs, which makes RBC removal from the product a greater challenge.

Reports of unmobilized MNC collections from healthy donors report CEs ranging from 44% to 62% on multiple devices.[17–19] For autologous collections for CAR T-cell therapy, CE ranged from <40% to >80%[2,6,20,21] as summarized in Table 2.4. However, most or all patients in these studies met the specified target yield, with sufficient cells for manufacture obtained in a single collection. Fortunately, with planning, most CAR T-cell therapy candidates undergo successful autologous MNC apheresis collections, achieving preset lymphocyte goals. The apheresis procedure can be extended if needed for patients with low ALC or CD3$^+$ counts to achieve target yields; however, the longer the procedure, the greater the RBC and platelet loss from the patient, and hence the greater the risk of citrate-related toxicity.

ADVERSE EVENTS DURING APHERESIS
The majority of donors and patients undergo apheresis safely. Overall, adverse events related to therapeutic apheresis (TA) for patients is higher than in apheresis

donors and has been reported in the range of 5% −12%.[22] The overall incidence of TA fatalities was reported as rare at 0.05%, but deaths may have been related to severe preexisting conditions.[23] A recent World Apheresis Association registry report indicated there were no deaths in >50,000 patients.[24] Specifically in relation to MNC collections for CAR T-cell production, the adverse event rate in two studies performed in predominantly pediatric and young adult patients was 9.8%−15%, with only two events considered severe among the cumulative patient total of 170 from both studies; one patient had an allergic reaction to apheresis tubing,[6] and another patient with progressive ALL developed hypoxia and seizures ascribed to his underlying disease rather than to apheresis.[2]

The most common adverse events are associated with citrate AC, including decreasing ionized calcium, magnesium, hypokalemia, and transient metabolic alkalosis, and can be anticipated and managed. Citrate toxicity is usually mild and includes symptoms such as perioral tingling and paresthesias. Moderate symptoms include nausea and vomiting, abdominal cramping, hypotension, and carpopedal spasm; while severe symptoms include tetany, cardiac arrhythmias, and seizures.[25] If a patient has symptomatic hypocalcemia, the apheresis operator can pause the procedure, slow the inlet WB flow rate and AC pump rate, or increase the WB AC ratio. Most of these interventions will effectively prolong the procedure for the patient. In very small pediatric patients (<20 kg), to limit citrate exposure and shorten the length of the procedure, a reduced amount of ACD-A supplemented by unfractionated heparin may be used. However, since heparin carries additional risk such as bleeding and HIT, it is often avoided. To proactively prevent and manage

---

TABLE 2.5
Information Affixed or Attached to Mononuclear Cell Apheresis Product.

1. Donation identification number (permanently affixed to container)
2. Name of product (affixed or attached)
3. Donor identification (internal protocols only), (affixed or attached)
4. Date of collection
5. Time of completion of collection
6. Name of facility/donor registry
7. Approximate product volume or weight
8. Names and volumes of anticoagulants and other additives
9. For patient-specific product, recipient name and/or identifier
10. Recommended storage temperature
11. "For Autologous use only" or "For Intended Recipient only" (affixed or attached)

---

hypocalcemia in patients, prophylactic continuous IV calcium infusions are routinely used in large-volume apheresis[26]; IV magnesium infusions can also be considered in pediatric patients (<40 kg) and patients with renal impairment or diabetes.[27] Hypotensive reactions may be due to a vasovagal event, fluid shifts, or hypocalcemia, and bedside clinical assessment is necessary. Bleeding, hematoma, and other complications associated with vascular access insertion are uncommon.

After the apheresis procedure, patient vital signs are taken and laboratory data are evaluated, such as a CBC to evaluate for postprocedure anemia or thrombocytopenia. Patients should be given routine postapheresis instructions to drink plenty of fluids, restrict strenuous exercise for 24 hours, and elevate feet if feeling dizzy or lightheaded. Patients may require transport by wheelchair. A clinician should document a summary of the procedure in the patient's medical record and describe any complications, along with actions taken as necessary. If a temporary CVC was placed, it should be flushed and capped with an infusion plug and removed by trained personnel if there is no need for a further day of collection.

APHERESIS PRODUCT TRANSPORT AND HANDLING

Once the procedure is completed, the apheresis nurse must disconnect the bag containing collected product from the remainder of the kit and heat-seal the tubing to achieve sterile product closure. The nurse then assesses the product appearance, integrity of all ports, and seals; confirms the accuracy of the label; and ensures the chain of custody is preserved. The product should be labeled in accordance with International Society of Blood Transfusion (ISBT) Cellular Therapy Nomenclature specifications. The clinical protocol group or manufacturing company may require additional product labeling. The label contains an individual identification number, which is to be used throughout the chain of custody.

The original collection container label must be placed on the container at the time of collection. The label must include, at a minimum, the name of product (ISBT code) and a unique identifier (donation identification number, DIN). Additional labeling information may be attached to the collection before the product is removed from the immediate vicinity of the donor, as listed in Table 2.5. After labeling the apheresis product, the accuracy of the label and donor identification should be verified and documented.

SUMMARY AND FUTURE DIRECTIONS

MNC leukapheresis is a vital early step in CAR T-cell manufacture and treatment of the patient. Apheresis procedures, in the hands of trained, knowledgeable personnel, are safe and effective to collect starting material. While early trials are investigating the possibility of using off-the-shelf third-party collections from healthy donors, at this point, CAR T-cells are manufactured using autologous lymphocytes from patients; therefore, conscientious patient care is needed during the apheresis procedure. In children and adults, collection of adequate CD3$^+$ lymphocytes from heavily pretreated lymphopenic patients can be difficult but may be possible with planning and ongoing evaluation of the procedure.

CONFLICTS OF INTEREST

The authors have no conflicts of interest to declare. The views expressed are the authors' own and do not represent the National Institutes of Health, the Department of Health and Human Services, or the US Federal government.

REFERENCES

1. Freireich EJ, Judson G, Levin RH. Separation and collection of leukocytes. *Cancer Res.* 1965;25:1516–1520.
2. Allen ES, Stroncek DF, Ren J, et al. Autologous lymphapheresis for the production of chimeric antigen receptor T cells. *Transfusion.* 2017;57:1133–1141.
3. Leberfinger DL, Badman KL, Roig JM, Loos T. Improved planning of leukapheresis endpoint with customized prediction algorithm: minimizing collection days, volume of blood processed, procedure time, and citrate toxicity. *Transfusion.* 2017;57:685–693.
4. American Society for Apheresis. Guidelines for therapeutic apheresis clinical privileges. *J Clin Apher.* 2007;22:181–182.
5. Chibber V, King KE. Management of the therapeutic apheresis patient. In: McLeod BC, Weinstein R, Winters JL, Szczepiorkowski ZM, eds. *Apheresis: Principles and Practice.* 3rd ed. Bethesda, Maryland: AABB Press; 2010:240–241.
6. McGuirk J, Waller EK, Qayed M, et al. Building Blocks for institutional preparation of CTL019 delivery. *Cytotherapy.* 2017;19:1015–1024.
7. Ceppi F, Rivers J, Annesley C, et al. Lymphocyte apheresis for chimeric antigen receptor T-cell manufacturing in children and young adults with leukemia and neuroblastoma. *Transfusion.* 2018;58:1414–1420.
8. Elavia N, McManus A, Highfill SL, et al. The post-thaw recovery of cryopreserved chimeric antigen receptor (CAR) T-cells during manufacture is better than that of cryopreserved peripheral blood CD3$^+$ cells. *Blood.* 2017;130(Suppl. 1):4475.
9. Padmanabhan A. Cellular collection by apheresis. *Transfusion.* 2018;58(Suppl. 1):598–604.
10. Meisenberg BR, Callaghan M, Sloan C, Sampson L, Miller WE, McMillan R. Complications associated with central venous catheters used for the collection of peripheral blood progenitor cells to support high-dose chemotherapy and autologous stem cell rescue. *Support Care Cancer.* 1997;5:223–227.
11. Styczynski J, Balduzzi A, Gil L, et al. European group for blood and marrow transplantation pediatric diseases working party. Risk of complications during hematopoietic stem cell collection in pediatric sibling donors: a prospective European group for blood and marrow transplantation pediatric diseases working party study. *Blood.* 2012;119:2935–2942.
12. Michon B, Moghrabi A, Winikoff R, et al. Complications of apheresis in children. *Transfusion.* 2007;47:1837–1842.
13. To LB, Haylock DN, Thorp D, et al. The optimization of collection of peripheral blood stem cells for

14. Kolb HJ, Mittermüller J, Clemm C, et al. Donor leukocyte transfusions for treatment of recurrent chronic myelogenous leukemia in marrow transplant patients. *Blood.* 1990;76:2462–2465.
15. Deneys V, Fabry A, Van Hooydonk M, et al. Efficiency of autologous stem cell collection: comparison of three different cell separators. *Transfus Apher Sci.* 2017;56:35–38.
16. Cancelas JA, Scott EP, Bill JR. Continuous CD34+ cell collection by a new device is safe and more efficient than by a standard collection procedure: results of a two-center, crossover, randomized trial. *Transfusion.* 2016;56:2824–2832.
17. Schulz M, Bialleck H, Thorausch K, et al. Unstimulated leukapheresis in patients and donors: comparison of two apheresis systems. *Transfusion.* 2014;54:1622–1629.
18. Steininger P, Zimmermann R, Eckstein R, Strasser E. Possible reasons for variable leukapheresis collection outcomes with automated apheresis systems. *Transfusion.* 2014;54:2584–2585.
19. Anyanwu A, Sitzmann N, Hetjens S, Klüter H, Wuchter P. Low-volume leukapheresis in non-cytokine-stimulated donors for the collection of mononuclear cells. *Transfus Med Hemother.* 2018;45:323–330.
20. Even-Or E, Di Mola M, Ali M, et al. Optimizing autologous nonmobilized mononuclear cell collections for cellular therapy in pediatric patients with high-risk leukemia. *Transfusion.* 2017;57:1536–1542.
21. Tuazon SA, Li A, Gooley T, et al. Factors affecting lymphocyte collection efficiency for the manufacture of chimeric antigen receptor T cells in adults with B-cell malignancies. *Transfusion.* 2019;59:1773–1780.
22. Okafor C, Ward DM, Mokrzycki MH, Weinstein R, Clark P, Balogun RA. Introduction and overview of therapeutic apheresis. *J Clin Apher.* 2010;25:240–249.
23. Kaplan A. Therapeutic apheresis for nephrologists. Complications of apheresis. *Semin Dial.* 2012;25:152–158.
24. Henricksson MM, Newman E, Witt V, et al. Adverse events in apheresis: an update of the WAA registry data. *Transfus Apher Sci.* 2016;54:2–16.
25. Lee G, Arepally GM. Anticoagulation techniques in apheresis: from heparin to citrate and beyond. *J Clin Apher.* 2012;27:117–125.
26. Bolan CD, Cecco SA, Wesley RA, et al. Controlled study of citrate effects and response to i.v. calcium administration during allogeneic peripheral blood progenitor cell donation. *Transfusion.* 2002;42:935–946.
27. Haddad S, Leitman SF, Wesley RA, et al. Placebo-controlled study of intravenous magnesium supplementation during large-volume leukapheresis in healthy allogeneic donors. *Transfusion.* 2005;45:934–944.

autotransplantation in acute myeloid leukaemia. *Bone Marrow Transplant.* 1989;4:41–47.

CHAPTER 3

CAR T-Cell: Cell Processing Laboratory Considerations*

DAVID STRONCEK, MD • SANDHYA RAMANATHAN PANCH, MD, MPH • PING JIN, PHD • STEVEN L. HIGHFILL, PHD

INTRODUCTION

Chimeric antigen receptor (CAR) T-cells are one of the most rapidly growing cancer immunotherapies, particularly for B-cell malignancies.[1-9] While the manufacturing of CAR T-cells is relatively straightforward,[10] there are many barriers associated with the manufacturing process. Additionally, most CAR T-cells are produced from a patient's own or autologous lymphocytes, which creates many unique cell production and logistical challenges. Many patients receiving CAR T-cells have life-threatening cancers, and the progression of their disease may not allow for the manufacturing of another CAR T-cell product, should the first manufacturing attempt not yield sufficient quantities of cells.

An important goal for manufacturing all cell therapies is to consistently produce high-quality products. This is especially true for CAR T-cells. Factors that can cause or contribute to manufacturing failure include inability to collect sufficient quantities of T-cells, microbial contamination, low levels of T-cell transduction, insufficient expansion of T-cells in culture, and low levels of CD3+ T-cells in the final CAR T-cell product. Occasionally, CAR T-cells do not meet lot release criteria and cannot be used.[11,12] Although generally not a release criteria, skewing of CD4 and CD8 T-cells within the culture may have unintended clinical consequences and should be considered. The critical need for patients to receive CAR T-cells along with the possibility of poor manufacturing outcomes makes it important for healthcare professionals involved with cellular immunotherapy to understand the CAR T-cell manufacturing processing.

Some CAR T-cells are being manufactured commercially,[6,8,9,13] and many others are in early-phase clinical trials.[4,5] The commercial development of CAR T-cells has led to centralization of CAR T-cell manufacturing in large cell processing facilities. Although CAR T-cells are increasingly being manufactured in centralized current good manufacturing practice (cGMP) cell manufacturing facilities, academic hospital-based cell processing laboratories continue to manufacture CAR T-cells. In addition, academic medical centers that do not manufacture CAR T-cells may be involved with many aspects of CAR T-cell therapy. Hospital-based cell processing laboratories may ship the autologous cells used as starting material in the manufacturing process and receive, store, thaw, and issue the CAR T-cells. For commercially manufactured CAR T-cells, the details of the manufacturing process may not be available, but the processing laboratory will have access to the results of analysis of the final CAR T-cell product performed by the manufacturing facility, which the lab staff can help clinical care teams interpret. The cell processing laboratory staff can also address questions related to the CAR T-cell infusion and reactions associated with their infusion. This chapter will provide a general overview of manufacturing CAR T-cells as well as specific issues of importance to clinical care teams involved with treatment of patients with CAR T-cells.

GENERAL CONSIDERATIONS

Nature of the Cells Used to Produce CAR T-Cells

The manufacturing of any cellular therapy is highly dependent on the source of the cellular material used to manufacture the product. Genetically engineered cell therapies that must be HLA compatible with the recipient, such as CAR T-cells, are generally produced from

---

*Role of the Local Cytotherapy Lab contributed by David Stroncek, Sandhya Ramanathan Panch, Ping Jin & Steven L. Highfil is under Public domain as the contributors are US Government employee.

Chimeric Antigen Receptor T-Cell Therapies for Cancer. https://doi.org/10.1016/B978-0-323-66181-2.00003-2

the patient's own, or autologous, cells. Cell therapies that do not require HLA matching can be manufactured from any person willing to donate cells. In the latter scenario, cell therapies made from any healthy donor cells can be produced in large batches or lots, which may contain enough cells to treat hundreds of patients. In contrast, for CAR T-cells, an individual autologous cell therapy must be produced for each unique patient treated. Since each cell therapy lot manufactured must undergo in-process and lot release testing and quality review, producing autologous cell therapies is more resource-intensive and costly.

Currently, almost all CAR T-cells are being manufactured from autologous leukocytes. Efforts are underway to produce CAR T-cells using T-cells from healthy subjects, which have been engineered to no longer express T-cell receptor (TCRs) and major histocompatibility complex (MHC) molecules.[14–16] CAR T-cells that lack TCRs and MHC molecules could be used to treat any patient without causing graft-versus-host disease or being subject to immune-mediated rejection. The development of such a "universal donor" CAR T-cells would have several advantages over autologous CAR T-cells (Table 3.1). They could be produced in large quantities, which would allow cells from one lot to be used to treat many patients. This would eliminate many of the logistical problems related to manufacturing CAR T-cells and would allow for the distribution of the cost of in-process and lot release testing, and GMP manufacturing across many CAR T-cells doses rather than just one autologous lot. Overall, the cost of producing one dose of universal donor CAR T-cells would be much less than that of one autologous CAR T-cell product. In addition, an inventory of universal donor CAR T-cells could be developed. These cells would be available for immediate administration and hence would be an "off-the-shelf" therapy.

Manufacturing Facilities and Closed-System Processing

Since the media and conditions used to culture T-cells can promote the growth of microbes and any microbial contamination of the cells at any point in the collection and manufacturing process may result in microbial growth and cause serious harm to the recipient, considerable effort is taken to maintain sterility. The manufacturing process takes place in a highly controlled facility specifically designed to maintain an environment with minimal quantities of microbes. In addition, whenever possible, cells are cultured in vessels that are closed to the environment. T-cells can be expanded in a variety of different culture systems. Classically, T-cells have been expanded in flasks. However, standard laboratory culture flasks, such as

		TABLE 3.1 Comparison of Autologous and Universal Donor Chimeric Antigen Receptor T-Cells.	
Considerations	**Autologous**	**Universal Donor**
Lot size	A separate lot is required for each patient	One lot for many patients
Product testing	In-processing and lot release testing is performed on cells for every patient	In-process and lot release testing is performed on each lot
Consistency	High variability among products given to each patient	Same or similar product given to each patient
Time required to provide cells	Cells must be collected, manufactured, and tested	Cells can be given immediately
Manufacturing failures	Common	Rare
Consequence of manufacturing failure	Repeat manufacturing or no treatment	Provide cells from a different lot
Possible immune rejection	Low	High unless genetically modified
Possibility of causing graft-versus-host disease	Rare observance in patients with previous allogeneic hematopoietic stem cell transplantation	Possible unless genetically modified

T-flasks, are open to the environment and hence are subject to microbial contamination. The simplest closed culture systems are cell culture bags. Bags that are specifically designed for cell culture are available in a variety of sizes, which allows bag culture systems to easily accommodate a wide variety of culture volumes. Culturing T-cells in bags is limited by the relatively low T-cell concentration that must be maintained. Closed-system flasks specifically designed for T-cell growth[17,18] and closed-system bioreactors are also available and are being used for CAR T-cells production in several early phase clinical trials.[19,20] The impact of manufacturing methodologies on CAR T-cell function will be important to study.

Cells collected in bags can be sterilely connected to cell culture bags or closed-system culture flasks and bioreactors. In addition, culture media and other reagents can be purchased in bags, which can be sterilely connected to maintain the closed nature of these culture systems. Cells and culture media can also be removed sterilely from these closed-system bags, flasks, and bioreactors.

Automation

Automation of the CAR T-cell manufacturing process is highly desirable (Table 3.2). Automated instruments are available for cell separation, washing, concentration, and culture. Automation reduces the amount of staff time required in the manufacturing process. Manual processing is also associated with some variability due to differences among staff, and automation reduces this variability. In general, the time required to train staff to operate automated instruments is less than the time required to train staff to perform similar operations manually. Automated instruments developed more recently are likely to be more highly automated and to electronically document important elements of the procedure.[19]

There are some disadvantages to automation. Most instruments are designed for a specific range of cell quantities and culture media volume, and it may be difficult to work with quantities of cells and media outside this range. In addition, some automated culture systems provide limited measures of culture conditions, and it may be difficult to change these conditions. From more of a logistical perspective, many of the automated devices currently on the market require specific tubing

sets and reagents that are only available from the vendor that manufactures the instrument. Therefore, manufacturing facilities with these types of instruments run the risk of halting cell production if there are issues with a particular vendor. With the growth of cancer cellular immunotherapy, it is expected that the number and types of automated instruments available will grow and their quality and capabilities will improve.

Chain of Custody

As autologous cells used to manufacture CAR T-cells move from the collection center to the manufacturing facility and back to the medical center that administers the cells, it is critical to be sure that the cells can be linked to the patient throughout this process. Typically, to maintain this "chain of custody," the cells are labeled with a unique identification number that is assigned by the collection center and with patient identifiers such as name, date of birth, and medical record number. Whenever the cells are manipulated in a way that requires changing the container or vessel holding the cells, the unique identifiers are added to the new container or vessel. Each CAR T-cell product is labeled with patient identifiers, the product name, number of cells, and name of the manufacturing site. The label also includes the date of product manufacture and the product expiration date.

Regulatory Considerations

Medical facilities that treat patients with CAR T-cells, in general, are experienced with allogeneic and/or autologous hematopoietic stem cell (HSC) transplantation. However, the regulations concerning CAR T-cell manufacturing and HSCs processing differ greatly. All CAR T-cells are regulated much like drugs, vaccines, and other biologics and must be manufactured as a licensed biologic or under an investigational new drug (IND) application. If under an IND, they must contain the following statement, "Caution: New Drug—Limited by Federal Law to Investigational Use." HSCs are considered minimally manipulated cell therapies and are not subject to these regulations. CAR T-cells are expected to be manufactured using cGMPs. The number of air exchanges, level of air filtration, and staff and material flow requirements for the facilities used to manufacture CAR T-cells exceed those required for processing HSCs.

OVERVIEW OF CHIMERIC ANTIGEN RECEPTOR T-CELL MANUFACTURING

The manufacturing of CAR T-cells requires several separate processes or unit operations (Fig. 3.1). Typically,

TABLE 3.2
Comparison of Manual and Automated Processing Operations.

Considerations	Manual	Automated
Labor requirements	High	Low
Training requirements	High	Low
Processing closed to the environment	Possibly	Usually
Consistency of outcomes	Variable	High
Documentation of results	Manual entry	Electronic
Scalability	High	Limited

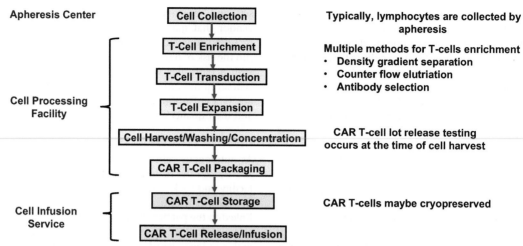

FIG. 3.1 **Steps in manufacturing chimeric antigen receptor (CAR) T-cells.** Several steps are involved with providing autologous CAR T-cell therapies. The peripheral blood mononuclear cells (PBMNCs) are generally collected from the patient by apheresis. Although the PBMNC concentrates collected by apheresis contain large quantities of lymphocytes, they must be enriched for T-cells. Several methods are being used for T-cell enrichment including density gradient separation, counterflow elutriation, and antibody selection. The T-cells are then placed in culture with factors that stimulate T-cell growth such as anti-CD3 plus IL-2 or anti-CD3/anti-CD28 beads plus IL-2. After a day or two in culture, the cells are transduced with retroviral or lentiviral vectors. The T-cells are then allowed to expand in culture for several days. At the end of the culture period, the CAR T-cells are harvested, washed, concentrated, and packaged. The cells are stored until they are issued and infused. If the CAR T-cells must be stored for more than a few hours, they are cryopreserved

CAR T-cells are manufactured from peripheral blood lymphocytes. Most are manufactured from autologous T-cells, but for recipients of allogeneic HSC transplants, CAR T-cells may still be collected from the patient who is now tolerated to the prior HSCT, or have been produced from T-cells collected from the HLA-matched related or unrelated HSC donor.[2] The autologous or healthy donor lymphocytes are collected as mononuclear cell concentrates from the blood using a blood cell separator. The first step in the manufacturing process involves enriching the peripheral blood mononuclear cell (PBMNC) concentrates collected by apheresis for lymphocytes or T-cells. The enriched leukocytes are then placed in culture, transduced, and expanded. The resulting CAR T-cells are harvested, tested, packaged, and stored. Most CAR T-cells are cryopreserved. When CAR T-cells are manufactured at a centralized facility, the CAR T-cells must be shipped to the center where the patient will be treated.

Collection of Leukocytes

While some patients have an adequate quantity of lymphocytes for autologous CAR T-cell manufacturing in as little as a few hundred milliliters of blood, the quantity of circulating lymphocytes is highly variable and is often low due to the patient's disease and prior chemotherapy. Consequently, autologous lymphocytes are typically collected using blood cell separators that are specifically designed to collect blood cells and are operated using instrument setting, which optimize the collection of mononuclear leukocytes.[21] They draw whole blood from a vein or venous access port, separate mononuclear leukocytes from other blood cells based on cell density, and return red blood cells (RBCs), platelets, and plasma back to the patient through another vein or venous access port.

It is desirable to begin CAR T-cell manufacturing with T-cells; however, because the size and density of T-cells is similar to that of B-cells, monocytes, and natural killer (NK) cells, the leukocytes collected by apheresis are enriched in T-cells, B-cells, monocytes, and NK cells and are known as PBMNC concentrates. When PBMNCs are collected by apheresis from patients with leukemia, the PBMNC concentrate may also contain leukemic blast cells. PBMNC concentrates also contain some platelets, RBCs, and granulocytes. The degree of platelet and RBC contamination is, generally, consistent, but the granulocyte content is variable. Some PBMNC concentrates contain few if any granulocytes, whereas others contain large quantities. The collection of T-cells by apheresis for CAR T-cell manufacturing is reviewed in detail in Chapter 2 of this guide.

T-Cell Enrichment

The enrichment of the PBMNC concentrate for lymphocytes or T-cells is an important step in the CAR T-cell manufacturing process. Since it is costly to produce clinical grade viral vector, it is important to start the manufacturing process using a relatively small quantity of T-cells of high purity to reduce the quantity of vector that is needed to obtain a sufficient quantity of transduced T-cells. There are other benefits to enriching the PBMNC concentrates for T-cells. Lymphocyte enrichment eliminates monocytes and granulocytes that may include myeloid-derived suppressor cells with monocytic or granulocytic phenotypes, which can inhibit T-cell expansion.[11] The presence of large quantities of monocytes in PBMNC concentrates and the material used to start CAR T-cell manufacturing has been associated with reduced T-cell expansion during the manufacturing process.[11,12] Some T-cell enrichment methods will also remove leukemia blast cells from the PBMNC concentrate. The end result of having an enriched population of T-cells as a starting material also improves the consistency of stimulation using activator reagents, given that the elimination of contaminating cells would reduce the potential for non—T-cell-specific binding of these activators. In addition, the presence of platelets and RBCs with the T-cells used to start CAR T-cell manufacturing can affect T-cell expansion and the T-cell phenotype (unpublished observation).

Several methods can be used for T-cell enrichment including density gradient separation, counterflow elutriation, and monoclonal antibody selection. All of these methods have been used for manufacturing clinical CAR T-cells.[10,12,20,22] All are associated with some T-cell loss, but the proportion of cells lost is dependent on the specific enrichment process.

Density gradient separation using Ficoll can reduce the quantity of granulocytes and RBCs, but it does not separate T-cells from B-cells, monocytes, and NK cells. If blast cells are present in the PBMNC concentrate, density gradient separation will not separate T-cells from most types of blast cells. Classically, density gradient separation has been performed using tubes, and the liquid gradients and cell suspensions are added manually. Density gradient separation using manual tube methods is still being used by some clinical cell processing laboratories; however, automated instruments are available for closed-system density gradient separation. Some of these instruments are modified cell washers,

but others are made specifically for density gradient enrichment of PBMNC concentrates, bone marrow, and cord blood.[23] These automated instruments make use of single-use closed-system sterile disposable sets or kits. Cells only come in contact with the disposable kit. Since a new kit is used for each procedure, there is no risk of cross-contaminating cells from one patient with cells from another or spreading an infectious agent among patients. The disposable nature of the kits makes preparing the instrument for processing cells from a new patient relatively quick and easy.

Counterflow elutriation separates cells based on size, and it provides good separation of lymphocytes from monocytes, granulocytes, and platelets, but the lymphocytes may be contaminated with RBCs.[24] The fraction of cells enriched for lymphocytes by elutriation is also rich in B, NK, and blast cells. Instruments and single-use disposable kits are available for closed-system counterflow elutriation, and they have been used to manufacture of CAR T-cells.[12,25—27]

Monoclonal antibodies linked to magnetic beads can be used to isolate T-cells and T-cell subsets. Selection or depletion of PBMNC concentrates with monoclonal antibodies is very effective and typically results in leukocyte population that has a high proportion of T-cells with very little contamination with RBCs or platelets. Monoclonal antibody-based closed-system automated cell selection systems are available. While monoclonal antibody selection is very effective, it is more expensive than other T-cell enrichment methods. Monoclonal antibody selection systems also make use of sterile closed-system disposable sets.[20,28,29]

T-Cell Transduction

CAR T-cells have typically been transduced with integrating retroviral and lentiviral vectors. Generally, the vectors are manufactured at a site separate from the cell manufacturing center, and centers that produce clinical CAR T-cells often purchase vectors from facilities or commercial groups that specialize in manufacturing viral vectors. The T-cells are transduced once or twice, which results in expression of the CAR construct in 50% or more of the T-cells.[10,30] Retroviral vector transduction requires T-cell division. Therefore, T-cells are stimulated or activated for 2 or 3 days prior to transduction. In addition, retroviral vectors and cells are typically centrifuged to increase transduction efficiency. This process that is known as spinoculation is generally performed in plates. The vessel containing cells to be transduced is coated with RetroNectin. The plates must be opened to add RetroNectin, vector, and cell suspension. Spinoculation can be performed in bags, which significantly reduces the risk of microbial contamination and increases the volume and number of cells transduced.[30] Lentiviral vector transduction does not require T-cell stimulation, spinoculation, or RetroNectin coating, but typically T-cells are stimulated for a day prior to lentiviral transduction in the presence of positively charged polycations, such as polybrene or protamine sulfate. Lentiviral vector transduction of T-cells can also be performed in bags, enhancing the safety and number of cells transduced.

Gene editing using CRISPR/Cas 9 can be used to produce CAR T-cells. This system requires no retro- or lentiviral vectors and thus avoids the concern about recombinant retro- and lentiviruses. Gene editing also allows for targeted CAR insertion. Preclinical studies have shown that targeting a CD19-CAR to the T-cell receptor α constant (TRAC) locus enhances tumor rejection that resulted in less tonic signaling and thus less exhaustion and increases the therapeutic potential over cells that had the same CAR transduced with viral vectors.[14] Furthermore, the targeted insertion into the endogenous TRAC locus would minimize the risk of insertional oncogenesis and alloreactivity.

While retro- and lentivirus vector transduction and gene editing results in integration of vector in the T-cell genome, long-term presence of T-cells expressing the CAR vector may not be necessary for clinically effective therapy. In vivo the levels of circulating CAR T-cells are transiently elevated. After infusion, CAR T-cells expand greatly and reach peak levels after 7−14 days.[3−6] While CAR T-cells may be present in the blood for months or years, their levels are generally far below peak levels 30−60 days after infusion.[6] Since the long-term presence of circulating CAR T-cells may not be needed, some clinical trials are making use of nonintegrated plasmids or mRNA encoding the CAR construct. CAR T-cells produced with transiently expressed constructs can be given on multiple occasions if needed.

T-Cell Culture and Expansion

Classically, T-cells have been cultured in T-flasks, but the culture of cells in T-flasks is not suited for GMP cell culture. The flasks must be opened to the environment numerous times during culture to add or remove cells or media. In addition, for culturing large quantities of T-cells, many flasks are needed, which increases the labor required for maintaining the culture and the risk of microbial contamination.

T-cells can also be cultured in gas-permeable bags, which are better suited for GMP manufacturing. The use of bags is advantageous since cells and media can be added without opening the bags to the environment.

Consequently, cells cultured in bag systems are less likely to become contaminated with bacteria or fungi than cells cultured in flasks.

Cell culture bags are much like the bags used for collecting and processing blood. They have integral tubes that can be used to add or remove media or cells in suspension. The tubes from two bags can be connected sterilely. The ability to sterile connect tubes from two bags allows for the sterile transfer of fluid from one bag to another. This allows for media to be added or changed, for cell suspensions to be transferred to a larger bag or for cells to be sampled, washed, or concentrated while maintaining a closed system.

One limitation of bags is that the maximum concentration of T-cells in culture is limited to about 2×10^6 cells per mL. However, recently, closed-system gas-permeable flasks have been developed, which can be used to culture T-cells at several-fold higher concentrations.[17,18] Some of these gas-permeable flasks are manufactured with tubes, which can be used to sterilely add and remove media and cells in suspension.

Several automated commercially closed-system instruments are available for T-cell culture, including bag-based systems and hollow fiber bioreactors.[17] One of these systems allows for closed-system T-cell selection, transduction, and expansion.[19,20]

Culture media designed for T-cell culture and produced specifically for cGMP manufacturing of T-cell therapies are available commercially. These media can be packaged in bags of various sizes that can be sterilely connected to culture bags or other culture systems. T-cell culture media are generally supplemented with serum, cytokines, and other factors to stimulate T-cell growth.

Classically, the media used for T-cell culture were supplemented with 5%−10% fetal bovine serum (FBS). However, FBS is no longer used for clinical CAR T-cell expansion. FBS may transmit infectious agents such as prions. In addition, residual bovine proteins may be present in the final T-cell preparation that could cause an immune reaction in the cell therapy recipient. Clinical T-cell cultures are supplemented with up to 10% human serum that has been heated to inactivate complement. Media made up of defined factors, which require no serum supplementation, are being developed.

The cytokine most commonly used for T-cell culture is IL-2. While IL-2 is an effective T-cell growth factor, it has some limitations. Prolonged expansion of T-cells in the presence of IL-2 can result in a T-cell population with a terminally differentiated effector cell phenotype,[31] which has a limited ability to expand in vivo. In addition, IL-2 also promotes the expansion of CD8+ cells.[31] Other cytokines used for T-cell expansion include IL-7, IL-15, and IL-21, which are more likely to maintain a more immature T-cell phenotype.[32,33]

T-cell culture media are also supplemented with factors that stimulate the TCR and possibly a costimulatory receptor such as CD28. Anti-CD3 antibodies are often used to stimulate the TCR. An alternative to the use of soluble anti-CD3 stimulation with anti-CD3 and anti-CD28 attached to magnetic beads. These beads stimulate the TCR and the CD28 costimulatory molecule, allowing the beads to act as artificial antigen presenting cells. Different types of anti-CD3/anti-CD28 beads are available. Some have both antibodies on the same bead, and others have the antibodies on separate beads. At the end of the cell culture period, the beads will need to be removed from the CAR T-cells prior to infusion.

Different sources of reagents used in T-cell culture may yield T-cells with different phenotypes or potency. The phenotype of T-cells in the final CAR T-cell product is an important factor in the clinical effectiveness of the CAR T-cells, and culture conditions can impact the phenotype of the T-cells. Both cytotoxic, CD8+, T-cells and helper, CD4+, T-cells are required for optimal in vivo immune responses.[34,35] Prolonged stimulation of mixed populations of CD4+ and CD8+ T-cells can skew the final product toward CD4+ cells or CD8+ cells. To avoid this issue, some groups make two types of CAR T-cells: CD4+ CAR T-cells and CD8+ CAR T-cells, and these groups prepare a final CAR T-cell product, which contains equal proportions of CD4+ and CD8+ CAR T-cells.[36,37]

Circulating T-cells have a mixture of phenotypes including naïve, stem memory, central memory, effector memory, and effector phenotypes. Prolonged culture is also associated with the production of a larger proportion of T-cells with an effector phenotype. Preclinical studies have shown that genetically engineered T-cells with a stem memory or central memory phenotype persist longer in vivo and are more effective as a cancer immunotherapy than genetically engineered T-cells with effector phenotype.[38] Clinical trials are underway, which use CAR T-cells with a T stem memory phenotype.

POSTMANUFACTURING OR DOWNSTREAM PROCESSING

At the conclusion of the CAR T culture period, additional processing is required. Postmanufacturing processing or downstream processing involves preparing cells for clinical use. The CAR T-cells must be washed to remove culture media and factors used as media supplements, such as cytokines and antibodies. Culture media, in general, are not meant to be given intravenously, and the cytokines

used as culture media supplements may be toxic if given intravenously. If the cells have been manufactured in the presence of anti-CD3/anti-CD28 magnetic beads, it may be necessary to remove the beads. In addition, the volume of culture media is usually much greater than the volume that can be given intravenously over a short period of time. Consequently, the CAR T-cells must be concentrated. Following washing and concentration of the CAR T-cells, they are resuspended in an infusible liquid if administered fresh and in a cryoprotectant if they are to be cryopreserved and stored.

Cryopreservation

CAR T-cells are often cryopreserved after manufacturing is complete. After the cells are washed and concentrated, they are aliquoted into the appropriate dose, a cryoprotectant is added, and the cells are cryopreserved. The purpose of the cryoprotectant is to prevent damage to the cells by ice crystal formation during the freeze-thaw process. To further improve the recovery of cells at the time of thaw and infusion, cells are typically cryopreserved using a programmable freezer, which controls the rate of cooling and freezing. A wide variety of formulations of cryoprotectants are used, but most contain dimethyl sulfoxide (DMSO). Commercially prepared cryoprotectants are available, but many laboratories prepare their own.

Following cryopreservation, the cells are generally stored in liquid nitrogen or the vapor phase of liquid of nitrogen. It is preferred to store cells in liquid nitrogen tanks rather than mechanical freezers since liquid nitrogen storage tanks will maintain their temperature for days or even weeks if there is a loss of electrical power. In contrast, when there is a loss of electrical power, the temperature of mechanical freezers will begin to rise within hours, which may compromise any products that are stored there.

Laboratory Testing of Chimeric Antigen Receptor T-Cells

The cells produced each time CAR T-cells are manufactured are considered a new lot of cells. Each lot of CAR T-cells is tested during and at the end of manufacturing. The testing of CAR T-cells during processing is known as in-process testing. In-process testing typically includes cell counts and phenotype to evaluate the progress of the manufacturing process. Testing at the end of manufacturing is known as lot release testing.

Lot release testing includes testing for CAR T-cell safety, identity, purity, and potency (Table 3.3). The CAR T-cells are tested for bacteria and fungus in culture assays; cultures are typically incubated for 14 days

TABLE 3.3
Typical Lot Release Testing for Chimeric Antigen Receptor (CAR) T-Cells.

Assay	Method	Acceptable Result
Sterility—bacteria	Culture	No growth
Sterility—fungus	Culture	No growth
Sterility—mycoplasma	PCR	None detected
Transduction efficiency	Flow	>10%–20%
Vector copy number	PCR	<5 copies per cell
T-cell phenotype	Flow cytometry	Presence of some CD4+ and CD8+ T-cells
Purity	Flow cytometry	>80% T-cells
Viability	Dye exclusion	>70% viable cells
Identity	Flow or PCR	Correct CAR vector present
Potency	Cytokine release or cell proliferation; targeted cell killing	Variable

PCR, polymerase chain reaction.

before concluding that no organisms are present. The CAR T-cells are also tested for mycoplasma contamination, usually with a PCR assay.

Evaluation of the CAR-transduced T-cells for replication competent of retrovirus (RCR)/lentivirus (RCL) is a required safety assay. The standard cell culture–based RCL assay takes more than 8 weeks to perform, and results are not available at the time of release of CAR T-cells for administration to the patient. PCR-based assays for (RCR/RCL) are sensitive assays, can be completed within 2 days, and provide preliminary results for the release of the CAR T-cells for administration. In a recent study by Cornetta et al., 460 transduced products from 26 different clinical trials from six institutions were evaluated for potential RCL, and all products were negative. In addition, of the 296 patients screened 1 month post-CAR infusion, no research subject has shown evidence of RCL infection.[39] With the high cost of the 8-week

assay, and no added value to increasing patient safety using this assay, it is likely that the requirements at least for the cell-based assay may be relaxed in the near future.

T-cell transduction efficiency is measured using flow cytometry. The range of acceptable transduction efficiencies varies with each type of CAR T-cell product, but it typically ranges from about 20% to 80%. If a facility is manufacturing more than one type of CAR T-cell, the cells must be tested to ensure that correct vector was used. If the flow cytometry assay that measures transduction efficiency makes use of a labeled molecule that specifically targets the expressed CAR construct, then the flow cytometry assay can be used for assessing both transduction and vector identity. If the flow cytometry assay used to measure transduction efficiency makes use of a molecule that binds nonspecifically to the CAR construct, then it cannot be used for identity testing. In this case, PCR assays that target a unique portion of the CAR vector can be used for identity testing. In addition to measuring transduction efficiency, vector copy number is often measured by PCR. For CAR T-cells, the Food and Drug Administration (FDA) currently recommends that the integration copy number should be less than five copies per cell.

The proportion of T-cells in the final product and their phenotype are measured by flow cytometry. Typically, more than 80% of CAR T-cells express CD3. Generally, the proportion of CD4+ and CD8+ cells are also measured. While the general consensus is that it is important to have both CD4+ and CD8+ T-cells in the CAR T-cell product, their proportion is variable.

CAR T-cell viability is also measured and is required to have a passing criterion of 70% viability. Viability can be measured manually using a microscope and trypan blue exclusion or by flow cytometry using propidium iodide or 7-aminoactinomycin D (7AAD) staining. The CAR T-cells also need to be evaluated, usually by visual microscopy, to ensure that an adequate quantity of beads has been removed.

CAR T-cells may also tested for potency as a measure of CAR T-cell in vivo effectiveness. It may be measured using a cell function assay or a surrogate analytical assay that is associated with cell function, such as transduction efficiency. Potency testing is not required for CAR T-cells manufactured for early-phase clinical trials, but it is for CAR T-cells used in late-phase clinical trials and for CAR T-cells that have been licensed by the FDA. Many different assays can be used to assess CAR T-cell potency. Typically, these assays involve the stimulation of CAR T-cells with cells expressing the antigen targeted by the CAR T-cells and the measurement of target cytotoxicity, T-cell proliferation, or T-cell cytokine production such as IFN-γ.[40]

CENTRALIZED MANUFACTURING

Most CAR T-cells are currently manufactured from autologous leukocytes. For early-phase clinical trials, the cells are often collected, manufactured, and infused at the same center where the patient is being treated. For late-phase clinical trials and licensed products, patients are typically treated at multiple medical centers, and the cells are manufactured in a single or a few centralized facilities (Fig. 3.2). The lymphocytes used for manufacturing the CAR T-cells are collected at an apheresis or medical center convenient for the patient to be treated. The cellular starting material is shipped to the central site where the CAR T-cells are manufactured. When manufacturing is complete, the final CAR T-cell product is shipped to the medical center where the patient will be treated. Centralized manufacturing allows for more efficient use of labor and cGMP cell processing facilities. It also allows for more uniform manufacturing and greater consistency among products. However, centralized manufacturing creates some logistical challenges associated with the scheduling of manufacturing and cell shipping.

Shipping of Apheresis Concentrates and Chimeric Antigen Receptor T-Cells

The process used to ship PBMNC concentrates and the manufactured CAR T-cells must be highly reliable. The CAR T-cell recipient's underlying medical condition may make collecting autologous cells by apheresis difficult, and if the cells are lost or damaged during shipping, it may not be possible to replace the cells. The acute nature of their underlying disease may not allow enough time to manufacture another CAR T-cell product. Consequently, the shipping process must be highly reliable. The starting material collected by apheresis may be shipped immediately after collection at room temperature or 4°C or after cryopreservation. If the PBMNC concentrate is stored at room temperature or 4°C for a prolonged period of time, it may be necessary to dilute the cells with autologous plasma, plasmalyte A, or another infusible liquid. Although dilution and 4°C storage helps to preserve cells, processing should begin as soon as possible after collection. In some cases, the PBMNC concentrates are cryopreserved immediately after collection and are shipped frozen. Shipping containers are available, which will maintain cells at room temperature, 4°C, or cryopreserved for several days.

When cells are manufactured centrally, they are cryopreserved at the end of manufacturing. This allows for the cells to be stored for 7 or more days required for the completion and evaluation of lot release assays. Containers called dry shippers are available, which, when charged with liquid nitrogen, can maintain cells cryopreserved for several days. Dry shippers have been used successfully for many years to ship cryopreserved cord blood products for HSC transplantation.

To ensure that the appropriate storage temperature has been maintained during shipping and whether the

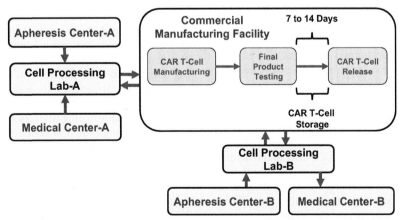

FIG. 3.2 **Centralized manufacturing of chimeric antigen receptor (CAR) T-cells.** Manufacturing CAR T-cells commercially for late-phase multiple-center clinical trials or as a licensed cell therapy often involves centralized manufacturing. Autologous peripheral blood mononuclear cells are collected at an apheresis center, and they are shipped to a centralized manufacturing center. On completion of manufacturing, the CAR T-cells are cryopreserved. After lot release testing is complete and if the test results meet release criteria, the CAR T-cells are shipped to the healthcare center treating the patient where they are infused

cells are cryopreserved or are at 4°C in a liquid state, the temperature of the containers is monitored during shipping using a portable temperature monitoring device. Sometimes, devices are added to the shipping container that allows their location to be tracked during shipping.

Receiving Chimeric Antigen Receptor T-cells

When the CAR T-cell product is received by the medical center that will infuse the product, the shipping container and CAR T-cell product are inspected to be sure that the product has arrived at the appropriate temperature and in good condition. The bag or vessel containing the CAR T-cells should be intact and free of cracks, breaks, or other defects. The product label is also reviewed to be sure that the correct product has been received. The product also comes with a Certificate of Analysis and circular of information.

THE CELL THERAPY INFUSION

Before the CAR T-cells are administered to the patient, they must be thawed and issued to the patient care unit. After the cells are infused, the patient must be monitored for infusion- and cell expansion—associated reactions.

Storage, Thawing, and Infusion

Typically, the CAR T-cell product is stored in the cell processing laboratory at the medical center that will be infusing the cells for at least a day. The storage conditions are specified by the manufacturer, but they are typically stored in a liquid nitrogen storage tank. The method of thawing and infusing the CAR T-cells is also specified by the manufacturer. They are generally thawed rapidly and, once thawed, are infused as soon as possible since most cryoprotectants are toxic to cells. The product must be infused within the duration of time specified by the manufacturer and using the infusion set specified by the manufacturer. For early-phase clinical trials, the center infusing the CAR T-cells may thaw and wash the cells and, after measuring cell viability, adjust the dose of viable CAR T-cells to a specific dose per kg of patient weight. However, for late-phase studies involving CAR T-cells manufactured centrally, all of the cells received are typically thawed and infused. The cell processing laboratory documents the time the cells are thawed. Generally, the cells are infused within an hour or two after thawing.

Infusion Reactions

Anytime a cellular product is administered, the patient may have a reaction. Since many reactions associated with the infusion of cell therapies occur within a few

hours of the infusion, it is important to document the patient's vital signs immediately before the infusion and at defined interval after the infusion. The time at which the infusion begins and ends should also be documented.

One of the most serious potential adverse reactions is associated with microbial agents in the cell therapy. All CAR T-cells are tested for sterility, but if the cells are contaminated during shipping, storage, thawing, or infusion, the recipient could experience fever, chills, and hypotension. They could also develop sepsis.

The infusion of DMSO, which is present in most cryoprotectants, can cause nausea, vomiting, and flushing. The infusion of dead cells or cellular debris with the thawed CAR T-cells can result in a fever. If the CAR T-cells contain RBCs, some may lyse during thawing, and the free hemoglobin released by hemolyzed cells can cause a reaction.

Following the infusion of CAR T-cells, patients may develop reactions due to cytokines produced during CAR T-cell in vivo expansion. These cytokines can result in reactions known as cytokine release syndrome (CRS) and less commonly neurologic toxicities.[41,42] CRS and neurologic toxicities generally occur 1—14 days following the infusion of CAR T-cells and are discussed in detail in Chapters 6—9.

SUMMARY

CAR T-cells are an effective and growing cellular immunotherapy. Providing this promising immunotherapy is complicated by the fact that the CAR T-cells are manufactured from leukocyte collected from the patient receiving the CAR T-cells, multiple steps are involved with cell manufacturing and the cells may be shipped. The provision of autologous CAR T-cells requires commitment and coordination among the teams collecting, manufacturing, and administering the cells. The development of universal CAR T-cells produced using cells from healthy donors would simplify this process and make it significantly more affordable. Since patients treated with CAR T-cells may have serious and often life-threatening diseases and providing these cells can be complicated, it is beneficial for healthcare professionals involved with CAR T-cell therapy to be familiar with the manufacturing process.

REFERENCES

1. Kochenderfer JN, Wilson WH, Janik JE, et al. Eradication of B-lineage cells and regression of lymphoma in a patient treated with autologous T cells genetically engineered to recognize CD19. *Blood*. 2010;116(20):4099—4102.
2. Brudno JN, Somerville RP, Shi V, et al. Allogeneic T cells that express an anti-CD19 chimeric antigen receptor

induce remissions of B-cell malignancies that progress after allogeneic hematopoietic stem-cell transplantation without causing graft-versus-host disease. *J Clin Oncol.* 2016;34(10):1112−1121.

3. Lee DW, Kochenderfer JN, Stetler-Stevenson M, et al. T cells expressing CD19 chimeric antigen receptors for acute lymphoblastic leukaemia in children and young adults: a phase 1 dose-escalation trial. *Lancet.* 2015;385(9967):517−528.

4. Fry TJ, Shah NN, Orentas RJ, et al. CD22-targeted CAR T cells induce remission in B-ALL that is naive or resistant to CD19-targeted CAR immunotherapy. *Nat Med.* 2018;24(1):20−28.

5. Brudno JN, Maric I, Hartman SD, et al. T cells genetically modified to express an anti-B-cell maturation antigen chimeric antigen receptor cause remissions of poor-prognosis relapsed multiple myeloma. *J Clin Oncol.* 2018. JCO2018778084.

6. Neelapu SS, Locke FL, Bartlett NL, et al. Axicabtagene ciloleucel CAR T-cell therapy in refractory large B-cell lymphoma. *N Engl J Med.* 2017;377(26):2531−2544.

7. Schuster SJ, Svoboda J, Chong EA, et al. Chimeric antigen receptor T cells in refractory B-cell lymphomas. *N Engl J Med.* 2017;377(26):2545−2554.

8. Maude SL, Laetsch TW, Buechner J, et al. Tisagenlecleucel in children and young adults with B-cell lymphoblastic leukemia. *N Engl J Med.* 2018;378(5):439−448.

9. Park JH, Riviere I, Gonen M, et al. Long-term follow-up of CD19 CAR therapy in acute lymphoblastic leukemia. *N Engl J Med.* 2018;378(5):449−459.

10. Tumaini B, Lee DW, Lin T, et al. Simplified process for the production of anti-CD19-CAR-engineered T cells. *Cytotherapy.* 2013;15(11):1406−1415.

11. Stroncek DF, Ren J, Lee DW, et al. Myeloid cells in peripheral blood mononuclear cell concentrates inhibit the expansion of chimeric antigen receptor T cells. *Cytotherapy.* 2016;18(7):893−901.

12. Stroncek DF, Lee DW, Ren J, et al. Elutriated lymphocytes for manufacturing chimeric antigen receptor T cells. *J Transl Med.* 2017;15(1):59.

13. Locke FL, Ghobadi A, Jacobson CA, et al. Long-term safety and activity of axicabtagene ciloleucel in refractory large B-cell lymphoma (ZUMA-1): a single-arm, multicentre, phase 1-2 trial. *Lancet Oncol.* 2019;20(1):31−42.

14. Eyquem J, Mansilla-Soto J, Giavridis T, et al. Targeting a CAR to the TRAC locus with CRISPR/Cas9 enhances tumour rejection. *Nature.* 2017;543(7643):113−117.

15. MacLeod DT, Antony J, Martin AJ, et al. Integration of a CD19 CAR into the TCR alpha chain locus streamlines production of allogeneic gene-edited CAR T cells. *Mol Ther.* 2017;25(4):949−961.

16. Poirot L, Philip B, Schiffer-Mannioui C, et al. Multiplex genome-edited T-cell manufacturing platform for "Off-the-Shelf" adoptive T-cell immunotherapies. *Cancer Res.* 2015;75(18):3853−3864.

17. Jin J, Sabatino M, Somerville R, et al. Simplified method of the growth of human tumor infiltrating lymphocytes in gas-permeable flasks to numbers needed for patient treatment. *J Immunother.* 2012;35(3):283−292.

18. Lapteva N, Vera JF. Optimization manufacture of virus- and tumor-specific T cells. *Stem Cells Int.* 2011;2011:434392.

19. Lock D, Mockel-Tenbrinck N, Drechsel K, et al. Automated manufacturing of potent CD20-directed chimeric antigen receptor T cells for clinical use. *Hum Gene Ther.* 2017;28(10):914−925.

20. Zhu F, Shah N, Xu H, et al. Closed-system manufacturing of CD19 and dual-targeted CD20/19 chimeric antigen receptor T cells using the CliniMACS Prodigy device at an academic medical center. *Cytotherapy.* 2018;20(3):394−406.

21. Allen ES, Stroncek DF, Ren J, et al. Autologous lymphapheresis for the production of chimeric antigen receptor T cells. *Transfusion.* 2017;57(5):1133−1141.

22. Mock U, Nickolay L, Philip B, et al. Automated manufacturing of chimeric antigen receptor T cells for adoptive immunotherapy using CliniMACS prodigy. *Cytotherapy.* 2016;18(8):1002−1011.

23. Lu TL, Pugach O, Somerville R, et al. A rapid cell expansion process for production of engineered autologous CAR-T cell therapies. *Hum Gene Ther Methods.* 2016;27(6):209−218.

24. Stroncek DF, Fellowes V, Pham C, et al. Counter-flow elutriation of clinical peripheral blood mononuclear cell concentrates for the production of dendritic and T cell therapies. *J Transl Med.* 2014;12:241.

25. Kim S, Kim HO, Baek EJ, Choi Y, Kim HS, Lee MG. Monocyte enrichment from leukapheresis products by using the Elutra cell separator. *Transfusion.* 2007;47(12):2290−2296.

26. Lemarie C, Sugaye R, Kaur I, et al. Purification of monocytes from cryopreserved mobilized apheresis products by elutriation with the Elutra device. *J Immunol Methods.* 2007;318(1−2):30−36.

27. Perseghin P, D'Amico G, Dander E, et al. Isolation of monocytes from leukapheretic products for large-scale GMP-grade generation of cytomegalovirus-specific T-cell lines by means of an automated elutriation device. *Transfusion.* 2008;48(8):1644−1649.

28. McNiece IK, Stoney GB, Kern BP, Briddell RA. CD34+ cell selection from frozen cord blood products using the Isolex 300i and CliniMACS CD34 selection devices. *J Hematother.* 1998;7(5):457−461.

29. Schumm M, Lang P, Taylor G, et al. Isolation of highly purified autologous and allogeneic peripheral CD34+ cells using the CliniMACS device. *J Hematother.* 1999;8(2):209−218.

30. Jin J, Gkitsas N, Fellowes VS, et al. Enhanced clinical-scale manufacturing of TCR transduced T-cells using closed culture system modules. *J Transl Med.* 2018;16(1):13.

31. Zhang X, Lv X, Song Y. Short-term culture with IL-2 is beneficial for potent memory chimeric antigen receptor T cell production. *Biochem Biophys Res Commun.* 2018;495(2):1833−1838.

32. Crompton JG, Sukumar M, Restifo NP. Uncoupling T-cell expansion from effector differentiation in cell-based immunotherapy. *Immunol Rev.* 2014;257(1):264−276.

33. Lugli E, Gattinoni L, Roberto A, et al. Identification, isolation and in vitro expansion of human and nonhuman primate T stem cell memory cells. *Nat Protoc.* 2013;8(1):33—42.

34. Janssen EM, Lemmens EE, Wolfe T, Christen U, von Herrath MG, Schoenberger SP. CD4+ T cells are required for secondary expansion and memory in CD8+ T lymphocytes. *Nature.* 2003;421(6925):852—856.

35. Wang JC, Livingstone AM. Cutting edge: CD4+ T cell help can be essential for primary CD8+ T cell responses in vivo. *J Immunol.* 2003;171(12):6339—6343.

36. Sommermeyer D, Hudecek M, Kosasih PL, et al. Chimeric antigen receptor-modified T cells derived from defined CD8+ and CD4+ subsets confer superior antitumor reactivity in vivo. *Leukemia.* 2016;30(2):492—500.

37. Turtle CJ, Hanafi LA, Berger C, et al. CD19 CAR-T cells of defined CD4+:CD8+ composition in adult B cell ALL patients. *J Clin Invest.* 2016;126(6):2123—2138.

38. Gattinoni L, Lugli E, Ji Y, et al. A human memory T cell subset with stem cell-like properties. *Nat Med.* 2011; 17(10):1290—1297.

39. Cornetta K, Duffy L, Turtle CJ, et al. Absence of replication-competent lentivirus in the clinic: analysis of infused T cell products. *Mol Ther.* 2018;26(1):280—288.

40. Rossi J, Paczkowski P, Shen YW, et al. Preinfusion polyfunctional anti-CD19 chimeric antigen receptor T cells are associated with clinical outcomes in NHL. *Blood.* 2018;132(8):804—814.

41. Brudno JN, Kochenderfer JN. Toxicities of chimeric antigen receptor T cells: recognition and management. *Blood.* 2016; 127(26):3321—3330.

42. Mahadeo KM, Khazal SJ, Abdel-Azim H, et al. Management guidelines for paediatric patients receiving chimeric antigen receptor T cell therapy. *Nat Rev Clin Oncol.* 2019; 16(1):45—63.

CHAPTER 4

Peri-CAR T-Cell Management

KARLO PERICA, MD, PHD • KEVIN J. CURRAN, MD • JAE H. PARK, MD

SCREENING

Once identified as a candidate for chimeric antigen receptor (CAR) T-cell therapy, patients must undergo screening for eligibility. Prediagnostic evaluations are required to assess patient candidacy to undergo CAR treatment, fulfill regulatory criteria for cell product collection, and satisfy insurance standards for reimbursement.[1]

Patient's disease burden should be reevaluated per usual practice prior to receiving CAR T-cell therapy. Target antigen expression should be assessed by tissue biopsy prior to initiation of collection or treatment. This is particularly important if patients have received prior therapies sharing the same antigen specificity as the CAR T-cell, such as blinatumomab prior to CD19-targeted CARs, which may predispose to escape mutations, leading to loss of antigen expression.[2]

Interestingly, there has been evidence of CAR T-cell activity in antigen-negative disease; for example, in the phase II study of CD19-targeted axicabtagene ciloleucel (Yescarta),[3] eight patients with CD19-negative disease were treated with no suggestion of reduced efficacy. As a result, there is no absolute requirement for CD19 expression prior to treatment with axicabtagene. However, based on the mechanism of action of CAR T-cells, it is unlikely that CAR T-cells can recognize truly CD19 negative tumors, and "CD19-negative" responders likely express low levels of CD19 below the detectable level of the diagnostic assay. Therefore, the decision to treat an "antigen-negative" tumor should be made cautiously and only after discussion with pathology and CAR T-cell experts.

Location of disease is also important, as the successful use of cellular therapy is predicated on the ability of infused cells to traffic to the disease site. Regarding CD19 CAR T-cells, it has been shown that cells will penetrate the central nervous system (CNS) and mediate CNS lymphoma regression.[4] However, all large trials of currently available, commercially developed CAR products have excluded *active* CNS disease (e.g., CNS 3 in B-cell acute lymphoblastic leukemia [ALL] or radiographic evidence of disease for B-cell non-Hodgkin's lymphoma [NHL]). Patients previously and successfully treated for CNS disease have generally not been excluded on these trials. However, it is currently not well characterized what role CNS disease has on the occurrence or severity of postinfusion neurologic toxicity. Physicians should consider precollection and/or pretreatment diagnostics for CNS disease such as brain MRI or lumbar puncture as clinically appropriate. Future clinical trials and/or next-generation CAR T-cell designs may target patients with active CNS lesions.

Patient screening also involves a detailed clinical history including recent travel, immunizations, transfusion history, and infectious disease exposure. Basic screening laboratory testing including infectious disease markers (IDMs) should be obtained prior to collection. Additional diagnostics including echocardiogram and 12-lead electrocardiogram (Table 4.1) should be obtained when clinically indicated. Organ function assessment should confirm patient suitability to withstand potential adverse events following treatment including cytokine release syndrome (CRS) or other target organ toxicity. A pregnancy test for females of reproductive potential should be confirmed negative prior to collection and treatment.

Regulatory standards for IDMs are set by federal agencies such as the Food and Drug Administration,[5] accrediting organizations such as the Foundation for the Accreditation of Cell Therapy (FACT),[1,6] and the American Association of Blood Banks (AABB), as well as state and local agencies. The timing of IDM testing varies in these standards between 7 to 30 days prior to collection. Clinicians should check with national, local, and institutional regulatory agencies to determine additional testing requirements.

Critical to successful use of CAR T-cell therapy is the patient's ability to withstand any potential postinfusion toxicity such as CRS and/or end organ toxicity. To this end, organ function criteria to qualify for treatment can be extrapolated from the relevant clinical trials of

TABLE 4.1
Screening Diagnostics.
Complete blood count with differential
comprehensive metabolic panel
PT/PTT/INR
Urinalysis
Type and screen
Pregnancy test for females of child-bearing age
Hepatitis B core antibody
Hepatitis B surface antigen
Hepatitis C antibody
HIV 1/2 antibody
Echocardiogram (as clinically indicated and to confirm ability to withstand post infusion toxicity)
Electrocardiogram (as clinically indicated)

PT, Prothrombin time; *PTT*, Partial thromboplastin time; *INR*, International normalization ratio; *HIV*, Human immunodeficiency virus.

commercially approved CAR T-cell products, which are described in Table 4.2. Of note, all trials required robust performance status (ECOG of ≤ 1 or Karnofsky/Lansky $\geq 60\%$). Additional studies in populations that would not have met eligibility criteria for the registration trials are ongoing.

INFORMED CONSENT

Informed consent is a required element for institutions in compliance with FACT Immune Effector Cell (IEC) guidelines.[6] Due to the complexity and potential toxicity of CAR T-cell therapy, we recommend the development of institution-specific consent procedures for all patients treated outside of a clinical trial. Informed consent should explain the rationale for the use of CAR T-cells in terms the patient can understand including clinical benefit of therapy, risk of toxicities,

and alternative treatment options. Long-term toxicity (e.g., long-term B-cell aplasia with CD19-specific CAR T-cells) should also be described, including theoretical adverse events such as insertional oncogenesis, when appropriate.

Consent should be documented per institutional guidelines. Any additional investigational protocols or biospecimen banking will require separate consents, as will central line placement and leukapheresis. Practical requirements, such as the need for a caregiver and need to reside in proximity to the treatment facility, should also be highlighted.

COLLECTION

Most commonly, T-cells for CAR modification are harvested from leukapheresis of peripheral blood mononuclear cells. Leukapheresis involves removal of whole

TABLE 4.2 Key Clinical Trial Exclusion Criteria.		
Tisagenlecleucel in Pediatric/ Young Adult ALL	**Tisagenlecleucel in NHL**	**Axicabtagene Ciloleucel in NHL**
Age ≤ 3 or ≥ 21 years (label is ≤ 25)	ECOG ≥ 2	ECOG ≥ 2
Karnofsky or Lansky $< 50\%$	Active CNS disease[b]	Active CNS disease[b]
Active CNS disease[a]	Creatinine clearance < 60 mL/min	AST or ALT $> 2.5 \times$ normal
ALT > 5 times normal for age	ALT $> 5\times$ normal	Creatinine > 1.5 mg/dL
Bilirubin >2.0	LV-EF $< 45\%$	Bilirubin >1.5 mg/dL
LV-EF $< 45\%$		LV-EF $< 50\%$

ALL, Acute lymphoblastic leukemia; *NHL*, Non-Hodgkin's lymphoma; *CNS*, Central nervous system; *ALT*, Alanine aminotransaminase; *LV-EF*, Left ventricular ejection fraction; *AST*, Aspartate aminotransferase; *NCCN*, National Comprehensive Cancer Network.
[a] Defined as CNS-3 by NCCN guidelines. Treated CNS disease eligible.
[b] Defined as any active CNS disease. Treated CNS disease eligible.

blood, separation of peripheral blood mononuclear cells, and reinfusion of unselected components. Compared with peripheral blood stem cell collection, which typically takes 4–6 hours per day over several days, collection of mononuclear cells for CAR T-cell manufacture is quicker, usually requiring a single 2–3 hour collection.[8]

Standards for the necessary personnel, physical space, and organization of apheresis facilities are provided by regulatory agencies including FACT.[1] In addition, for the initial development of commercial CAR T-cell products, manufacturers have required a standardization and assessment process of apheresis facilities, which is required prior to selection as a treatment site.[9] These protocols may change as CAR T-cell commercial products are brought to a wider group of facilities.

Leukapheresis is generally well tolerated, and the rate of serious adverse events is extremely low. Commonly reported low-grade adverse effects include fatigue, nausea, dizziness, cold sensation, and tingling in the fingers and mouth. More serious adverse events include pre-syncopal and syncopal reactions, as well as citrate-related hypocalcemia, which are rare, reported at 0.37% in one series.[10] ACE inhibitors should be held for 24 hours prior to collection to reduce the risk of bradykinin-mediated reactions. Most pediatric and adult patients will require a dedicated apheresis catheter. At our center, the decision as to whether a large bore, nontunneled catheter is placed is made in discussion with transfusion medicine physicians, nurses, and as per institutional guidelines developed for IEC collection.

Since the desired cells are lymphocytes, no myeloid growth factors, mobilization factors, or chemotherapy is given to enhance collection. In fact, patients require a washout period without any active treatment to optimize lymphocyte counts.[8] The tisagenlecleucel trials advised 2 weeks without cytotoxic chemotherapy prior to collection (Table 4.3). Pegylated asparaginase was held at least 4 weeks prior to collection, and therapeutic doses of steroid were held for at least 72 hours prior to collection. Since peripheral lymphocyte count is predictive of CD3+ T-cell harvest and ultimate CAR T-cell dose generated, the axicabtagene ciloleucel trial in NHL required a minimum absolute lymphocyte count (ALC) of 100 cells/μL, whereas the tisagenlecleucel trial suggested a minimum ALC of 500 cells/μL and/or a

---

TABLE 4.3
Guidelines for Drug Discontinuation Prior to Cell Collection.

8 Weeks Prior to Collection
- Anti-T-cell antibodies
- CNS radiation
- Anti-T-cell serotherapy (e.g., antithymocyte globulin, alemtuzumab)
- Donor lymphocyte infusion
- Clofarabine

4 weeks prior to collection
- Pegylated asparaginase

2 weeks prior to collection
- High-dose salvage chemotherapy (e.g., cytosine arabinoside >100 mg/m^2, anthracycline-based leukemia regimens, high-dose methotrexate (>1000 mg/m^2), platinum-based lymphoma regimens)
- Radiation therapy at a non-CNS site
- Systemic drug used for GVHD (e.g., calcineurin inhibitors)
- Antitumor antibodies (e.g., rituximab)

1 week prior to collection
- Maintenance-type chemotherapy (e.g., vincristine, 6-mercaptopurine)
- Low-to-moderate dose methotrexate (<1000 mg/m^2)
- Tyrosine kinase inhibitors (TKIs)[a]

72 hours prior to collection
- Therapeutic systemic doses of steroids
- Hydroxyurea
- CNS disease prophylaxis

CNS, Central nervous system; *GVHD*, Graft-versus-host disease.
[a] Some centers do not hold TKIs before leukapheresis.

minimum CD3+ cell count of 150 cells/μL. Thus, acceptable cutoffs vary by trials and products.

For patients receiving CAR T-cells after allogeneic stem cell transplantation, immunosuppressive drugs (e.g., calcineurin inhibitors) that suppress T-cell expansion and function must be held for at least 2 weeks prior to leukapheresis. Additionally, CAR T-cell candidates who have had a prior allogeneic transplant cannot have active graft-versus-host disease or be in the early posttransplant period where immunosuppression is required or lymphopenia is expected. Clinical trials typically required a period of at least 3 months between transplant and CAR therapy, but the period required will depend on immune reconstitution, graft-versus-host disease, and ability to wean from immunosuppression.

Numerous product-specific factors can affect the quality of leukapheresis. For example, the amount of circulating T-cells is predictive of yield,[11] whereas other cells in the collection product, particularly myeloid cells, can inhibit subsequent T-cell growth.[12,13] Furthermore, the identity and composition of the T-cells themselves can affect quality. In pediatric ALL and NHL, patients with a higher proportion of "early lineage" T-cell phenotypes such as T central memory and T stem cell memory cells[14] had better in vitro CAR expansion.[15] This mirrors data that suggest effector differentiation *after* T-cell manufacturing and expansion leads to impaired proliferation and efficacy.[16,17]

MANUFACTURING

Following apheresis, T-cells must be selected, genetically modified, and expanded to produce CAR T-cells. The manufacturing process for both academic medical centers and commercial manufacturers is reviewed in depth by Wang and Riviere,[18,19] Levine et al.,[20] and Roberts et al.[21] and will be discussed only briefly here. The initial step for CAR T-cell manufacturing includes the isolation, activation, and expansion of the target T-cell population. Several methodologies are utilized, including the commercial expansion platforms such as Life Sciences/Invitrogen Dynabeads and Miltenyi TransAct beads, which stimulate T-cells via CD3 and CD28. Other platforms such as soluble CD3 antibodies are also utilized, and the optimal method is still an area of active research.

Viral and nonviral methods are next used to genetically modify the targeted T-cell population for CAR expression. Most commonly, gamma retroviral and/or lentiviral vectors are utilized to introduce the CAR vector into the target T-cell population, as this method allows for stable integration of the CAR into the T-cell

genome. The transduction and expansion process takes place in a bioreactor culture system to avoid contamination and adhere to good manufacturing practice (GMP) requirements.

Prior to release, cell products must meet release criteria including (1) dose threshold with predetermined minimum viability, (2) identity criteria such as percentage of cells expressing the CAR construct, and (3) safety criteria such as Gram stain, endotoxin, and mycoplasma levels. Assays to determine potency may also be performed at this time. A major commercial innovation has been the development of shipping and logistics infrastructure necessary to produce and track cell products. Failure to fulfill predefined release criteria is a major obstacle to the utilization of this therapy, as those products may be rendered unusable (e.g., manufacture failure), though release criteria standards and the use of "out-of-specification" products are under investigation.

BRIDGING

The need for individualized CAR T-cell manufacturing creates a "bridging" period that is unique to cell therapies. During this period, patients are vulnerable to disease progression, infection, and other complications of active malignancy. The length of the bridging period, which begins following leukapheresis and lasts until the initiation of lymphodepleting chemotherapy, varies by product but is typically on the order of 2–4 weeks, not accounting for delays due to logistics, insurance approval, and treatment complications.

The median time from initial apheresis to return of cells to the clinical site for axicabtagene ciloleucel was 17 days in the ZUMA-1 trial of adult NHL patients, with a low manufacturing failure rate of less than 1% (1 out of 110 enrolled patients).[3] The median time from apheresis to return of cells to the clinical site for tisagenlecleucel was 23 days (range, 21–37 days) in the JULIET and ELIANA trials. The manufacturing failure rate for tisagenlecleucel was 7%, predominantly occurring in patients with ALC <300 cells per cubic millimeter.[22]

Since leukemia and lymphoma patients can have rapidly progressive disease, they often require bridging therapy to stabilize and control disease while cells are manufactured. We define bridging therapy as any treatment given between the decision to proceed with CAR therapy and CAR T-cell infusion. Patients who have a large disease burden, disease at sites of potential organ compromise, or disease that has rapidly progressed through prior treatment will require a careful evaluation to determine the optimal bridging therapy and appropriate timing of CAR T-cell infusion. As with all hematologic malignancies, close monitoring and supportive care are paramount. Patients should be assessed frequently during the bridging period, and prophylactic antibiotics, transfusions, and diagnostic studies should be provided per institutional guidelines and standard clinical practice.

If patients experience complications or are hospitalized during the bridging period, infusion may be delayed while patients recover. Aside from disease progression, the duration of maximum allowable delay is predicated on the validated time each specific CAR T-cell product can be stored. Typical storage periods are 9–12 months from time of cryopreservation; however, these times can be extended if the manufacturer validates extended expiration dates. Clinicians should understand the duration of storage to help guide any bridging strategies and to time optimal treatment initiation.

Acute Lymphoblastic Leukemia

Bridging chemotherapy is a key component of the therapeutic strategy in patients with relapsed/refractory ALL receiving CAR T-cells. The goal of bridging therapy is to stabilize the patient and reduce disease burden without inducing any short-term toxicity that would preclude a patient from receiving CAR T-cell therapy.

The choice and intensity of bridging chemotherapy depends on the patient's prior treatment history, disease burden, age, and comorbidities. Clinical trials in patients with relapsed/refractory ALL list a wide range of "acceptable" bridging chemotherapeutic options. Table 4.4 suggests a wide variety of overlapping regimens, stratified as low or high intensity, which can be employed. However, it is most critical to recognize that the goal of bridging chemotherapy is not to achieve a remission, but rather to allow a safe transition to CAR T-cell infusion. Overly aggressive bridging therapy in refractory ALL patients is likely to be of little clinical benefit and will likely cause additional treatment-related toxicities that may prohibit administration of CAR T-cells.

In the ELIANA pediatric study,[23] bridging therapy was given in 58 patients of the 68 infused (85%). Investigators stratified regimens as salvage type (including cytarabine, cyclophosphamide, etoposide, high-dose methotrexate, high-dose cytarabine, inotuzumab) and maintenance type (vincristine, 6-meracaptopurine (6-MP), 6-thioguanine, low-dose methotrexate, low-dose cytarabine, and hydroxyurea). Steroids, pegasparaginase, intrathecal chemotherapy, and vincristine were used in both salvage and maintenance therapies. Similarly, in a recent pediatric cohort reported at the American Society of Hematology Annual Meeting in

TABLE 4.4
Bridging Regimens in Acute Lymphoblastic Leukemia.

Low Intensity	High Intensity
POMP maintenance regimen (6-MP, vincristine, methotrexate, and prednisone)[30] or any combination of these drugs	Hyper CVAD (cyclophosphamide, vincristine, doxorubicin, dexamethasone)
Liposomal vincristine (weekly) (+/− steroids)[31]	High-dose cytarabine (including HiDAC and MEC-type regimens[32])
MinihyperCVD (reduced cyclophosphamide and dexamethasone, cytarabine)	Attenuated FLAG/FLAG-IDA (reduced fludarabine, cytarabine, G-CSF +/− idarubicin)
Blinatumomab[a]	Four-Drug pediatric-type induction (vincristine/steroids/asparaginase/anthracycline)
Inotuzumab	Cyclophosphamide/etoposide
Hydroxyurea	
Three-drug pediatric-type induction (vincristine/steroids/asparaginase)	

6-MP, 6-mercaptopurine.
[a] CD19-targeted therapy, see discussion in text.

2018, investigators stratified regimens into low and high intensity, with no evidence of benefit and a higher rate of infectious complications for high-intensity regimens in this limited single-center experience.[24]

In the Memorial Sloan-Kettering Cancer Center adult ALL study,[25] bridging therapy was left to the investigator's discretion. In a few cases, patients without morphologic evidence of disease were able to proceed to treatment without bridging therapy. Patients more commonly received bridging, which most commonly consistented of a low-intensity, maintenance-type regimen utilizing 6-MP, vincristine, methotrexate, or combinations thereof (Table 4.4), though high-intensity, salvage-type regimens were also used. Patients with Philadelphia chromosome–positive disease taking tyrosine kinase inhibitors (TKI) typically continued treatment through leukapheresis and the bridging period, though other trials required patients hold TKIs for at least 1 week prior to leukapheresis. TKIs were discontinued at the start of the conditioning regimen (see subsequent sections) and resumed (if necessary due to persistent disease or perceived high relapse risk) 3–4 weeks after infusion. Patients received CNS prophylaxis in the bridging period as per usual care, with some patients requiring multidrug intrathecal therapy to achieve remission in the CNS prior to CAR treatment.

Blinatumomab deserves special consideration, as it targets the same CD19 molecule as commercially available CAR T-cell products. While blinatumomab has activity in the minimal residual disease[26] and relapsed setting,[27] there is concern that exposure to a CD19-directed therapy may increase the possibility of antigen loss and tumor escape. Initial assessments of adult and pediatric patients with prior blinatumomab exposure suggest that treatment with CD19-directed CARs after blinatumomab therapy is effective,[28] but that CD19-low populations in previously treated patients may predispose to CD19-negative relapse.[2] However, these data do not necessarily apply to the limited use of blinatumomab as a bridging treatment, and further study of mechanisms of antigen loss and escape[29] is required.

B-Cell Lymphoma

Commercial CAR T-cell products for lymphoma are approved for large-cell lymphomas refractory or relapsed after two or more lines of therapy, and patients therefore generally have chemorefractory disease.[33] The CORAL analysis[34] demonstrated low rates of response to third-line chemotherapy in this setting, motivating the need for novel therapies such as CARs, and also informing the judicious use of combination chemotherapy as a bridging agent.

Comparison of study design in the two largest lymphoma trials, ZUMA-1 and JULIET, provides insight into bridging strategies. The JULIET study of tisagenlecleucel in diffuse large B-cell lymphoma (DLBCL) was designed such that 92% of patients received a bridging chemotherapy regimen,[35] including regimens utilizing rituximab (54%), gemcitabine (40%), etoposide (26%), cisplatin (19%), and cytarabine (19%). Of 165 enrolled patients, 67% (111) ultimately received CAR treatment, with a large proportion of untreated patients having poor performance status and disease refractory to the last line of therapy. This experience highlights the challenge of maintaining patient fitness in a highly refractory population.

In the ZUMA-1 study of axicabtagene ciloleucel, systemic bridging therapy was not allowed between leukapheresis and infusion. Of 111 patients, 101 received CAR treatment, with 1 manufacturing failure, 5 adverse events, 2 deaths, and 2 patients with nonmeasurable disease prior to infusion.[3] The lack of bridging may be in part due to more rapid time to infusion, which was a median of 17 days in this study compared with 23 days in the tisagenlecleucel study. However, patient selection and study design also likely contributed. Furthermore, in a real-world experience with commercial axicabtagene ciloleucel, slightly more than half of patients (52%) did receive some form of bridging therapy,[36] which may be due to treatment of patients with more aggressive disease, as well as logistical and planning delays in routine practice.

Regimen selection can be guided by prior therapy and disease subtype as per usual lymphoma care. Sample chemotherapy regimens are described in Table 4.5. The benefit of chemotherapy must be weighed against the risk of complications that can delay infusion; therefore, clinicians should exercise caution with intensive regimens and in patients at higher risk of complications. If possible, one cycle is given, with the goal of maintaining clinical stability for 2–4 weeks during cell manufacturing and allowing bone marrow recovery prior to lymphodepletion (see below).

Novel drugs such as lenalidomide,[37,38] ibrutinib, and PD-1 inhibitors are potentially attractive bridging agents for several reasons: (1) activity in specific lymphoma subtypes, such as ibrutinib in the ABC subtype[39] or PD-1 inhibitors in primary mediastinal B-cell lymphoma[40]; (2) less severe bone marrow suppression and associated complications requiring prolonged recovery prior to infusion; and (3) the potential for synergy with CAR T-cell therapy. For example, ibrutinib has been utilized to improve safety[41] and enhance efficacy[42,43] of CAR T-cells, whereas PD-1 inhibitors have been used to restore CAR T-cell function after exhaustion.[44,45]

Experience with these agents as bridging therapies is limited. For example, only 9% of patients in JULIET

TABLE 4.5
Selected Bridging Regimens for Lymphoma.
GemOx[47] (gemcitabine, oxaliplatin ± rituximab)
DHAP[48] (dexamethasone, cytarabine, cisplatin ± rituximab)
DHAX[49] (dexamethasone, cytarabine, oxaliplatin ± rituximab)
Lenalidomide[37,38] (lenalidomide ± rituximab)
Prednisone

were bridged with ibrutinib and 7% with lenalidomide.[35] Key questions remain, including how to best incorporate CAR T-cells if patients have a response to bridging therapy. We anticipate upcoming clinical trials will address how best to use these agents as bridging, combination, and/or maintenance therapy with CAR T-cells.

Finally, patients with stable and indolent disease can be either observed or treated with low-dose steroids that are typically held at least 3 days prior to infusion. Palliative radiation therapy is frequently useful to control symptoms and disease at sites of functional compromise.[46]

In summary, there is no universal bridging strategy in lymphoma, and the type and intensity of bridging will vary by patient and product. Patients with rapidly progressive disease that may cause clinical deterioration within 2–3 weeks are more likely to benefit from bridging compared with patients with indolent disease. A single cycle of systemic chemotherapy is often sufficient, but many patients will not require bridging. Agents such as ibrutinib and lenalidomide are being increasingly studied, and radiation and steroids are appropriate for selected patients. Finally, the need for bridging will depend in large part on the turnaround time between leukapheresis and product delivery, which can vary by product and can be delayed by patient complications and administrative barriers.

Multiple Myeloma

At the time of writing, numerous cellular therapies targeting multiple myeloma are in development, with the majority targeting B-cell maturation antigen.[50–52] As no products are commercially available, the approach to bridging therapy is in flux and dictated by research protocols. Further complicating the choice of therapy is the extensive treatment history and resistance of many myeloma patients enrolled on CAR T-cell trials.

Many protocols allow high-intensity, chemotherapy-based regimens for patients with rapidly progressive and aggressive disease. These include dexamethasone, cyclophosphamide, etoposide, and cisplatin (DCEP) or bortezomib, dexamethasone, cisplatin, doxorubicin, cyclophosphamide, and etoposide (VD-PACE), typically given as one cycle immediately following leukapheresis. Ongoing trials will provide information on the benefit patients with aggressive disease derived from CAR T-cell therapy and the risk of complications that delay CAR T-cell infusion.

Alternatively, some protocols allow bridging with a less intense, two-drug regimen such as Vd (bortezomib/dexamethasone) or Kd (carfilzomib/dexamethasone). Regimens employing commonly used monoclonal antibodies require more study due to antibody persistence and potential interactions with CAR T-cells. For example, daratumumab has numerous effects on T-cells, both indirectly and directly as CD38 is expressed on certain lymphocyte subsets.[53] Similarly, CS1 expression on lymphocytes may complicate the use of CS1-targeted agents such as elotuzumab.[54] However, these interactions are pleiotropic and require further study before recommendations can be made.

Chronic Lymphocytic Leukemia

CAR T-cells have had comparatively lower rates of activity in chronic lymphocytic leukemia (CLL).[55–57] However, a subset of patients have experienced long-term durable responses, with remissions more likely in those with "higher-quality" T-cells, such as a higher proportion of phenotypically memory-like lymphocytes.[58] As in myeloma, trials for CAR T-cell therapy are ongoing, and no universal recommendations for bridging therapy can be made. However, there is emerging evidence that ibrutinib prior to CAR T-cell therapy[42,57,59] can enhance efficacy, perhaps in part by modulating T-cell quality and phenotype.

LYMPHODEPLETING CHEMOTHERAPY

Several days prior to CAR T-cell infusion, patients receive a conditioning or lymphodepleting chemotherapy regimen to enhance engraftment and activity. This is a separate treatment than the bridging regimen described above. The rationale and benefit of chemotherapeutic conditioning prior to cell infusion was initially developed for autologous and allogeneic hematopoietic stem cell transplantation.[60] Regimens in this setting are selected for disease activity and at least partial myeloablation to enhance stem cell engraftment.

The role of conditioning chemotherapy prior to tumor-specific cellular therapy was subsequently advanced by tumor infiltrating lymphocyte (TIL) experiments performed at the National Cancer Institute. In these studies, the activity of melanoma-specific TILs was significantly enhanced by aggressive conditioning with total body irradiation and cyclophosphamide in mouse models[61,62] and clinical trials.[63]

Conditioning chemotherapy has numerous theoretical benefits. First, chemotherapy can have a direct antitumor cytotoxic effect, although the regimens and doses typically used are not highly active in this setting. Chemotherapy can also have indirect immune enhancing effects[64] such as (1) depletion of immunosuppressive cells including myeloid suppressor cells[65] and regulatory T-cells (particularly for low-dose cyclophosphamide),[66]

(2) release of tumor antigens and danger signals through tumor killing,[67] and (3) enhancing trafficking to the tumor site through binding of SDF-1 with CXCR-4 expressed on the T-cell surface.[68] Perhaps most importantly, chemotherapy depletes host lymphocytes and thus reduces competition for homeostatic signals such as self-MHC and cytokines, increasing the proliferation and persistence of adoptively transferred cells.[69]

The optimal conditioning regimen has not been rigorously examined, but several experiences are illustrative. In NHL, Kochenderfer and colleagues initially used a high-dose chemotherapy regimen of cyclophosphamide (60–120 mg/kg once) and fludarabine (25 mg/m^2/day × 5 days).[70] Despite encouraging responses, significant hypotension and neurologic toxicities were reported, even at CAR T-cell doses as low as 1×10^6 cells/kg. When lower doses of cyclophosphamide (300 mg/m^2/day × 3 days) and fludarabine (30 mg/m^2/day × 3 days) were used, severe hypotension and severe neurotoxicity were eliminated, although less severe CRS and neurotoxicity were still observed.[71] In a subsequent study summarizing experience with the high- and low-dose regimens, the median time to an absolute neutrophil count of less than 500/uL was 0 days (0–6 days) with the low-dose chemotherapy versus 5 days (0–16 days) with the high-dose regimen, with most patients in the latter group requiring platelet transfusion.[72] Further attempts to refine the regimen by increasing cyclophosphamide from 300 to 500 mg/kg again suggested increased toxicity, and the dose was reverted.[73]

Severe neurotoxicity, including deaths from cerebral edema in the JCAR015 ROCKET trial,[74,75] led to concerns regarding fludarabine, which has historically been associated with neurologic toxicity.[76] Unfortunately, cerebral edema also occurred in a cyclophosphamide-only conditioning cohort, suggesting fludarabine is not solely responsible for severe neurotoxicity. In fact, severe neurotoxicities and fatal cerebral edema have been observed in other studies using different conditioning and various CAR T-cells containing either 4-1BB and CD28 costimulatory domains.[3,7,77,78]

In a study by Turtle et al. in patients with NHL,[79] combining fludarabine and cyclophosphamide conditioning chemotherapy was associated with higher complete response (CR) rates than regimens without fludarabine (50% vs. 8%), higher serum levels of IL-15 and IL-7 on the day of cell infusion and a greater degree of subsequent CAR T-cell expansion. However, a separate study of pediatric ALL patients using the same construct reported a higher peak CAR T-cell expansion but could not detect a difference in the CR rate and persistence of B-cell aplasia with the addition of fludarabine.[17] Therefore, the optimal choice of conditioning chemotherapy may depend on the cell product and disease subtypes.

Currently, the most commonly used conditioning chemotherapy regimen includes low-dose cyclophosphamide and fludarabine, as utilized in the multicenter JULIET,[35] TRANSCEND,[7] and ZUMA-1[3] trials, though the dose and regimens used in different trials and regimens are slightly different (Table 4.6). Conditioning regimens are typically given 1–7 days prior to T-cell infusions. For axicabtagene ciloleucel, cyclophosphamide 500 mg/m^2 and fludarabine 30 mg/m^2 intravenously are given on the fifth, fourth, and third day prior to infusion. For tisagenlecleucel in pediatric ALL, fludarabine 30 mg/m^2 is given daily for 4 days and cyclophosphamide 500 mg/m^2 daily any time from 2 to 14 days prior to infusion. For adult DLBCL, fludarabine is given at 25 mg/m^2 daily for 3 days and cyclophosphamide 250 mg/m^2 daily for 3 days any time between 2 and 11 days before infusion.

However, there are certain conditions in which alternative regimens, or no conditioning at all, can be used. The University of Pennsylvania NHL study[22] allowed a number of conditioning regimens, and only one patient received a fludarabine-based treatment. The regimens were selected based on response history, blood counts, and organ function at investigator's discretion. As a result, a bendamustine regimen was permitted in the JULIET trial,[35] and therefore, the tisagenlecleucel label includes a preparative regimen with bendamustine at 90 mg/m^2 for 2 days. In some settings, particularly highly pretreated and lymphopenic patients, no conditioning may be necessary. For example, the tisagenlecleucel label recommends that lymphodepletion be omitted if the white blood cell count is less than or equal to 1×10^9/L within 1 week prior to cell infusion.

Finally, the optimal conditioning regimen is likely to vary by disease. For example, in the University of Pennsylvania single center experience with CLL, pentostatin was added to cyclophosphamide both as a lymphodepleting agent and due to its known activity in this disease.[80] More importantly, as the field expands to target other hematologic and nonhematologic malignancies, the optimal conditioning regimen may change.

CELL DOSE AND FORMULATION

The cell dose and formulation infused are product and disease dependent. Some trials have used weight-based dosing on the order $1-5 \times 10^6$ cells/kg,[70,81,83,84]

TABLE 4.6
Preparative/Lymphodepleting Regimens Used in Key CAR T-Cell Trials.

Study	Disease	Preparative/lymphodepleting Regimen
Axicabtagene ciloleucel,[3] multicenter	NHL	Fludarabine 30 mg/m^2/day and cyclophosphamide 500 mg/m^2/day each for 3 days
Park et al.,[25] Memorial Sloan Kettering	Adult ALL	Cyclophosphamide 3 g/m^2 for 1 day Or cyclophosphamide 3 g/m^2 × 1 day + fludarabine 25 –30 mg/m^2/day × 3 days
Tisagenlecleucel,[35] multicenter	NHL	Fludarabine 25 mg/m^2/day and cyclophosphamide 250 mg/m^2/day each for 3 days Or bendamustine 90 mg/m^2/day × 2 days
Schuster et al.,[22] Penn	NHL	Cyclophosphamide 1.8 mg/m^2 Or EPOCH Or cyclophosphamide 1 g/m^2 Or bendamustine 90 mg/m^2/day × 2 days Or radiation therapy (4000 cGy) + cyclophosphamide 750 mg/m^2 Or etoposide 50 mg/m^2/day × 4 days + cyclophosphamide 750 mg/m^2
Lisocabtagene maraleucel,[7] multicenter	NHL	Fludarabine 30 mg/m^2/day and cyclophosphamide 300 mg/m^2/day each for 3 days
Turtle et al.,[81] FHCRC	Adult ALL	Cyclophosphamide 30–60 mg/kg × 1 day and fludarabine 25 mg/m^2/day × 3–5 days
Turtle et al.,[79] FHCRC	NHL	Cyclophosphamide 2–4 g/m^2 × 1 day and etoposide 100 –200 mg/m^2/day × 3 days Or cyclophosphamide 60 mg/kg × 1 day ± fludarabine 25 mg/m^2/day on days 2–4 or 2–6
Porter et al.,[82] Penn	CLL	Pentostatin 4 mg/m^2 and cyclophosphamide 600 mg/m^2

NHL, Non-Hodgkin's lymphoma; *ALL*, Acute lymphoblastic leukemia; *CLL*, Chronic lymphocytic leukemia; *FHCRC*, Fred Hutchinson Cancer Research Center.

whereas studies at the University of Pennsylvania and with tisagenlecleucel have infused all available cells after expansion with natural variation between patients, ranging from 0.2 to 5.4 × 10^6 cells/kg in pediatric ALL[85] and 3 to 8.87 × 10^6 cells/kg in adult NHL.[22]

In the tisagenlecleucel studies, there was no correlation between dose infused and response. This lack of dose-response is explained by the log-fold expansion that CARs undergo after infusion. While peak expansion correlates with response (though not survival) for CD28[3,25,72] and 4-1BB constructs in pediatric ALL and CLL,[58] this relationship is not seen in NHL.[22]

However, cell dose, CAR construct activity, and disease burden can interact to impact safety and efficacy. For example, investigators at Memorial Sloan Kettering used a disease burden modified dosing regimen for adult ALL. Under conditions that promote aggressive CAR expansion, including a CD28 construct and high burden of disease (≥5% bone marrow blasts or extramedullary disease), we observed that disease burden correlates with CRS severity.[25] Therefore, investigators infused a lower dose of CAR T-cells (1 × 10^6 cells/kg) for patients with high disease burden, compared with 3 × 10^6 cells/kg for low disease burden patients, though this strategy has not formally been proven to reduce toxicity. Similarly, investigators at the Fred Hutchinson Cancer Center demonstrated a correlation between the onset of neurotoxicity and both tumor burden and cell dose in a cohort of 133 patients treated for NHL, ALL, and CLL.[86] In general, an emerging paradigm is that conditions that encourage robust CAR expansion, including high cell dose, a CD28 construct, and high burden of disease, increase the risk of both severe CRS and neurotoxicity.[77]

The two commercially approved CAR products are both provided as frozen suspensions for infusion. The label for tisagenlecleucel indicates that

$0.2 \times 10^6 - 5 \times 10^6$ cells/kg can be infused for pediatric patients <50 kg, and a flat dose of $0.1-6 \times 10^8$ cells for others. This should represent the contents of the bag. Axicabtagene ciloleucel is dosed at 2×10^6 cells/kg, up to 2×10^8 total cells, for adults.

Lisocabtagene maraleucel, Juno/Celgene's investigational product for adult NHL, is provided as two separate suspensions of CD4+ and CD8+ CAR T-cells. This split product is based on studies in NHL[79] and B-ALL[81] patients performed at Fred Hutchinson Cancer Research Center, where a defined composition of CD4+ and CD8+ CAR T-cells infused at a 1:1 ratio enhanced CAR function, with CD4+ cells providing help to CD8+ CAR T-cell killing.[16] Manufacturing techniques, in particular cytokines used in culture and the upfront isolation of central memory CD8+ T-cells, differ between the CAR T-cell subsets. The dose of CD8+ suspension cells is administered first, typically followed by CD4+ cells 10–15 minutes later. In case of delay for infusion reaction or other complication, the two products must be infused within 48 hours of each other.

INFUSION

It is important to develop institutional guidelines for safe, proper, and timely administration of immune effector cells.[9] These guidelines can be modeled after those used for autologous and allogeneic stem cell products and donor lymphocyte infusions. Critical issues include the need to verify patient and product identity, ensure cell product availability, and coordinate activity between the clinical team, cell laboratory, and pharmacy. The following timeline is modeled after guidelines for immune effector cell infusion at Memorial Sloan Kettering Cancer Center.

Prior to infusion, the attending physician is responsible for entering an order for cell preparation, stating the name of the patient, patient identification number, the type of product to be infused, the dose of product to be infused, and the date of requested infusion. This order notifies the respective groups involved in the administration of the cellular therapy. In the commercial setting, these include the cell laboratory (responsible for storage, delivery, and thawing of the product) and pharmacy (responsible to ensure two doses of the anti-IL6 receptor antibody, tocilizumab, are available as per FDA-mandated REMS programs).

On the day prior or day of infusion, communication between the cell laboratory staff and the treating physician is required to confirm the patient has maintained eligibility for infusion. The frozen cell product is hand delivered by a laboratory staff member to the patient's location. The clinical staff member receiving the product verifies the product identity with the laboratory staff member, confirming the patient identity with at least two patient-specific identifiers, as well as the identity of the cell product and the dose. Furthermore, prior to infusion, the attending physician is responsible for confirming the following:

1. Consent documented in chart
2. Order reviewed and confirmed as appropriate
3. Recipient and unit identity confirmed
4. Cell dose appropriate
5. Bag identification cross-checked
6. Product number confirmed
7. Product integrity inspected
8. Product characteristics, volume, and cell dose on the infusion slip are appropriate

Prior to administration, the medical team should also verify the central line is available, accessed, and patent with blood return. Prior to each CAR T-cell infusion, patients are given acetaminophen and diphenhydramine as prophylaxis against infusion-related reactions (see below). Steroids should not be given as premedication due to cytolytic and immunosuppressive effects but can be used in the context of adverse effects.

Each bag is thawed one at a time at 37°C and, once thawed, the labeled dose volume administered into the subject within the specified expiration time after removal from the shipping container, which is provided on the label. In the context of the commercial products, axicabtagene ciloleucel can be stored at room temperature for up to 3 hours; the tisagenlecleucel labels recommend infusion within 30 minutes.

A nurse should be present at bedside and is responsible for monitoring the patient throughout the infusion. Temperature, pulse, respirations, and blood pressure are measured and recorded in the patient's chart prior to infusion, at set intervals during infusion (e.g., every 15 minutes), and then subsequently measured following institutional guidelines for cellular therapy.

INFUSION REACTIONS

The rate of immediate hypersensitivity reactions during or after CAR T-cell infusion is extremely low (and to our knowledge has not been reported for any commercially available product).[87] There have, however, been case reports of severe reactions in specific investigational products. A patient treated with an investigational antimesothelin CAR developed anaphylaxis and cardiac arrest 1 minute after his third autologous CAR T-cell infusion, with elevated serum tryptase,[88] and may represent a hypersensitivity reaction in the setting of multiple CAR infusions.

The most commonly described postinfusion adverse effect is nausea, which is attributed to DMSO cryoprecipitate from the cell product and can be managed with antiemetics per institutional guidelines. Mild fatigue and hypotension are also common, which may be related to an infusion reaction, but are also commonly associated with diphenhydramine premedication.

Infusion reactions are managed according to severity using the hypersensitivity or infusion reaction management guidelines of the individual institution. Suggested guidelines are summarized in Table 4.7.

CRS is the most common toxicity observed after CAR T-cell infusion[89] and is characterized by an inflammatory syndrome with a wide spectrum of presentations, from transient fever to critical illness with hypotension, respiratory failure, and death. The management of CRS is discussed in Chapters 5 and 6. We note that there can be overlap between the symptoms of infusion reactions and initial presentation of CRS. However, the onset of CRS is later, at least 8–12 hours after infusion and more typically 1–5 days after infusion. Tachycardia and fever are the usual presenting symptoms of CRS, whereas infusion reactions are associated with skin reactions and bronchospasm.

SITE OF INFUSION: INPATIENT VERSUS OUTPATIENT

CAR T-cell products must be administered in a controlled clinical environment where infusions can be given and patients can be monitored. Several trials have demonstrated the feasibility of administering CAR T-cells in an outpatient setting in both children[85] and adults. Conditioning chemotherapy regimens can be safely administered in infusion centers that can accommodate daily treatment. Furthermore, as discussed above, infusion is generally well tolerated, and if patients are stable several hours after administration, they can be safely sent home or to local housing.

The primary concern for outpatient administration is the onset of CRS, which typically occurs 1–5 days following infusion. Tachycardia and fever are generally the first signs of CRS and require immediate evaluation. Since most patients have received conditioning chemotherapy with subsequent neutropenia, the evaluation and empiric treatment of febrile neutropenia must be included in any initial evaluation. Beyond CRS, neurotoxicity typically occurs later, approximately 4–10 days after infusion,[77,86] and can be marked by subtle changes such as aphasia prior to the onset of severe symptoms. Therefore, if infusion is given as an outpatient, patients must return for frequent assessments, which include monitoring for fever, testing biomarkers of CRS (e.g.,

TABLE 4.7
Suggested Management of Infusion Reactions.

CTCAE v5[90]	Grade 1	Grade 2	Grade 3	Grade 4	Grade 5
Definition	Mild transient reaction; infusion interruption not indicated; intervention not indicated	Therapy or infusion interruption indicated but responds promptly to symptomatic treatment; prophylactic medications indicated for <24 hours	Prolonged (not rapidly responsive to symptomatic medication and/or brief interruption of infusion); recurrence of symptoms following initial improvement; hospitalization indicated for clinical sequelae	Life-threatening consequences; urgent intervention indicated	Death
Management	Continue infusion at same rate; manage symptoms	Reduce infusion rate by 50%; manage symptoms	Interrupt infusion. Manage symptoms, consider steroids if necessary. Rechallenge at 50% rate	Discontinue infusion, treat reaction, and do not rechallenge	

CRP), and screening for signs or symptoms of neurologic toxicity. The overall side effect profile for each CAR T-cell product will dictate the frequency (daily vs. intermittent) and duration of frequent follow-up. In the setting of the currently available commercial CAR T-cells, daily follow-up during the first 1–2 weeks with gradual weaning until >4 weeks from infusion is recommended.

Additionally, in the setting of the currently available commercial CAR T-cells, there is a strict requirement that all patients live within 2 hours (preferably within 1 hour) of the treating center for the immediate pre- and posttreatment period. Furthermore, patients should have a caregiver who is present full time and can assist the patient and contact medical professionals at the first sign of fever, confusion, word finding difficulty, or other worrying symptoms. A CAR-trained provider should be on call at all times to evaluate patients.

Only fit patients with good performance status and few comorbidities should be considered for outpatient infusion, whereas older patients, patients with a history of severe infection, and patients with pertinent comorbidities such as neurologic disorders may be better suited for inpatient infusion, though more precise guidelines are still being developed. In addition, reimbursement practices differ between the outpatient and inpatient setting and between public and private payers in the United States and are currently in flux. Therefore, the exact criteria for inpatient versus outpatient infusion are still being developed, and institutions will need to develop stringent criteria that mirror any programs for the outpatient delivery of autologous and allogeneic transplantation.

ACKNOWLEDGMENTS

We thank ML Silverberg for assistance with development of nursing and postinfusion protocols.

REFERENCES

1. Maus MV, Nikiforow S. The why, what, and how of the new FACT standards for immune effector cells. *J Immunother Cancer.* 2017;5(1):36. https://doi.org/10.1186/s40425-017-0239-0.
2. Pillai V, Rosenthal J, Muralidharan K, et al. Correlation of pre-CAR CD19 expression with responses and relapses after CAR T cell therapy. *J Clin Oncol.* 2018;36(15_suppl l). https://doi.org/10.1200/JCO.2018.36.15_suppl.3051, 3051-3051.
3. Neelapu SS, Locke FL, Bartlett NL, et al. Axicabtagene ciloleucel CAR T-cell therapy in refractory large B-cell lymphoma. *N Engl J Med.* 2017. https://doi.org/10.1056/NEJMoa1707447. NEJMoa1707447.
4. Abramson JS, McGree B, Noyes S, et al. Anti-CD19 CAR T cells in CNS diffuse large-B-cell lymphoma. *N Engl J Med.* 2017;377(8):783–784. https://doi.org/10.1056/NEJMc1704610.
5. Food and Drug Administration. Guidance for industry: eligibility determination for donors of human cells. In: *Tissues and Cellular and Tissue-Based Products (HCT/Ps);* 2007. http://www.fda.gov/cber/guidelines.htm.
6. Foundation for the Accreditation of Cellular Therapy. *Standards for Immune Effector Cells.* first edition; 2017. Published http://www.factwebsite.org/Standards/.
7. Abramson JS, Palomba ML, Gordon LI, et al. High durable CR rates in relapsed/refractory (R/R) aggressive B-NHL treated with the CD19-directed CAR T cell product JCAR017 (TRANSCEND NHL 001). *Am Soc Hematol Annu Meet;* 2017. https://ash.confex.com/ash/2017/webprogram/Paper102372.html.
8. McGuirk J, Waller EK, Qayed M, et al. Building blocks for institutional preparation of CTL019 delivery. *Cytotherapy.* 2017;19(9):1015–1024. https://doi.org/10.1016/J.JCYT.2017.06.001.
9. Perica K, Curran KJ, Brentjens RJ, Giralt SA. Building a CAR garage: preparing for the delivery of commercial CAR T cell products at memorial Sloan Kettering cancer center. *Biol Blood Marrow Transplant.* March 2018. https://doi.org/10.1016/J.BBMT.2018.02.018.
10. Yuan S, Ziman A, Smeltzer B, Lu Q, Goldfinger D. Moderate and severe adverse events associated with apheresis donations: incidences and risk factors. *Transfusion.* 2010;50(2):478–486. https://doi.org/10.1111/j.1537-2995.2009.02443.x.
11. Allen ES, Stroncek DF, Ren J, et al. Autologous lymphapheresis for the production of chimeric antigen receptor T cells. *Transfusion.* 2017;57(5):1133–1141. https://doi.org/10.1111/trf.14003.
12. Stroncek DF, Ren J, Lee DW, et al. Myeloid cells in peripheral blood mononuclear cell concentrates inhibit the expansion of chimeric antigen receptor T cells. *Cytotherapy.* 2016;18(7):893–901. https://doi.org/10.1016/j.jcyt.2016.04.003.
13. Wang X, Qu J, Stefanski J, et al. Depletion of high-content CD14+ cells from apheresis products is critical for the successful transduction and expansion of CAR T cells during large-scale cGMP manufacturing. *Mol Ther.* 2015;23:S35. https://doi.org/10.1016/S1525-0016(16)33685-1, 80.
14. Gattinoni L, Lugli E, Ji Y, et al. A human memory T cell subset with stem cell-like properties. *Nat Med.* 2011; (September). https://doi.org/10.1038/nm.2446.
15. Singh N, Perazzelli J, Grupp SA, Barrett DM. Early memory phenotypes drive T cell proliferation in patients with pediatric malignancies. *Sci Transl Med;* 2018. http://stm.sciencemag.org/content/scitransmed/8/320/320ra3.full.pdf.
16. Sommermeyer D, Hudecek M, Kosasih PL, et al. Chimeric antigen receptor-modified T cells derived from defined CD8+ and CD4+ subsets confer superior antitumor reactivity in vivo. *Leukemia.* 2016;30(2):492–500. https://doi.org/10.1038/leu.2015.247.Chimeric.

17. Gardner RA, Finney O, Annesley C, et al. Intent to treat leukemia remission by CD19CAR T cells of defined formulation and dose in children and young adults. *Blood*. 2017; 129(25). https://doi.org/10.1182/blood-2017-02-769208. blood-2017-02-769208.

18. Wang X, Rivière I. Clinical manufacturing of CAR T cells: foundation of a promising therapy. *Mol Ther Oncolytics*. 2016;3(16015):1−7. https://doi.org/10.1038/mto.2016.15.

19. Wang X, Rivière I. Manufacture of tumor- and virus-specific T lymphocytes for adoptive cell therapies. *Cancer Gene Ther*. 2015;22(2):85−94. https://doi.org/10.1038/cgt.2014.81.

20. Levine BL, Miskin J, Wonnacott K, Keir C. Global manufacturing of CAR T cell therapy. *Mol Ther Methods Clin Dev*. 2017;4(March):92−101. https://doi.org/10.1016/j.omtm.2016.12.006.

21. Roberts ZJ, Better M, Bot A, Roberts MR, Ribas A. Axicabtagene ciloleucel, a first-in-class CAR T cell therapy for aggressive NHL. *Leuk Lymphoma*; 2017. Published http://www.tandfonline.com/action/journalInformation?journalCode=ilal20.

22. Schuster SJ, Svoboda J, Chong EA, et al. Chimeric antigen receptor T cells in refractory B-cell lymphomas. *N Engl J Med*. 2017. https://doi.org/10.1056/NEJMoa1708566. NEJMoa1708566.

23. Buechner J, Grupp SA, Maude SL, et al. Global registration trial of efficacy and safety of CTL019 in pediatric and young adult patients with relapsed/refractory (R/R) acute lymphoblastic leukemia (all): update to the interim analysis. In: *European Hematology Association Annual Meeting*; 2017. https://learningcenter.ehaweb.org/eha/2017/22nd/181763/stephan.a.grupp.global.registration.trial.of.efficacy.and.safety.of.ctl019.in.html?f=m3.

24. Gupta S, Alexander S, Zupanec S, Maude SL, Krueger J. *High vs. Low-Intensity Bridging Chemotherapy in Children with Acute Lymphoblastic Leukemia Awaiting Chimeric Antigen Receptor T-Cell Therapy*. Canada: A Population-Based Study From Ontario; December 2018. https://ash.confex.com/ash/2018/webprogram/Paper115593.html.

25. Park JH, Rivière I, Gonen M, et al. Long-term follow-up of CD19 CAR therapy in acute lymphoblastic leukemia. *N Engl J Med*. 2018;378(5):449−459. https://doi.org/10.1056/NEJMoa1709919.

26. Gökbuget N, Zugmaier G, Klinger M, et al. Long-term relapse-free survival in a phase 2 study of blinatumomab for the treatment of patients with minimal residual disease in B-lineage acute lymphoblastic leukemia. *Haematologica*. 2017;102(4):e132−e135. https://doi.org/10.3324/haematol.2016.153957.

27. Fielding AK, Schuh AC, et al. Blinatumomab versus chemotherapy for advanced acute lymphoblastic leukemia. *N Engl J Med*. 2017. https://doi.org/10.1056/NEJMoa1609783.

28. Shah BD, Oluwole OO, Baer MR, et al. Outcomes of patients (pts) treated with prior blinatumomab (Blin) in ZUMA-3: a study of KTE-C19, an anti-CD19 chimeric antigen receptor (CAR) t cell therapy, in adult pts with relapsed/refractory acute lymphoblastic leukemia (R/R ALL). *J Clin Oncol*. 2018;36(15_suppl l). https://doi.org/10.1200/JCO.2018.36.15_suppl.7006, 7006-7006.

29. Majzner RG, Mackall CL. Tumor antigen escape from CAR T-cell therapy. *Cancer Discov*. 2018:1219. https://doi.org/10.1158/2159-8290.CD-18-0442.

30. Kantarjian H, Thomas D, O'Brien S, et al. Long-term follow-up results of hyperfractionated cyclophosphamide, vincristine, doxorubicin, and dexamethasone (Hyper-CVAD), a dose-intensive regimen, in adult acute lymphocytic leukemia. *Cancer*. 2004;101(12):2788−2801. https://doi.org/10.1002/cncr.20668.

31. O'Brien S, Schiller G, Lister J, et al. High-dose vincristine sulfate liposome injection for advanced, relapsed, and refractory adult Philadelphia chromosome-negative acute lymphoblastic leukemia. *J Clin Oncol*. 2013;31(6): 676−683. https://doi.org/10.1200/JCO.2012.46.2309.

32. Liedtke M, Dunn T, Dinner S, et al. Salvage therapy with mitoxantrone, etoposide and cytarabine in relapsed or refractory acute lymphoblastic leukemia. *Leuk Res*. 2014; 38(12):1441−1445. https://doi.org/10.1016/J.LEUKRES.2014.09.018.

33. Perica K, Palomba ML, Brentjens RJ. *Dawn of Chimeric Antigen Receptor T Cell Therapy in non-Hodgkin Lymphoma*. 2018:1−10. https://doi.org/10.1002/acg2.23. June.

34. Van Den Neste E, Schmitz N, Mounier N, et al. Outcome of patients with relapsed diffuse large B-cell lymphoma who fail second-line salvage regimens in the International CORAL study. *Bone Marrow Transplant*. 2016;51(1): 51−57. https://doi.org/10.1038/bmt.2015.213.

35. Schuster SJ, Bishop MR, Tam CS, et al. Tisagenlecleucel in adult relapsed or refractory diffuse large B-cell lymphoma. *NEJM*. 2018:1−12. https://doi.org/10.1056/NEJMoa1804980.

36. Nastoupil L, Jain MD, Spiegel D, et al. Axicabtagene ciloleucel (Axi-cel) CD19 chimeric antigen receptor (CAR) T-cell therapy for relapsed/refractory large B-cell lymphoma: real world experience. *Ther Clin Risk Manag*; December 2018. https://ash.confex.com/ash/2018/webprogram/Paper114152.html.

37. Witzig TE, Vose JM, Zinzani PL, et al. An international phase II trial of single-agent lenalidomide for relapsed or refractory aggressive B-cell non-Hodgkin's lymphoma. *Ann Oncol*. 2011;22(7):1622−1627. https://doi.org/10.1093/annonc/mdq626.

38. Wang Y, Wagner-Bartak N, Zhou S, et al. Lenalidomide plus rituximab for relapsed or refractory diffuse large B-cell, follicular and transformed lymphoma: final data analysis of a phase 2 trial. *Blood*. 2015;126(23), 2018 http://www.bloodjournal.org/content/126/23/3969.

39. Wilson WH, Young RM, Schmitz R, et al. Targeting B cell receptor signaling with ibrutinib in diffuse large B cell lymphoma. *Nat Med*. 2015;21(8):922−926. https://doi.org/10.1038/nm.3884.

40. Zinzani PL, Ribrag V, Moskowitz CH, et al. Safety and tolerability of pembrolizumab in patients with relapsed/refractory primary mediastinal large B-cell lymphoma. *Blood*. 2017;130(3):267−270. https://doi.org/10.1182/blood-2016-12-758383.

41. Ruella M, Kenderian SS, Shestova O, et al. Kinase inhibitor ibrutinib to prevent cytokine-release syndrome after anti-CD19 chimeric antigen receptor T cells for B-cell neoplasms. *Leukemia.* 2017;31(1):246–248. https://doi.org/10.1038/leu.2016.262.

42. Gill S, Frey NV, Hexner EO, et al. CD19 CAR-T cells combined with ibrutinib to induce complete remission in CLL. *J Clin Oncol.* 2017;35(15_suppl):7509. https://doi.org/10.1200/JCO.2017.35.15_suppl.7509.

43. Fraietta JA, Beckwith KA, Patel PR, et al. Ibrutinib enhances chimeric antigen receptor T-cell engraftment and efficacy in leukemia. *Blood.* 2016;127(9):1117–1127. https://doi.org/10.1182/blood-2015-11-679134.

44. Chong EA, Melenhorst JJ, Lacey SF, et al. PD-1 blockade modulates chimeric antigen receptor (CAR)-modified T cells: refueling the CAR. *Blood.* 2017;129(8):1039–1041. https://doi.org/10.1182/blood-2016-09-738245.

45. Maude SL, Hucks GE, Seif AE, et al. The effect of pembrolizumab in combination with CD19-targeted chimeric antigen receptor (CAR) T cells in relapsed acute lymphoblastic leukemia (ALL). *J Clin Oncol.* 2017;35(15_suppl):103. https://doi.org/10.1200/JCO.2017.35.15_suppl.103.

46. Jain M, Chavez JC, Shah BD, et al. *Radiation Therapy as a Bridging Strategy for Refractory Diffuse Large B Cell Lymphoma Patients Awaiting CAR T Manufacturing of Axicabtagene Ciloleucel*; December 2018, 2019 https://ash.confex.com/ash/2018/webprogram/Paper117133.html.

47. Mounier N, El Gnaoui T, Tilly H, et al. Rituximab plus gemcitabine and oxaliplatin in patients with refractory/relapsed diffuse large B-cell lymphoma who are not candidates for high-dose therapy. A phase II lymphoma study association trial. *Haematologica.* 2013;98(11):1726–1731. https://doi.org/10.3324/haematol.2013.090597.

48. Velasquez WS, Cabanillas F, Salvador P, et al. Effective salvage therapy for lymphoma with cisplatin in combination with high-dose Ara-C and dexamethasone (DHAP). *Blood.* 1988;71(1):117–122, 2018 http://www.ncbi.nlm.nih.gov/pubmed/3334893.

49. Lignon J, Sibon D, Madelaine I, et al. Rituximab, dexamethasone, cytarabine, and oxaliplatin (R-DHAX) is an effective and safe salvage regimen in relapsed/refractory B-cell non-hodgkin lymphoma. *Clin Lymphoma Myeloma Leuk.* 2010;10(4):262–269. https://doi.org/10.3816/CLML.2010.n.055.

50. Smith EL, Staehr M, Masakayan R, et al. Development and evaluation of an optimal human single-chain variable fragment-derived BCMA-targeted CAR T cell vector. *Mol Ther.* 2018;26(6):1447–1456. https://doi.org/10.1016/j.ymthe.2018.03.016.

51. Carpenter RO, Evbuomwan MO, Pittaluga S, et al. B-cell maturation antigen is a promising target for adoptive T-cell therapy of multiple myeloma. *Clin Cancer Res.* 2013;19(8):2048–2060. https://doi.org/10.1158/1078-0432.CCR-12-2422.

52. Ghosh A, Mailankody S, Giralt SA, Landgren CO, Smith EL, Brentjens RJ. CAR T cell therapy for multiple myeloma: where are we now and where are we headed? *Leuk Lymphoma.* 2017;0(0):1–12. https://doi.org/10.1080/10428194.2017.1393668.

53. Krejcik J, Casneuf T, Nijhof IS, et al. Daratumumab depletes CD38+ immune regulatory cells, promotes T-cell expansion, and skews T-cell repertoire in multiple myeloma. *Blood.* 2016;128(3):384–394. https://doi.org/10.1182/blood-2015-12-687749.

54. Wu N, Veillette A. SLAM family receptors in normal immunity and immune pathologies. *Curr Opin Immunol.* 2016;38:45–51. https://doi.org/10.1016/J.COI.2015.11.003.

55. Porter DL, Levine BL, Kalos M, Bagg A, June CH. Chimeric antigen receptor-modified T cells in chronic lymphoid leukemia. *N Engl J Med.* 2011;365(8):725–733. https://doi.org/10.1056/NEJMoa1103849.

56. Brentjens RJ, Rivière I, Park JH, et al. Safety and persistence of adoptively transferred autologous CD19-targeted T cells in patients with relapsed or chemotherapy refractory B-cell leukemias. *Blood.* 2011;118(18):4817–4828. https://doi.org/10.1182/blood-2011-04-348540.

57. Geyer MB, Rivière I, Sénéchal B, et al. Autologous CD19-targeted CAR T cells in patients with residual CLL following initial purine analog-based therapy. *Mol Ther.* 2018;26(8). https://doi.org/10.1016/j.ymthe.2018.05.018.

58. Fraietta JA, Lacey SF, Orlando EJ, et al. Determinants of response and resistance to CD19 chimeric antigen receptor (CAR) T cell therapy of chronic lymphocytic leukemia. *Nat Med.* 2018;24(5):563–571. https://doi.org/10.1038/s41591-018-0010-1.

59. Gauthier J, Hirayama AV, Hay Kevin A, et al. Comparison of efficacy and toxicity of CD19-specific chimeric antigen receptor T-cells alone or in combination with ibrutinib for relapsed and/or refractory CLL. *Blood*; December 2018, 2019 https://ash.confex.com/ash/2018/webprogram/Paper111061.html.

60. Gyurkocza B, Sandmaier BM. Conditioning regimens for hematopoietic cell transplantation: one size does not fit all. *Blood.* 2014;124(3):344–353. https://doi.org/10.1182/blood-2014-02-514778.

61. Wrzesinski C, Paulos CM, Kaiser A, et al. Increased intensity lymphodepletion enhances tumor treatment efficacy of adoptively transferred tumor-specific T cells. *J Immunother.* 2010;33(1):1–7. https://doi.org/10.1097/CJI.0b013e3181b88ffc.

62. Gattinoni L, Finkelstein SE, Klebanoff C a, et al. Removal of homeostatic cytokine sinks by lymphodepletion enhances the efficacy of adoptively transferred tumor-specific CD8+ T cells. *J Exp Med.* 2005;202(7):907–912. https://doi.org/10.1084/jem.20050732.

63. Dudley ME, Yang JC, Sherry R, et al. Adoptive cell therapy for patients with metastatic melanoma: evaluation of intensive myeloablative chemoradiation preparative regimens. *J Clin Oncol.* 2008;26(32):5233–5239. https://doi.org/10.1200/JCO.2008.16.5449.

64. Gandhi L, Rodríguez-Abreu D, Gadgeel S, et al. Pembrolizumab plus chemotherapy in metastatic non–small-cell lung cancer. *N Engl J Med*. April 2018. https://doi.org/10.1056/NEJMoa1801005. NEJMoa1801005.

65. Wang Z, Till B, Gao Q. Chemotherapeutic agent-mediated elimination of myeloid-derived suppressor cells. *OncoImmunology*. June 2017. https://doi.org/10.1080/2162402X.2017.1331807. e1331807.

66. Le DT, Jaffee EM. Regulatory T-cell modulation using cyclophosphamide in vaccine approaches: a current perspective. *Cancer Res*. 2012;72(14):3439–3444. https://doi.org/10.1158/0008-5472.CAN-11-3912.

67. Bracci L, Schiavoni G, Sistigu A, Belardelli F. Immune-based mechanisms of cytotoxic chemotherapy: implications for the design of novel and rationale-based combined treatments against cancer. *Cell Death Differ*. 2014;21(1):15–25. https://doi.org/10.1038/cdd.2013.67.

68. Fierro FA, Brenner S, Oelschlaegel U, et al. Combining SDF-1/CXCR4 antagonism and chemotherapy in relapsed acute myeloid leukemia. *Leukemia*. 2009;23(2):393–396. https://doi.org/10.1038/leu.2008.182.

69. Klebanoff C a, Khong HT, Antony P a, Palmer DC, Restifo NP. Sinks, suppressors and antigen presenters: how lymphodepletion enhances T cell-mediated tumor immunotherapy. *Trends Immunol*. 2005;26(2):111–117. https://doi.org/10.1016/j.it.2004.12.003.

70. Kochenderfer JN, Dudley ME, Kassim SH, et al. Chemotherapy-refractory diffuse large B-cell lymphoma and indolent B-cell malignancies can be effectively treated with autologous T cells expressing an anti-CD19 chimeric antigen receptor. *J Clin Oncol*. 2015;33(6):540–549. https://doi.org/10.1200/JCO.2014.56.2025.

71. Kochenderfer J, Kassim S, Somerville R, et al. Treatment of chemotherapy-refractory B-cell malignancies with anti-CD19 chimeric antigen receptor T cells. In: *Molecular Therapy*. Vol. 22. 2014. https://doi.org/10.1016/S1525-0016(16)35778-1.

72. Kochenderfer JN, Somerville RPT, Lu T, et al. Lymphoma remissions caused by anti-CD19 chimeric antigen receptor T cells are associated with high serum interleukin-15 levels. *J Clin Oncol*. 2017;35(16):1803–1813. https://doi.org/10.1200/JCO.2016.71.3024.

73. Kochenderfer JN, Somerville RPT, Lu T, et al. Lymphoma remissions caused by anti-CD19 chimeric antigen receptor T cells are associated with high serum interleukin-15 levels. *J Clin Oncol*. 2017;35(16):1803–1813. https://doi.org/10.1200/JCO.2016.71.3024.

74. DeAngelo DJ, Ghobadi A, Park JH, et al. Clinical outcomes for the phase 2, single-arm, multicenter trial of JCAR015 in adult B-all (ROCKET study). *Soc Immunother Cancer Annu Meet*. 2017.

75. Torre M, Solomon IH, Sutherland CL, et al. Neuropathology of a case with fatal CAR T-cell-associated cerebral edema. *J Neuropathol Exp Neurol*. July 2018. https://doi.org/10.1093/jnen/nly064.

76. Warrell RP, Berman E. Phase I and II study of fludarabine phosphate in leukemia: therapeutic efficacy with delayed central nervous system toxicity. *J Clin Oncol*. 1986;4(1):74–79. https://doi.org/10.1200/JCO.1986.4.1.74.

77. Park JH, Santomasso B, Riviere I, et al. Baseline and early post-treatment clinical and laboratory factors associated with severe neurotoxicity following 19-28z CAR T cells in adult patients with relapsed B-ALL. *J Clin Oncol*. 2017;35(15 suppl):7024. https://doi.org/10.1200/JCO.2017.35.15_suppl.7024.

78. Schuster SJ, Bishop MR, Tam CS, et al. Primary analysis of Juliet: a global, pivotal, phase 2 trial of CTL019 in adult patients with relapsed or refractory diffuse large B-cell lymphoma. *Am Soc Hematol Annu Meet*; 2017. https://ash.confex.com/ash/2017/webprogram/Paper105399.html.

79. Turtle CJ, Hanafi L, Berger C, et al. Immunotherapy of non-Hodgkin's lymphoma with a defined ratio of CD8$^+$ and CD4$^+$ CD19-specific chimeric antigen receptor – modified T cells. *Sci Transl Med*. 2016;8(355).

80. Lamanna N, Kay NE. Pentostatin treatment combinations in chronic lymphocytic leukemia. *Clin Adv Hematol Oncol*. 2009;7(6):386–392, 2018 http://www.ncbi.nlm.nih.gov/pubmed/19606074.

81. Turtle CJ, Hanafi L-A, Berger C, et al. CD19 CAR–T cells of defined CD4$^+$:CD8$^+$ composition in adult B cell all patients. *J Clin Invest*. 2016;126(6):2123–2138. https://doi.org/10.1172/JCI85309.

82. Porter DL, Hwang W, Frey NV, et al. Chimeric antigen receptor T cells persist and induce sustained remissions in relapsed refractory chronic lymphocytic leukemia. *Sci Transl Med*. 2015;7(303):303ra139. https://doi.org/10.1126/scitranslmed.aac5415.

83. Brentjens R, Davila M, Riviere I, Park J, Wang X. CD19-targeted T cells rapidly induce molecular remissions in adults with chemotherapy-refractory acute lymphoblastic leukemia. *Sci Transl Med*. 2013;5(177). https://doi.org/10.1126/scitranslmed.3005930, 177ra38.

84. Lee DW, Kochenderfer JN, Stetler-Stevenson M, et al. T cells expressing CD19 chimeric antigen receptors for acute lymphoblastic leukaemia in children and young adults: a phase 1 dose-escalation trial. *Lancet*. 2015;385(9967):517–528. https://doi.org/10.1016/S0140-6736(14)61403-3.

85. Maude SL, Laetsch TW, Buechner J, et al. Tisagenlecleucel in children and young adults with B-cell lymphoblastic leukemia. *N Engl J Med*. 2018;378(5):439–448. https://doi.org/10.1056/NEJMoa1709866.

86. Gust J, Hay KA, Hanafi L-A, et al. Endothelial activation and blood–brain barrier disruption in neurotoxicity after adoptive immunotherapy with CD19 CAR-T cells. *Cancer Discov*. October 2017. https://doi.org/10.1158/2159-8290.CD-17-0698.

87. Cruz CR, Hanley PJ, Liu H, et al. Adverse events following infusion of T cells for adoptive immunotherapy: a 10-year experience. *Cytotherapy*. 2010;12(6):743–749. https://doi.org/10.3109/14653241003709686.

88. Maus MV, Haas AR, Beatty GL, et al. T cells expressing chimeric antigen receptors can cause anaphylaxis in

humans. *Cancer Immunol Res.* 2013;1:26–31. http://www.ncbi.nlm.nih.gov/pubmed/24432303.

89. Neelapu SS, Tummala S, Kebriaei P, et al. Chimeric antigen receptor T-cell therapy — assessment and management of toxicities. *Nat Rev Clin Oncol.* 2017. https://doi.org/10.1038/nrclinonc.2017.148.

90. US Department of Health and Human Services. Common Terminology Criteria for Adverse Events (CTCAE) v5.0. https://ctep.cancer.gov/protocolDevelopment/electronic_applications/ctc.htm#ctc_50.

CHAPTER 5

Management of Cytokine Release Syndrome

INDUMATHY VARADARAJAN, MBBS • TAMILA L. KINDWALL-KELLER, DO • DANIEL W. LEE, MD

INTRODUCTION

Chimeric antigen receptor (CAR) T-cell therapy has been shown to have antitumor activity in a variety of cancers including pediatric and adult acute lymphoblastic leukemia (ALL),[1,2,3] diffuse large B-cell non-Hodgkin's lymphoma (NHL),[4,5] multiple myeloma,[6] and chronic lymphocytic leukemia (CLL),[7,8] leading to the commercial approval of two CD19 CAR T-cell therapies, tisagenlecleucel and axicabtagene ciloleucel.

Cytokine release syndrome (CRS) is a constellation of symptoms resulting from supraphysiologic cytokine production that can begin within hours of infusion and last up to 30 days after the administration of CAR T-cell therapy.[9,10] Fever, hypotension, tachycardia, tachypnea, hypoxia and capillary leak, hypoalbuminemia, coagulopathy, and, in rare cases, multiorgan failure characterize CRS.[9,10] Presentation of CRS may vary depending on which CAR T-cell therapy or dose is given, on patient characteristics, and on disease burden. The symptoms associated with CRS are caused by a robust, rapid release of cytokines and chemokines from proliferating CAR T-cells as well as from the host immune response.[11]

In a recent systematic review and meta-analysis of CAR T-cell trials in hematologic malignancies and solid tumors, more than 50% of recipients experienced CRS. CRS prevalence did not differ between the hematologic cancers treated, costimulatory domains, or phase of the clinical trial.[12] While CRS can be mild in some patients, in others the reactions can be life-threatening or even result in death. While this study did not find an association between CRS incidence and severity and tumor efficacy,[12] several single studies have identified correlations between response and CRS incidence and severity within their patient population.[1,13] Since severity of CRS can be mitigated with anticytokine

therapies, such as tocilizumab or corticosteroids, and since the timing of such intervention has changed over time from later to earlier in the course, broad studies of correlations between CRS severity and outcome may not be valid. Grading of CRS was not uniform across all studies further complicating analysis.

With the anticipated adoption of the recently published CRS consensus definition and grading criteria sponsored by the American Society for Transplantation and Cellular Therapy (ASTCT),[14] future analyses across trials and products will be more robust. However, the field has yet to establish consensus management guidelines for CRS, which would allow for even better intraproduct comparisons. The ASTCT and other groups are actively pursuing a CRS management consensus, but at this time, it is not available. Therefore, this chapter will dissect the common clinical manifestations of CRS and suggest current best management approaches where data exist or expert opinion aligns. Importantly, practitioners should remain current with the latest data and practice in CRS management, as this is a rapidly evolving field. Furthermore, every clinical situation is unique, so practitioners should exercise their best judgment when interpreting or implementing suggestions contained herein. To begin, one should understand the pathophysiology and risk factors for CRS.

PATHOPHYSIOLOGY OF CYTOKINE RELEASE SYNDROME

CRS begins with the engagement of CAR T-cells to its corresponding antigen on both malignant and nonmalignant, antigen-expressing cells, releasing a large amount of inflammatory cytokines.[9] It is important to note that cytokine production is not restricted to CAR T-cells. CRS may occur with other agents that target

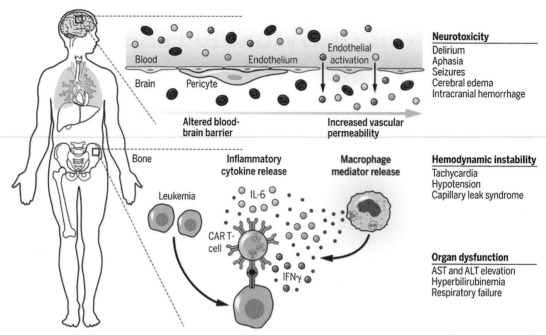

FIG. 5.1 Potential mechanisms of toxicity after chimeric antigen receptor (CAR) T-cell activation. CAR T-cells produce inflammatory cytokines, such as IFN-γ, which act in an autocrine and paracrine fashion to elevate the immune response through the recruitment of other immune mediators such as macrophages. Activated monocytes and macrophages release IL-6, among other molecules, which serve to feed-forward the inflammatory state, ultimately resulting in hemodynamic instability and compromised perfusion followed by organ dysfunction. Meanwhile, inflammatory mediators act on endothelium throughout the body, including the blood–brain barrier, increasing their permeability resulting in capillary leak and endothelial activation. Though less well characterized, CAR T-cell–associated neurotoxicity is thought to result from endothelium leak and activation in the central nervous system.

and engage T and/or B-cells, including rituximab and blinatumomab.[15,16]

Early insight into the pathophysiology of CRS was obtained when six healthy individuals were administered TGN1412—a superagonist monoclonal antibody to CD28.[17] Within 90 minutes of the infusion, all volunteers developed a systemic inflammatory response accompanied by headache, nausea, diarrhea, and hypotension and progressed rapidly (12–16 hours) to multiorgan failure requiring aggressive critical care support for recovery. Severe hypotension requiring vasopressors, capillary leak syndrome resulting in respiratory failure and acute kidney injury, coagulopathy, and neurological manifestations were all reported. C-reactive protein (CRP) was elevated, and retrospective analysis revealed marked elevations in IFN-γ, TNF-α, IL-6, IL-10, IL-2, and IL-1β, among others. High-dose corticosteroids were administered, and all patients eventually recovered.

Correlative studies in patients who develop CRS after CAR T-cell therapy have similar patterns of supraphysiologic cytokine production. The direct and indirect effects of such robust cytokine release are highly complex and have not been systematically evaluated. Though a small handful of molecules involved are shown in Table 5.1, this list is by no means exhaustive. The end result of this inflammatory milieu is endothelial injury and capillary leak, which contribute to the predominant clinical manifestations (Fig. 5.1). Such effects have recently been recapitulated in animal models.

MURINE MODELS OF CYTOKINE RELEASE SYNDROME

A humanized, leukemia-bearing mouse model developed by Norelli et al. demonstrates features of CRS when treated with murine-derived human CAR T-cells.[18] Mice experience weight loss, systemic inflammation, fever, and elevated IL-6, TNF-alpha, IL-1, and IL-10, all reminiscent of CRS in humans. As suspected, IL-1 and IL-6 were produced by monocytes in animals rather than the CAR T-cells themselves. Indeed, if monocytes are eliminated in this model, the clinical manifestations of CRS did not occur. Administration of tocilizumab, a monoclonal antibody that blocks the IL-6 receptor, also prevented CRS though it did not prevent CAR T-cell–associated neurotoxicity. Interestingly, anakinra, an IL-1 receptor small molecule antagonist, prevented both CRS and neurotoxicity in this mouse model[18] providing strong evidence for a clinical trial of this agent in managing CAR toxicities.

T. Giavridis et al. reported a mouse model with high intraperitoneal lymphoma burden, which develops CRS within 2–3 days after CD19 CAR T-cell infusion. Interestingly, the same mice when engrafted with leukemia in their marrow did not develop CRS.[19] Mice present with fatigue and weight loss, and if untreated, this syndrome resulted in mortality. IL-6, IL-1, and nitric oxide were produced extensively by host macrophages not CAR T-cells, and tocilizumab or anakinra abrogated CRS symptoms and prevented mortality, similar findings to Norelli's group. In contrast, Giavridis did not observe neurologic dysfunction in these animals, which do not bear a humanized immune system, suggesting one is required for neurotoxicity.

NONHUMAN PRIMATE MODELS OF CYTOKINE RELEASE SYNDROME

ROR1, a tyrosine kinase receptor, is a potential candidate for CAR T-cell therapy since it is expressed on the surface of many hematologic malignancies and may have a role in the survival of tumor cells.[20] Berger and colleagues evaluated ROR1-directed CAR T-cells in nonhuman primates (*Macaca mulatta*) and did not see any increased toxicity to low-level, transcript-expressing ROR1 organs of the macaques.[21] CAR T-cells were thought to be activated as IFN-gamma and IL-6 levels in circulation increased after CAR T-cell infusion. However, only one of two animals with B-cells that highly expressed ROR1 developed fever 12 days after infusion of the ROR1 CAR T-cells but no other signs of CRS. Though data are limited, this study, which did not use lymphodepletion prior to CAR T-cell infusion, suggests that nonhuman primates may be an adequate model to study CRS.

A different group infused three *M. mulatta* nonhuman primates with CD20-targeted CAR T-cells after lymphodepletion with cyclophosphamide.[22] CAR T-cells proliferated and were detectable for up to 43 days after the infusion. Approximately 5–7 days after CAR T-cell administration, subjects developed symptoms of CRS (fever and weight loss), which coincided with the proliferation and activation of the CAR T-cells. Similar to humans, CRP, ferritin, IL-6, IL-8, and IL-1β, among others, were elevated in CD20 CAR recipients but not controls and correlated to symptoms. Interestingly, elevated IL-6, IL-2, granulocyte-macrophage colony-stimulating factor (GM-CSF), and VEGF were found in the CSF of animals that also developed neurotoxicity.

These mouse and nonhuman primate models as well as correlative studies from patients receiving CAR T-cell therapy on clinical trials have improved our knowledge of the pathophysiology of CRS. Cytokines from host monocytes and macrophages as well as endothelial activation may contribute to CRS (Table 5.1). Clearly, IL-6 plays a key role in toxicity, as blockade of its signaling with tocilizumab can mitigate the clinical symptoms of CRS, but IL-6 and tocilizumab are not the only possible areas for intervention. As more preclinical data are

TABLE 5.1
Cytokines and Chemokines Involved in Cytokine Release Syndrome.

Year	Publication	Model	Cytokines	Responsible Cell
2018	M. Norelli et al.[18]	Mouse	IL-1, IL-6	Human monocytes
2018	T. Giavridis et al.[19]	Mouse	IL-1, IL-6, nitrous oxide	Host macrophages
2016	A. Taraseviciute et al.[22]	Monkey	IL-6, IL-8, ITAC	—
2018	J. Gust et al.[25]	Human	Endothelium-activating cytokines	Endothelial cell
2017	Hay et al.[10]	Human	IFN-γ, IL-6, IL8, IL-10, MCP-1, TNF p55, macrophage inflammatory protein 1β	—
2016	Teachey et al.[24]	Human	IFN-γ, IL-6, IL-8, sIL2Rα, sgp130, sIL6R, MCP1, MIP1α, GM-CSF	—

GM-CSF, Granulocyte-macrophage colony-stimulating factor.

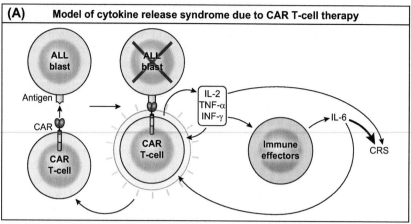

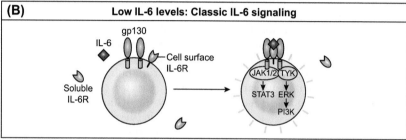

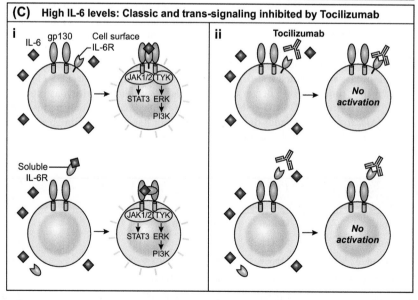

FIG. 5.2 **Cytokine release syndrome (CRS) is mediated principally by IL-6 and ameliorated by tocilizumab.** **(A)** Upon encountering its target, the chimeric antigen receptor (CAR) T-cell becomes activated and produces inflammatory cytokines (e.g., IL-2, TNF-α, and IFN-γ) that aid in maintaining CAR T-cell activation and recruits other immune effectors to produce IL-6. IL-6 also provides an activating signal to CAR T-cells and together with other inflammatory cytokines contributes to the clinical features of CRS. Activated CAR T-cells and their progeny are capable of killing additional tumor targets creating a feed-forward loop, potentially leading to an even greater degree of CRS. **(B)** During periods of low serum IL-6 levels, IL-6 signals its effectors via the classic pathway by binding to membrane-bound IL-6 receptor (IL-6R) followed by association

developed, clinical trials using other CRS inhibitors, such as anakinra, will be important to advance the field.

IMPORTANT BIOMARKERS OF CYTOKINE RELEASE SYNDROME

IL-6 is one of the central mediators of CRS. This cytokine can cause both proinflammatory and anti-inflammatory responses depending on its interaction with gp130 and the IL-6 receptor (IL-6R), respectively. CD130 (gp130) is expressed broadly on nonhematologic tissues, and the IL-6R is present on macrophages, neutrophils, hepatocytes, and T-cells. IL-6, when present at low concentrations, interacts primarily with the high-affinity, membrane-bound IL-6R and mediates anti-inflammatory properties. A soluble form of the IL-6R (sIL-6R) also exists.[23] During periods of higher IL-6 concentration (e.g., present during CRS), IL-6 will form a complex with the lower-affinity sIL-6R, which can then activate the trans signaling pathway through its binding to gp130 independent of the membrane-bound IL-6R, resulting in a proinflammatory response in a wider array of tissues[23] (Fig. 5.2). Understanding this pathophysiology has led to important therapeutic implications of using IL-6R inhibitors like tocilizumab[9] (Fig. 5.2) Indeed, serum IL-6 levels have been shown to correlate with CRS severity.[1]

Other groups have retrospectively mined clinical trials of CD19 CAR T-cells for correlations with other cytokines or chemokines in an effort to better characterize and perhaps predict severe CRS. Correlative studies performed by Hay et al. found that patients who developed > grade 4 CRS had higher levels of IFN-gamma, IL-6, IL-8, IL-10, IL-15, monocyte chemoattractant protein (MCP-1), tumor necrosis factor receptor p55, and macrophage inflammatory protein 1β within 36 hours after CAR T-cell infusion[10] (Table 5.1). For those patients with milder CRS, the levels took longer to increase. When compared with CRP, ferritin, or other cytokines, MCP-1 performed better at predicting patients with ≥ grade 4 CRS.[10] In another clinical trial, serum from 51 patients who received CD19 CAR T-cell therapy was analyzed serially for 43 cytokines that might predict CRS and compared with patients who

had severe CRS to those who did not. Twenty-four cytokines were associated with severe CRS, including IFN-gamma, IL-6, IL-8, sIL2Rα, sgp130, sIL6R, MCP1, MIP1α, and GM-CSF.[24] (Table 5.1)

The group at the Fred Hutchinson Cancer Research Center (FHCRC) made additional key discoveries. Analysis of samples from patients treated with CD19 CAR T-cell therapy at their center suggested that endothelial dysfunction may play a role in the hypotension, capillary leak syndrome, and coagulopathy associated with CRS.[25] An examination of angiopoietin-1 and angiopoietin-2 as well as von Willebrand factor levels in patients who received CAR T-cell infusions revealed that endothelial cell activation was seen in CRS (Table 5.1). Patients with severe CRS had higher levels of endothelium-activating cytokines and their serum activated human umbilical vein endothelial cells in the lab to a higher degree than controls. This led to the binding of von Willebrand factor and platelets. In some patients, the endothelial activation was even seen prior to the lymphodepleting chemotherapy for CAR T-cell therapy. A postmortem examination of a patient with fatal neurotoxicity after CAR T therapy revealed that the patient had had multifocal thrombotic microangiopathy.[25]

Much attention has been focused on IL-6 and CRP as possible biomarkers for real-time applications. Measuring IL-6 in real time is not widely available as a CLIA certified test and is expensive, which limits its usefulness as a biomarker at the present time. IL-6 signaling results in secretion of CRP from hepatocytes, and measuring CRP is, of course, readily available and inexpensive. However, CRP elevations are not specific to CRS, and changes in CRP tend to lag behind the clinical picture by as much as 24 hours. Therefore, CRP should not be relied upon to diagnose or manage CRS. Interestingly, CRP has been found to increase shedding of sIL-6R from neutrophils, possibly creating a feed-forward circuit of widespread cellular activation.[26]

RISK FACTORS FOR CYTOKINE RELEASE SYNDROME

Several clinical risk factors may predispose a patient to severe CRS (Table 5.2). In a phase I dose escalation trial

with two gp130 molecules. Formation of this complex leads to STAT3 and ERK/PI3K activation and immune activation. IL-6 in this state does not interact with soluble IL-6R. **(C) (i)** When high levels of IL-6 are present, the classic pathway is engaged, but IL-6 also signals through a trans approach since soluble IL-6R binds IL-6 in the serum, the complex of which can then associate two gp130 domains without aid from membrane-bound IL-6R and result in signaling. **(ii)** The anti-IL-6 receptor antibody tocilizumab blocks both the membrane-bound and soluble forms of the IL-6R, thereby preventing IL-6 from associating with gp130 and its subsequent activation signals.

TABLE 5.2
Clinical Risk Factors for Severe Cytokine Release Syndrome.

Clinical Risk Factors	Proposed Interventions
Increased CAR T-cell expansion	• Improve selection of ideal T-cell subset for CAR T-cell therapy • Continue dose finding studies to find ideal CAR T-cell dose to infuse
High disease burden in bone marrow	• Consider earlier treatment with CAR T-cell therapy (i.e.: prior to relapse) • Investigate strategies to reduce disease burden prior to CAR T-cell therapy
Thrombocytopenia	• Consider earlier treatment with CAR T-cell therapy (i.e.: prior to relapse)
Bulk CD8+ T-cells	• Improve selection of ideal T-cell subset for CAR T-cell therapy
Higher CAR T-cell dose infused	• Individualize dosing based on mathematical modeling (yet to be developed) balancing probability of toxicity and response
Lymphodepleting chemotherapy including fludarabine	• Evaluate other lymphodepleting regimens without fludarabine for efficacy

of CD19 CAR T-cell therapy in children and young adults with ALL, both CRS severity and probability of tumor response correlated with higher CAR T-cell expansion in blood after infusion. Not surprisingly, patients receiving higher CAR T-cell doses had more severe CRS[1,10]; thus, determining the ideal CAR T-cell dose to be infused (i.e., the biologically active dose rather than the maximally tolerated dose) is important to reducing CRS impact in CAR T-cell recipients. Along these lines, better selection of CAR T-cell subsets to be infused (i.e., selecting for central memory T-cells) may also be an important consideration in the management of CRS.[10]

Patients with higher disease burden tend to have more severe CRS.[1,8] This suggests that disease cytoreduction prior to treatment with CAR T-cells may reduce the incidence of severe CRS, though data are not yet available supporting this hypothesis and many patients are already refractory to conventional therapy, making this variable often difficult to modify.

In a study by Hay et al., authors looked at risk factors for CRS in 133 adult patients who received CD19 CAR T-cells for NHL, CLL, and B-cell ALL[10] (Table 5.2). Approximately 70% of the patients had CRS, and only 10 patients (3.8%) each had grade 4 or 5 CRS. By multivariate analysis, patient risk factors associated with CRS include higher CD19+ tumor burden in the bone marrow and severe thrombocytopenia. CAR T product risk factors for any grade CRS included using bulk CD8+ T-cells without selection of the central memory subset and higher CAR T-cell dose infused. The addition of fludarabine to the lymphodepleting chemotherapy regimen also increased the risk of developing severe CRS. Higher CAR T-cell dose and fludarabine/cyclophosphamide lymphodepleting chemotherapy were associated with grade 4 or higher CRS.[10] In a study of 32 patients with NHL treated with CD19 CAR T-cells by the same group, patients who were given fludarabine with their cyclophosphamide lymphodepleting regimen had increased expansion and persistence of CAR T-cells and higher complete response rates. However, lymphodepleting chemotherapy without fludarabine was determined to be less effective.[27]

CLINICAL PRESENTATION OF CYTOKINE RELEASE SYNDROME

Very early attempts to define and grade CRS described its constellation of symptoms including fever, hypotension, hypoxia, neurotoxicity and other end organ damage.[9] Transaminitis, for example, was specifically addressed. With continued experience, it became clear that these definitions and grading systems needed to be modified. CAR-associated neurotoxicity, now termed immune effector cell (IEC)—associated neurotoxicity syndrome (ICANS), can occur outside the temporal context of the other features of CRS suggesting a different pathophysiology. The most recent definition of CRS, arrived by a consensus of a large number of experienced investigators from all aspects of the CAR T-cell space, specifically identifies neurotoxicity and CRS as two distinct entities. The ASTCT consensus manuscript defines CRS as,

a supraphysiologic response following any immune therapy that results in the activation or engagement of endogenous or infused T-cells and/or other immune effector cells. Symptoms can be progressive, must include fever at the onset, and may include hypotension, capillary leak (hypoxia) and end organ dysfunction.[14]

Many early studies of CD19 CAR T-cells began to characterize the clinical course of patients experiencing CRS. It should be noted that most of these studies used varying criteria for grading CRS, as discussed in more detail below, so direct comparisons of one product or experience to another across these trials are impossible. However, we can begin to understand many key features of CRS from these studies.

First, for CRS to be diagnosed, symptoms must begin in a reasonable temporal association to the therapy given. Usually, this occurs rather rapidly and is limited in its duration. In a phase 2 study of axicabtagene ciloleucel in 111 patients with refractory NHL, 93% of patients experienced any grade CRS with 13% of patients experiencing grade ≥3 CRS with all patients in this latter group experiencing fever, hypoxia, and hypotension (Table 5.3). Median time to onset was 2 days with a range of 1−12 days and resolution taking a median of 8 days.[4] In a separate study, of 75 pediatric patients with ALL treated with tisagenlecleucel, CRS of any grade occurred in 77% with a median time of onset of 3 days, range of 1−22 days, and a median duration of 8 days. 46% of patients in this study experienced grade 3 or higher CRS[2] (Table 5.3).

This timecourse is not unique to CD19 CAR T-cells. A phase I CAR T-cell study targeting B-cell maturation antigen in multiple myeloma reported no grade 4 or higher CRS and only two recipients with grade 3 CRS despite 76% of the 33 treated patients experiencing any grade CRS (Table 5.3). Despite the lower CRS grade, median onset was 2 days, and the median duration was 5 days.[6]

It should be noted that very early onset of fever has been associated with more severe CRS in some studies.

For example, patients receiving CD19 CAR T-cells at FHCRC who developed grades 4−5 CRS had fever earlier (within 0.4 vs. 3.9 days), a higher temperature peak (40.4°C vs. 39.4°C), and longer duration (2.5 vs. 4.4 days) compared with those who developed grades 1−3 CRS.[10]

In addition to fever, hypotension, and hypoxia, patients with severe CRS can present with a host of other symptoms (Fig. 5.1). More common symptoms include tachycardia, tachypnea, hypoalbuminemia, and capillary leak syndrome, resulting in weight gain, respiratory insufficiency, and ultimately impaired hemodynamics.[9,10] Arrhythmias particularly in older patients have been noted. Many patients with grades 3−4 CRS will go on to develop organ dysfunction including acute kidney injury, coagulopathy, diarrhea, and hepatic injury manifested by transaminitis, hyperbilirubinemia, and elevated alkaline phosphatase.[10] Given the severity of CRS in many patients and the potential for long-term morbidity, identification, prevention, and treatment strategies for CRS are needed.

GRADING OF CYTOKINE RELEASE SYNDROME

The unique toxicities of adoptive T-cell therapies require standardizing their assessment and grading to diagnose and manage CRS properly. Previously, several different definitions and grading systems for CRS were used in medical centers utilizing CAR T-cell therapies, making comparisons of toxicity between CAR T-cell products, clinical trials, and centers increasingly difficult. These systems include the National Cancer Institute's

TABLE 5.3
Selected Incidence and Clinical Presentation of Cytokine Release Syndrome (CRS).

Author	Year	Phase Trial	# Of Pts	Disease	CRS Any Grade	CRS ≥ Grade 3	Symptoms
Neelapu et al.[4]	2017	II	111	Adult large B-cell NHL	93%	13%	Fever, hypoxia, hypotension
Maude et al.[2]	2018	II	75	Pediatric ALL	77%	46%	Fever, hypoxia, hypotension
Hay et al.[10]	2017	I/II	133	Adult ALL, CLL, NHL	70%	12%	Fever, hypoxia, hypotension, tachycardia
Raje et al.[6]	2019	I	33	Multiple myeloma	76%	6%	—
Lee et al.[1]	2014	I	21	Pediatric ALL, DLBCL	76%	32%	Fever, hypoxia, hypotension, tachycardia

CRS Grading scales used differed between studies. Please see primary reference for details.
ALL, Acute lymphoblastic leukemia; *NHL*, Non-Hodgkin's lymphoma; *DLBCL*, Diffuse large B-cell lymphoma; *CLL*, Chronic lymphocytic leukemia.

TABLE 5.4
Published CRS Grading Systems.

Grading System	Grade 1	Grade 2	Grade 3	Grade 4
CTCAE Version 4.03	Mild reaction; infusion interruption not indicated; intervention not indicated	Therapy or infusion interruption indicated but responds promptly to symptomatic treatment (antihistamines, NSAIDs, narcotics, IV fluids); prophylactic medications indicated for ≤ 24 hours	Prolonged (e.g., not rapidly responsive to symptomatic medication and/or brief interruption of infusion); recurrence of symptoms following initial improvement; hospitalization indicated for clinical sequelae (such as renal impairment, pulmonary infiltrate)	Life-threatening consequences; pressor or ventilatory support indicated
CTCAE Version 5.0	Fever, with or without constitutional symptoms	Hypotension responding to fluids. Hypoxia responding to <40% FiO$_2$	Hypotension managed with one pressor. Hypoxia requiring ≥40% FiO$_2$	Life-threatening consequences; urgent intervention needed
2014 Lee criteria[9]	Symptoms are not life-threatening and require symptomatic treatment only (fever, nausea, fatigue, headache, myalgias, malaise)	Symptoms require and respond to moderate intervention: • Oxygen requirement <40% FiO$_2$ or • Hypotension responsive to IV fluids or low dose of one vasopressor or • Grade 2 organ toxicity[a]	Symptoms require and respond to aggressive intervention: • Oxygen requirement ≥40% FiO$_2$ or • Hypotension requiring high dose or multiple vasopressors or • Grade 3 organ toxicity[a] or grade 4 transaminitis	Life-threatening symptoms: • Requirement for ventilator support or • Grade 4 organ toxicity[a] (excluding transaminitis)
Penn criteria	Mild reaction: Treated with supportive care such as antipyretics, antiemetics	Moderate reaction: Some signs of organ dysfunction (grade 2 creatinine or grade 3 LFTs) related to CRS and not attributable to any other condition Hospitalization for management of CRS-related symptoms, including neutropenic fever and need for IV therapies (not including fluid resuscitation for hypotension)	More severe reaction: Hospitalization required for management of symptoms related to organ dysfunction, including grade 4 LFTs or grade 3 creatinine, related to CRS and not attributable to any other condition Hypotension treated with multiple fluid boluses or low-dose vasopressors Coagulopathy requiring fresh frozen plasma, cryoprecipitate, or fibrinogen concentrate Hypoxia requiring supplemental oxygen (nasal cannula oxygen, high-flow oxygen, CPAP, or BiPAP)	Life-threatening complications such as hypotension requiring high-dose vasopressors Hypoxia requiring mechanical ventilation

	Grade 1	Grade 2	Grade 3	Grade 4
MSKCC criteria	Mild symptoms requiring observation or supportive care only (e.g., antipyretics, antiemetics, pain meds, etc.)	Hypotension requiring any vasopressors <24 hours; Hypoxia or dyspnea requiring supplemental oxygen <40%	Hypotension requiring any vasopressors ≥24 hours; Hypoxia or dyspnea requiring supplemental oxygen ≥40%	Life-threatening symptoms; Hypotension refractory to high-dose vasopressors; Hypoxia or dyspnea requiring mechanical ventilation
CARTOX criteria	Temperature ≥38°C; Grade 1 organ toxicity[b]	Hypotension responds to IV fluids or low-dose vasopressor; Hypoxia requiring $FiO_2 < 40\%$; Grade 2 organ toxicity[b]	Hypotension needing high-dose or multiple vasopressors; Hypoxia requiring $FiO_2 \geq 40\%$; Grade 3 organ toxicity[b] or grade 4 transaminitis	Life-threatening hypotension; Needing ventilator support; Grade 4 organ toxicity[b] except grade 4 transaminitis

NSAIDs, Nonsteroidal antiinflammatory drugs; *LFTs*, Liver function tests; *CPAP*, Continuous positive airway pressure; *BiPAP*, Bilevel positive airway pressure.

[a] As per CTCAE Version 4.03.

[b] Cardiac (tachycardia, arrhythmias, heart block, low ejection fraction), respiratory (tachypnea, pleural effusion, pulmonary edema), GI (nausea, vomiting, diarrhea), hepatic (increased serum ALT, AST, or bilirubin levels), renal (acute kidney injury, increased serum creatinine, decreased urine output), dermatological (rash), coagulopathy (disseminated intravascular coagulation).

Adapted from Lee et al. [14].

Common Terminology Criteria for Adverse Events (CTCAE; versions 4.03, 5.0),[28,29] the 2014 Lee criteria,[9] the Penn criteria,[30] the Memorial Sloan Kettering Cancer Center criteria (MSKCC criteria),[3] and the CARTOX criteria[31] (Table 5.4).

In June 2018, an international group of experts in CAR T-cell and other IEC engaging therapies met to establish consensus definitions and grading scales for CRS and ICANS. Sponsored by the American Society for Transplantation and Cellular Therapy (ASTCT), the resulting consensus manuscript was published shortly thereafter[14] (Table 5.5). The group determined that while patients can certainly experience end organ toxicities as a result of CRS, the pattern of such damage is highly variable. What is consistent between patients of all ages, diagnoses, and products received is the presence of fever at the onset followed, sometimes rapidly, by varying degrees of hypotension and/or hypoxia in more severe cases. Therefore, the severity of CRS is determined by the presence and degree of hypotension and hypoxia.

Fever is defined as a temperature ≥38.0°C, and hypotension is defined as a blood pressure that is below the normal expected for the individual in a given environment. Hypoxia is defined as present when oxygen is required to overcome a perceived deficit in oxygenation. It should be noted that while fever is required to diagnose CRS initially, it does not need to persist for a practitioner to determine that CRS is ongoing, particularly when antipyretics and/or anticytokine therapies (e.g., tocilizumab, corticosteroids, etc.) have been administered. In such a case, CRS is ongoing in a patient until all features that led to that diagnosis (i.e., hypotension, hypoxia) have fully resolved. Furthermore, for CRS to be diagnosed, the symptoms in question must be reasonably attributable to the IEC therapy given in terms of an expected temporal relationship between the therapy and toxicity and the absence of any other identifiable cause.

The simple, clinically based, and easily verifiable ASTCT consensus grading for CRS is presented in Table 5.5. Grade 1 CRS includes fever with or without systemic symptoms and requires the absence of both hypotension and hypoxia. Mild hypotension not requiring vasopressors and/or hypoxia requiring ≤6 L/minute of oxygen by nasal cannula (or blow-by oxygen in the case of pediatric patients) in addition to a fever is classified as grade 2 CRS. Grade 3 CRS is defined as a fever with hypotension requiring one vasopressor (with or without vasopressin) and/or hypoxia requiring high-flow oxygen > 6 L/minute by high-flow nasal cannula, face mask, nonrebreather mask, or Venturi mask. Hypotension requiring multiple vasopressors (excluding vasopressin) and/or hypoxia requiring positive pressure ventilation (CPAP, BiPAP, mechanical

TABLE 5.5
ASTCT Consensus Grading Scale for Cytokine Release Syndrome.

CRS Parameter	Grade 1	Grade 2	Grade 3	Grade 4
Fever[a]	Temperature ≥38°C	Temperature ≥38°C	Temperature ≥38°C	Temperature ≥38°C
		With:		
Hypotension	None	Not requiring vasopressors	Requiring a vasopressor with or without vasopressin	Requiring multiple vasopressors (excluding vasopressin)
		And/or[b]		
Hypoxia	None	Requiring low-flow nasal cannula[c] or blow-by	Requiring high-flow nasal cannula[c], facemask, nonrebreather mask, or Venturi mask	Requiring positive pressure (e.g., CPAP, BiPAP, intubation, and mechanical ventilation)

Organ toxicities associated with CRS may be graded according to CTCAE v5.0, but they do not influence CRS grading.
CPAP, Continuous positive airway pressure; *BiPAP*, Bilevel positive airway pressure.
[a] Fever is defined as temperature ≥38°C not attributable to any other cause. In patients who have CRS and then receive antipyretics or anticytokine therapy such as tocilizumab or steroids, fever is no longer required to grade subsequent CRS severity. In this case, CRS grading is driven by hypotension and/or hypoxia.
[b] CRS grade is determined by the more severe event: hypotension or hypoxia not attributable to any other cause. For example, a patient with temperature of 39.5°C, hypotension requiring one vasopressor, and hypoxia requiring low-flow nasal cannula is classified as having grade 3 CRS.
[c] Low-flow nasal cannula is defined as oxygen delivered at ≤ 6 L/minute. Low flow also includes blow-by oxygen delivery, sometimes used in pediatrics. High-flow nasal cannula is defined as oxygen delivered at > 6 L/minute.
Adapted from Lee et al. [14].

ventilation) with a fever is grade 4 CRS. Grade 5 is death due to CRS and not another cause by convention.[14]

For the remainder of this chapter, any mention of CRS grade refers to the ASTCT consensus grading unless otherwise indicated.

SUGGESTED MANAGEMENT OF CYTOKINE RELEASE SYNDROME

There is very little evidence-based data regarding the management of CRS. What follows will serve as recommended management strategies produced by a small group of individuals, albeit with extensive experience. It is anticipated that a consensus management strategy will be developed soon, and indeed, such consensus and, later, clinical trials comparing CRS interventions are welcomed. The reader should always maintain an up-to-date knowledge base and adjust his/her practice accordingly as new data, new drugs, and new approaches to managing CRS will no doubt be developed in the coming years. Finally, practitioners should always exercise their best clinical judgment even if it conflicts with the content of this chapter.

SUPPORTIVE CARE OF CYTOKINE RELEASE SYNDROME–RELATED TOXICITIES BY ORGAN SYSTEM

It is simplistic to rely solely on anticytokine therapies, herein defined as a medication given to directly counteract the effects of CRS such as tocilizumab or corticosteroids, for the management of CRS. CRS is a multiorgan dysfunction syndrome, even though grading is only based on a limited subset of them. Equally as important as knowing when to intervene with anticytokine therapies is implementing high-quality, often aggressive supportive care in a timely manner. Doing so will minimize complications related to extrinsic compounding forces, such as infections, as well as iatrogenic forces, such as fluid overload from aggressive IV fluid resuscitation in the presence of worsening capillary leak. For these reasons, we will discuss the important supportive care measures by organ systems first followed by a more detailed discussion of when and how to intervene with anticytokine therapies.

Patients with CRS at first glance present as one with sepsis might present. However, CRS is managed very differently than sepsis. Fundamentally, CRS is a toxicity that will resolve on its own once all target antigen is eliminated so long as high-quality supportive care and timely anticytokine therapy is provided. This is in stark contrast to sepsis and should create a shift in the practitioner's approach to management.

CONSTITUTIONAL: FEVER AND HYPOTHERMIA

Fever is the hallmark of CRS and is defined as a temperature $\geq 38.0°C$. Fever resulting from CRS will not occur during the product infusion but may occur within the first 24 hours and up to 3 weeks postinfusion (Fig. 5.3). A new fever outside this window is unlikely to be related to CRS, and other causes should be investigated. In general, fever occurs more quickly in patients receiving CD28 costimulatory domain containing CD19 CARs, such as axicabtagene ciloleucel, compared to those with the 4-1BB costimulatory domain, such as tisagenlecleucel.[22,10] While the precise mechanisms for fever production (or really any toxicity) after CAR T-cell therapy have not been elucidated fully, it is likely related to the robust production of inflammatory cytokines. Such a state also occurs in the presence of most infections, so differentiating between fever caused by CRS and fever caused by an infection is impossible.

The fever that occurs with CRS, particularly in patients with very low disease burden, can be relatively mild for a brief period of time (<24 hours). However, as many as 40%–80% of patients receiving CD19 CAR T-cell therapy will have grade 3–4 fever (>40°C) perhaps lasting days[1,32,33] (Fig. 5.3). The temperature curve will often vacillate throughout the day as much as 2°C or 3°C. Patients with low-grade fevers may have periods of normothermia, so continued close

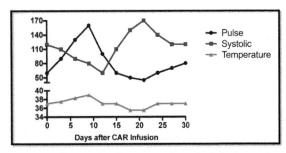

FIG. 5.3 Representative examples of vital signs after chimeric antigen receptor (CAR) T-cell therapy. During the acute phase of cytokine release syndrome (CRS), patients develop tachycardia and fever and may develop hypotension, all of which resolve with time, supportive care, and anticytokine therapy. The typical temporal relationship between these is shown. After CRS resolves, some patients may experience hypothermia, bradycardia, and hypertension that may require intervention. (Reproduced from: Varadarajan I, Lee DW. Management of T-cell engaging immunotherapy complications. Cancer J. 2019.)

observation is warranted, and such a presentation does not exclude the possibility of higher-grade fever developing even days later.

Interestingly, a period of hypothermia (temperature $\leq 35°C$) may occur days after a fever and other symptoms of CRS have resolved (Fig. 5.3). Due to its timing, this may occur after a patient has been discharged from the hospital, so continued and frequent monitoring of temperature as an outpatient is warranted. Hypothermia has been described to coincide with bradycardia and hypertension and may be the first objective sign of this trio to be noted by the patient. In such cases, the patient should notify the on-call provider for immediate evaluation as some patients have required continuous administration of vasoactive medications to control blood pressure. Symptomatic bradycardia may also require intervention. Anecdotal evidence suggests that this "anti-CRS" (i.e., symptoms are opposite from what is expected with CRS) is related to a shift in the cytokine milieu, but this is not well characterized.[11]

Management: Since it is impossible to differentiate between CRS and a new infection, any new onset fever warrants an immediate clinical evaluation by the healthcare team. All patients should have blood cultures obtained (including from any indwelling central venous catheters [CVCs]) and started empirically on broad-spectrum antibiotics including coverage for *Pseudomonas* species when neutropenia (absolute neutrophil count < 500 cells/uL) is present. Continuation of antibiotic therapy is recommended until fever and neutropenia resolve. Continuing antibiotics beyond the febrile period should be considered if anticytokine therapies are used, as these may mask a fever from an infectious source. Currently, there is no established role for prophylactic antibiotics prior to CAR infusion.

Given the lack of predictive factors for CRS severity and kinetics, patients with a new fever should be admitted to the hospital if not already. Initial assessment of newly febrile patients, administration of antibiotics, etc. should be performed rapidly. Institutions should have standard operating procedures in place that involve the emergency department (ED), pharmacy, and other necessary personnel so that these patients can be rapidly assessed and managed without waiting in the usual ED queue.

Suggested initial labs to obtain include a blood culture from each lumen of a CVC if present or percutaneously if not, complete blood count with differential (CBCdiff), complete metabolic panel with phosphorus and magnesium, CRP, ferritin, and a coagulation panel (PT/PTT) with fibrinogen. Imaging should be based on localizing symptoms. Symptomatic relief can be provided by acetaminophen and other supportive measures such as ice packs. Fever is often accompanied by myalgias, headache, tremulousness, and arthralgias—so called constitutional symptoms—and may be helped by nonsteroidal anti-inflammatory drugs (NSAIDs). These should be used with caution in the setting of renal hypoperfusion and thrombocytopenia. They should not be used when platelets are less than 50,000.

Importantly, there are currently no data supporting the use of tocilizumab or corticosteroids for fever alone, even persistent fever, in a normotensive patient without hypoxia and without any other signs of significant organ dysfunction.

CARDIOVASCULAR: ARRHYTHMIAS, HYPOTENSION, AND CARDIAC FAILURE

Cardiac arrhythmias, particularly in adults, have been reported during CRS. Sinus tachycardia is the most commonly seen clinical abnormality and is often accompanied by fever. In fact, sinus tachycardia is often the first presenting sign of developing CRS, even before the onset of fever (Fig. 5.3). Other supraventricular tachyarrhythmias such as atrial fibrillation and atrial flutter can also occur. Most arrhythmias resolve after CRS subsides. Heart block has also been described. Standard-of-care interventions should be employed to address the particular arrhythmia or heart block. In cases where perfusion is compromised or likely to be compromised or in case of other complicating factors putting the patient at greater risk, use of tocilizumab and/or corticosteroids is recommended.

Hypotension due to CRS most often is accompanied by fever and tachycardia. Grades 3–4 hypotension (as per CTCAEv5.0) has been reported in 22%–38% of patients receiving CAR T-cell therapy.[34,1,3] Hence, immediate clinical evaluation and intervention is warranted. It can occur as early as the onset of the first febrile episode or several days later (Fig. 5.3). Like fever, it is impossible to determine in the moment whether hypotension is related to CRS, sepsis, or both, so both possibilities should be addressed and treated simultaneously.

Persistent hypotension despite intervention can lead to rapid deterioration. Reduced left ventricular ejection fraction (LVEF) followed by left and then right ventricular cardiac failure can occur with severe or prolonged CRS. However, independent of hypotension, patients may develop diminished LVEF that is only compounded once hypotension develops.[35] The pathophysiology of decreased cardiac output is thought to be similar to stress cardiomyopathy. Cardiac arrests have been reported in as few as 7 days[1] and as late as 2 months[35] following CAR T-cell infusion. Most patients with diminished LVEF regain normal function after CRS resolves, though this may take some time. Asymptomatic prolongation of the QTc interval has also been reported.[1,36,32,37] Finally, after resolution of CRS, some patients develop asymptomatic bradycardia and hypertension (Fig. 5.3). Most often, this does not require any active intervention and resolves with supportive care. For these reasons, it is reasonable to closely follow patients who develop CRS for cardiac toxicities, even in the absence of hypotension.

Management: It is important to determine an individual's baseline blood pressure prior to cell infusion. The ASTCT CRS consensus criteria do not define hypotension with a particular systolic or diastolic blood pressure. Rather, it defines hypotension as a blood pressure (systolic, diastolic, or mean arterial pressure) that is below the normal expected for the individual in a given environment. So, the diagnosis of hypotension will vary from patient to patient, and it is up to the practitioner to determine when hypotension is present. Objectively establishing a patient's baseline blood pressure is immensely helpful.

In general, the first confirmed decrease of 20% or greater from baseline systolic, diastolic, or mean arterial pressure or evidence of worsening perfusion requires immediate intervention with an IV fluid bolus (20 mL/kg up to 1 L). Blood pressure and perfusion should be reassessed frequently. If no improvement is noted or if the patient has a subsequent drop in blood pressure or worsening perfusion, a second IV fluid bolus should be given. In this case, consideration should be given to transferring the patient to the intensive care unit (ICU) particularly if there is no response to the initial bolus or there is a short interval (e.g.,: <4 hours) between needed boluses. In these cases, the likelihood of requiring vasopressors is high.

Since CRS results in vasodilatation and capillary leak, practitioners should avoid multiple IV fluid boluses when at all possible, instead shifting management to vasopressors as early as possible. Good practice will involve starting a vasopressor no later than after the third IV fluid bolus. Reliance solely on crystalloid to maintain perfusion, as is often employed in the setting of bacterial sepsis, will result in pulmonary edema, hypoxia, and increased right heart strain (already occurring due to CRS), which sets up a feed-forward cycle of events (worsening pulmonary edema, worsening hypoxia, worsening right heart strain, and so on) that will

ultimately result in loss of cardiac output and potential cardiac arrest. As this cycle becomes more established, it is increasingly difficult to abort. This cycle can be prevented through the early employment of vasopressors in lieu of crystalloid and the timely use of tocilizumab and/or corticosteroids. Norepinephrine with or without vasopressin is often the preferred first-line pressor, as most patients have peripheral vasodilation. Vasopressor use is discussed in more detail in Chapter 6.

Particularly in older patients, arrhythmias and heart block have been described during CRS, but prolonged QTc is a common occurrence across age groups. A 12-lead electrocardiogram at baseline, when patients are admitted to the ICU for cardiovascular compromise, and in response to significant changes in rate or waveform should be obtained. Electrolytes should be corrected empirically to minimize the risk of arrhythmia.

In similar fashion, transthoracic echocardiogram (ECHO) should be obtained at baseline and upon admission to the ICU for cardiovascular compromise. Since diminished LVEF has been described even in the absence of hypotension as well as while hypotension is resolving, obtaining screening ECHOs every 48 hours while the patient is in the ICU is not unreasonable. Particular attention should be paid to cardiac strain, which is often affected first.[35] The aim is to identify a developing problem early and intervene promptly so as to diminish the probability of severe or life-threatening toxicities. Anticytokine therapy is indicated for unstable arrhythmias or significant (grade 3 or higher) drop in LVEF. The cardiology team should be consulted for tachyarrhythmias, other than sinus tachycardia, and for a reduction in LVEF. Since CRS is self-limited, maximal supportive therapy should be offered in the ICU, including extracorporeal membrane oxygenation if needed.

PULMONARY—HYPOXIA AND PULMONARY EDEMA

Pulmonary complications after CAR T-cell therapy are one of the main determinants of CRS severity. Most commonly, patients become tachypnic and/or dyspneic. Pulmonary edema may develop as capillary leak worsens in particular if aggressive IV fluid resuscitation is used. This may result in hypoxia and the need for supplemental oxygen. Grade 3—4 hypoxia has been reported in about 6%—15% of patients[1,3,32,33] and is usually a late manifestation of CRS-induced pulmonary toxicity. Most of the time, it is transient and has no known long-term consequences to lung function.

Pleural effusions may also develop or existing effusions may be exacerbated with the onset of CRS.

Percutaneous drainage may be necessary but is a procedure that may carry significant risk in patients with severe CRS and compromise of other organ systems. This underscores the importance of careful and judicious use of IV fluids in patients where effusions are known to be present before CAR T-cell infusion.

Management: Chest imaging, such as chest X-ray or a CT scan, should be considered in every patient receiving CAR T-cell therapy who develops hypoxia or tachypnea. The most common finding will be pulmonary edema, but consolidative pneumonia, pneumothorax, and pleural effusions should also be ruled out. Hypoxia should be corrected through the use of whatever oxygen delivery device is necessary, and CRS graded accordingly (Table 5.5). If there is a concern for hypoventilation, an arterial blood gas may be helpful, and if confirmed, positive pressure ventilation via BiPAP, CPAP, or intubation with mechanical ventilation should be provided. In general, diuresis should be avoided during the period of worsening CRS.

RENAL AND ELECTROLYTE DERANGEMENTS

Acute renal failure following CAR T-cell therapy is usually multifactorial and fortunately not common. Though renal toxicity from tumor lysis syndrome (TLS) is possible with bulk disease, it is surprisingly not commonly reported even in patients with bulk disease. However, together with nephrotoxic antibiotics, it may compound the renal injury caused by compromised renal perfusion related to CRS. Capillary leak and peripheral vasodilatation contribute to poor renal perfusion, and in later stages, diminished cardiac output from cardiac intrinsic damage or arrhythmias only intensify the renal injury. Therefore, the aim of supportive care is to prevent or minimize renal injury by mitigating the factors leading to it.

TLS is classically characterized by hyperkalemia, hyperphosphatemia, and hyperuricemia. However, the most common electrolyte derangements reported after CD19 CAR T-cell therapy are hypokalemia, profound hypophosphatemia, and hypomagnesemia. We hypothesize that the incredibly rapid, exponential expansion of the highly active CAR T-cell pool in vivo requires significant metabolic resources including intracellular potassium and phosphorous for ATP production to make new CAR T-cells and carry out their cytolytic and proliferative activities. If not proactively and aggressively managed, electrolyte concentrations can quickly fall to dangerous levels.

Management: A baseline comprehensive metabolic panel with uric acid, phosphorous, magnesium, and lactate dehydrogenase (if appropriate) will identify any preexisting electrolyte derangements that may need correction prior to beginning therapy. In addition, patients with bulky disease should be started on allopurinol prior to starting the lymphodepleting regimen. If hyperuricemia is noted after CAR T-cell infusion despite allopurinol, rasburicase may be required.

Adequate hydration should be maintained during the preparative regimen phase and until cells are infused, but hyperhydration should, in general, be avoided outside the period required for chemotherapy being administered (e.g., cyclophosphamide) unless laboratory findings of TLS are noted. This will minimize complications of capillary leak, should the patient develop rapid-onset CRS. As described previously, IV fluid boluses may be required if hypotension and/or hypoperfusion is noted during CRS. This along with early use of vasopressors is important to help maintain renal perfusion and prevent renal injury. Occasionally, this is unavoidable, and dialysis is needed. Institutional practices guiding indications for and method of dialysis should be followed. Fortunately, even when dialysis is required, renal injury is typically reversible.

Aggressive electrolyte repletion, particularly with phosphorous, is frequently required. Labs should be checked several times a day once abnormalities are noted even when electrolytes are being repleted, as patients often need multiple replacement doses each day. Finally, where possible, nephrotoxic agents such as NSAIDs should be avoided.

HEPATIC AND GASTROINTESTINAL

Diarrhea is a frequent symptom of CRS and can be clinically significant. It appears to be cytokine-mediated though the exact mechanisms have not been elucidated. Nausea and vomiting can occur and may be related to the chemotherapy preparative regimen or may be a feature of CRS itself. Colitis may also develop and may be particularly challenging to manage in the setting of neutropenia. Infection with *Clostridium difficile* should be assessed and managed aggressively. Colitis, in general, can exacerbate capillary leak and in severe cases can lead to bowel perforation, which in the setting of CRS can be devastating.

Elevated transaminases (liver function tests [LFTs]) and hyperbilirubinemia have also been described and can be mild or severe. Currently, there is no way to predict or mitigate LFT elevation. Fortunately, these often resolve spontaneously with supportive care.[3,7,38] Occasionally, this can be a symptom of hemophagocytic lymphohistiocytosis or macrophage activation syndrome (HLH/MAS) if it is accompanied by other features of that syndrome. This is addressed in further detail in Chapter 8.

Management—High-quality supportive care is essential to prevent or mitigate gastrointestinal and hepatic complications of CAR T-cell therapy. Judicious but appropriate use of antibiotics will minimize the risk of *C. difficile*. Careful fluid replacement for copious diarrhea aimed to maintain intravascular volume sufficient for adequate perfusion while balancing complications of capillary leak is essential. Hepatotoxic drugs should be avoided where possible, should LFTs be significantly elevated.

HEMATOLOGIC DISORDERS

Cytopenias, marked hypofibrinogenemia, and disseminated intravascular coagulation have been commonly described after CAR T-cell therapy. These complications and their management are discussed in more detail in Chapter 8.

ANTICYTOKINE THERAPY FOR CYTOKINE RELEASE SYNDROME

Tocilizumab

Tocilizumab, a humanized monoclonal immunoglobulin G1k antibody that binds to soluble and membrane-bound IL-6 receptors thereby inhibiting IL-6 signaling, is the only FDA-approved drug for the treatment of severe or life-threatening CRS. Dosing is provided in Table 5.6. In a retrospective analysis of 60 patients treated with either tisagenlecleucel or axicabtagene ciloleucel and received tocilizumab for CRS, approximately 65% had a response to tocilizumab within 14 days of the first dose. The median time from first dose to response was 4—4.5 days depending on the CAR T-cell product received.[39] Though tocilizumab was well tolerated in the series of patients presented, several significant side effects have been attributed to tocilizumab in clinical trials for rheumatologic conditions, including serious sometimes fatal infections, neutropenia, thrombocytopenia, elevated liver enzymes, and lipid dysregulation.[40] Whether any of these complications occur after use in patients with CRS remains an unanswered question.

Corticosteroids

Corticosteroids are lymphocytotoxic and can ameliorate the symptoms of CRS.[9,3] They have the advantage of being nonspecific, in contrast to tocilizumab, so their anti-inflammatory effects bridge a wide range of activated cellular immunity. There are reasonable data suggesting that monocytes and/or macrophages are the principle producers of IL-6 and other cytokines and chemokines that serve to further activate both the CAR T-cells and the global immune environment.[18] Unlike tocilizumab, steroids have the potential to inhibit these cells and limit further immune activation. Dosing for commonly used steroids is provided in Table 5.6.

GENERAL APPROACH TO USING ANTICYTOKINE THERAPY IN PATIENTS WITH CYTOKINE RELEASE SYNDROME

Prompt initiation of high-quality supportive care, with early use of vasopressor(s), in combination with the timely use of anticytokine therapy(ies) is the cornerstone for the successful management of CRS. The overarching goal is to prevent the development of life-threatening (grade 4—5) CRS. Investigators in the first CD19 CAR T-cell trials were initially hesitant to use anticytokine therapies early in the CRS course. They were treating patients with highly refractory disease with limited life expectancies, and no one knew how the use of tocilizumab or corticosteroids would impact the CAR T-cells and by extension their chance at achieving a response to the therapy.

As experience grew, investigators realized that earlier/timely use of tocilizumab could prevent patients from developing life-threatening CRS. This led to the publication of a manuscript authored by investigators from several institutions that redefined CRS, its grading, and suggested a treatment algorithm for when to intervene with tocilizumab and/or corticosteroids.[9] Since then, the field has shifted toward intervening even earlier in the CRS course. Today, practices are still quite variable as a consensus guideline for managing CRS has not yet been established. As such, what follows may need to be reassessed when such a guideline is published.

INITIATE ANTICYTOKINE THERAPIES IN A TIMELY MANNER

At present, there is no evidence that antitumor response is affected by tocilizumab or corticosteroids once CRS is established.[41] However, there is also no published experience regarding antitumor response and the *prophylactic* use of tocilizumab or steroids, so such a strategy is not recommended as the production of cytokines early might be necessary for proper CAR T-cell proliferation and activity. Once CRS is diagnosed, early and aggressive supportive therapy with the use of vasopressors and timely use of anticytokine therapy(ies) can mitigate potential life-threatening CRS.

At present, initiation of anticytokine therapy(ies) is absolutely indicated for grade 2 CRS when patients

TABLE 5.6
Recommended Anti-Cytokine Agents and Dosing (Where Reasonable Data are Available).

Drug	Dose	Route	Comments
Tocilizumab[40]	8 mg/kg/dose (max 800 mg/dose) over 60 minutes	IV	Premedicate with acetaminophen and diphenhydramine May repeat q6–8 hours; Give steroids with second dose Decreased utility with >3 doses
Dexamethasone	1 mg/kg/dose (max 10 mg/dose)	IV	Preferred if concurrent ICANS Consider over methylprednisolone due to improved CNS penetration even in absence of neurotoxicity May dose q6-24 hours depending on clinical response/needs Rapid (5–7 day) wean once CRS ≤ grade 1
Methylprednisolone	1 mg/kg/dose (max 100 mg/dose) q4–6 hours Or 30 mg/kg/dose (max 1000 mg/day)	IV	Consider dexamethasone due to improved CNS penetration Use lower doses for stable-appearing patient Use high dose for unstable patients Rapid (5–7 days) wean once CRS ≤ grade 1
Siltuximab	11 mg/kg/dose	IV	Third-line agent Premedicate with acetaminophen and diphenhydramine
Anakinra[44]	2–4 mg/kg/day (may increase to 8 mg/kg/day)	SC	Third-line agent
Cyclophosphamide	Variable	IV	Third-line agent

Dosing applies to pediatric patients.
IV, Intravenous; *SC*, Subcutaneous; *ICANS*, Immune effector cell–associated neurotoxicity syndrome; *CRS*, Cytokine release syndrome.

have additional comorbidities that put them at increased risk and for grade 3 and 4 CRS for all patients (Table 5.7). However, many practitioners will choose to intervene earlier. For example, an elderly patient with a fever for more than 72 hours or a very high fever (>40.5°C) may not tolerate the resulting sinus tachycardia as well as a younger patient, so tocilizumab may be indicated. A shift toward intervening with anticytokine therapy at grade 2 may be forthcoming, even in young, fit patients, as we gain more confidence that such a maneuver does not decrease the efficacy of the CAR T-cell therapy. Every clinical situation is unique. The practitioner must use his or her best clinical judgment when deciding when to employ anticytokine therapy.

Tocilizumab is the only FDA-approved therapy for severe or life-threatening CRS and as such should be given as first-line therapy (Table 5.6). However, some practitioners will concurrently give at least one dose of

TABLE 5.7
Recommended Timing of Initial Intervention With Tocilizumab and Corticosteroids Based on Grade of Cytokine Release Syndrome.

Grade CRS (as per ASTCT consensus criteria)	Tocilizumab	Steroids
1	No	No
2—no comorbidities	No	No
2—with comorbidities	Yes	Consider
3	Yes	Consider
4	Yes	Yes

steroids (Table 5.6) with the first dose of tocilizumab. The theory behind this practice is that steroids may help offset any increased risk of developing ICANS in patients treated with tocilizumab for CRS. No published data exist, and good outcomes have certainly been documented with tocilizumab monotherapy alone. For higher grades of CRS, simultaneous use of steroids with tocilizumab is indicated (Table 5.7). The choice of coadministering steroids with tocilizumab at lower CRS grades remains with the clinician.

EVALUATING RESPONSE TO FIRST TOCILIZUMAB/STEROID DOSE

After anticytokine therapy is employed, practitioners should evaluate whether the symptoms triggering the intervention improved. Tocilizumab tends to normalize body temperature rapidly with a resulting rapid improvement in heart rate. Improvements in perfusion or blood pressure often take more time, but so long as the general trend is in a positive direction, patients can continue to be monitored. If there is no improvement in symptoms within 6 hours of the initial tocilizumab dose or if patients begin to deteriorate after an initial improvement, a second dose of tocilizumab should be given along with a dose of corticosteroids. In general, all patients requiring a second dose of tocilizumab should also be given corticosteroids. There is limited utility in giving more than three doses of tocilizumab to a patient. In such a situation, alternative (third-line) agents should be considered (Table 5.6).

Choice of steroid to use is still controversial unless patients have concurrent ICANS. In this case, dexamethasone is preferred and is reviewed in more detail in Chapter 7. Otherwise, since the risk for developing ICANS in patients with severe CRS is higher than in patients with mild CRS, many practitioners prefer dexamethasone over methylprednisolone due to the former's superior penetration into the CNS. In addition, as there is anecdotal evidence suggesting tocilizumab may increase the probability of a patient subsequently developing ICANS,[1,42,22] other practitioners will use dexamethasone in all cases when tocilizumab is given.

Dosing of steroids is also controversial. Some take a graduated approach, basing dose on severity of symptoms, while others are aggressive upfront giving a high dose initially and then performing a rapid wean once symptoms subside. In general, dosing should at least be commensurate with CRS severity and ICANS, if present. Suggested dosing and intervals are given in Table 5.6.

PATIENTS MAY BE REFRACTORY TO TOCILIZUMAB AND STEROIDS

Should a patient continue to deteriorate despite multiple doses of tocilizumab and high-dose corticosteroids,

additional anticytokine therapies should be considered (Table 5.6). Use of these is entirely anecdotal and, as such, is entirely at the discretion of the treating physician.

Siltuximab is a monoclonal antibody that is indicated for the treatment of multicentric Castleman's disease. It binds IL-6 itself rather than its receptor, so it can potentially be complementary to tocilizumab, but it has not been formally evaluated in CAR T-cell patients with CRS. In a clinical trial of patients with Castleman's disease, common grade 3 adverse events were fatigue, night sweats, anemia, thrombocytopenia, neutropenia, and infection.[43]

Serum and CSF IL-6 levels have been shown to rise at least temporarily after tocilizumab administration since the only method of clearance of IL-6, via endocytosis with its receptor, is blocked.[1,42,22] Given the often delayed presentation of ICANS relative to CRS, it has been hypothesized that IL-6 may play a role in ICANS. If true, siltuximab has the theoretical benefit, unlike tocilizumab, of possibly preventing or mitigating ICANS since it removes IL-6 from circulation and, as a bulky antibody-IL-6 conjugate, prevents it from crossing the blood–brain barrier (BBB).

Anakinra is a 153 amino acid protein antagonist to the IL-1 receptor used to treat rheumatoid arthritis. Given to more than 1300 patients on clinical trials, neutropenia occurred in 8% of patients with the number of serious infections not significantly different than patients who received placebo.[44] Anakinra competitively inhibits the binding of IL-1 to the IL-1 receptor. In a recent manuscript where investigators developed a humanized mouse model of CRS and a form of neurotoxicity that developed after CAR T-cell administration, both CRS and neurotoxicity were prevented by the prophylactic administration of anakinra.[18] Furthermore, anakinra has been shown to cross the BBB in rhesus macaques,[45] suggesting it may play a role in treating or preventing ICANS. Clinical trials investigating the use of siltuximab and anakinra are sorely needed to determine what role these agents may have in managing CRS and ICANS.

Activated, replicating T-cells are known to be exquisitely sensitive to cyclophosphamide. Though its use would have the potentially negative effect of eliminating CAR T-cells, as opposed to other agents that modulate the immune environment, cyclophosphamide may be necessary in critically ill patients not responding to other interventions.

Sarilumab is a monoclonal antibody with high affinity for the membrane-bound and soluble IL-6 receptors and is FDA approved for use in patients with rheumatoid arthritis.[46] Despite its similarity to tocilizumab, sarilumab has not been evaluated formally in patients with CRS after CAR T-cell therapy.

Other non—FDA-approved drugs and CAR T-cell suicide strategies may have an impact in mitigating CRS in the future. Monocytes and macrophages are the principle source of IL-6 and IL-1 in humanized mouse models of CRS.[18] Sterner and colleagues used a neutralizing antibody to GM-CSF, lenzilumab, to prevent CRS and neurotoxicity in humanized mice. CAR T-cell activity was not impacted. In fact, CAR T-cell proliferation increased.[47] Clinical trials of lenzilumab in humans undergoing CAR T-cell therapy are no doubt under development.

Several CAR T-cell designs have incorporated suicide vectors that when triggered by an exogenous agent result in the controlled elimination of CAR T-cells. Inducible caspase 9, truncated epidermal growth factor receptor, and herpes simplex virus (HSV) thymidine kinase (tk) genes can be cotransduced into CAR T-cells and activated using rimiducid (AP1903), cetuximab, and ganciclovir, respectively.[48,49,50] Though these strategies are all investigational at the present time, they portend a possible future where additional functionality is incorporated in the CAR T-cell, allowing them to autoregulate in response to any number of factors.

CONCLUSIONS AND FUTURE DIRECTIONS

Even severe and life-threatening CRS is usually completely reversible with aggressive supportive therapy and timely anticytokine therapy. With the elimination of CAR-specific target antigen, inflammation will subside, leading to resolution of CRS unlike sepsis and other inflammatory states that are often irreversible.

Effective management and prevention of CAR T-cell therapy—associated CRS remains an evolving field. It is extremely important to identify symptoms of CRS at the earliest onset, rapidly initiate aggressive supportive care, and administer anticytokine therapy(ies) in a timely fashion. Using this approach will provide the patient the best chance at a positive outcome. For those who are refractory to initial interventions, additional off-label use of immune modulators may be necessary.

ACKNOWLEDGMENTS

COI disclosures: Dr. Lee serves on the external advisory board for Juno Therapeutics/Celgene, has provided ad hoc consulting to Harpoon Therapeutics, and has received clinical trial research support from Kite/Gilead.

REFERENCES

1. Lee DW, Kochenderfer JN, Stetler-Stevenson M, et al. T cells expressing CD19 chimeric antigen receptors for acute lymphoblastic leukaemia in children and young adults: a phase 1 dose-escalation trial. *Lancet.* 2015; 385(9967).
2. Maude SL, Laetsch TW, Buechner J, et al. Tisagenlecleucel in children and young adults with B-cell lymphoblastic leukemia. *N Engl J Med.* 2018;378(5):439—448.
3. Davila ML, Riviere I, Wang X, et al. Efficacy and toxicity management of 19-28z CAR T cell therapy in B cell acute lymphoblastic leukemia. *Sci Transl Med.* 2014;6(224), 224ra25.
4. Neelapu SS, Locke FL, Bartlett NL, et al. Axicabtagene ciloleucel CAR T-cell therapy in refractory large B-Cell lymphoma. *N Engl J Med.* 2017;377(26):2531—2544.
5. Schuster SJ, Svoboda J, Chong EA, et al. Chimeric antigen receptor T Cells in refractory B-Cell lymphomas. *N Engl J Med.* 2017;377(26):2545—2554.
6. Raje N, Berdeja J, Lin Y, et al. Anti-BCMA CAR T-cell therapy bb2121 in relapsed or refractory multiple myeloma. *N Engl J Med.* 2019;380(18):1726—1737.
7. Porter DL, Levine BL, Kalos M, Bagg A, June CH. Chimeric antigen receptor-modified T cells in chronic lymphoid leukemia. *N Engl J Med.* 2011;365(8):725—733.
8. Turtle CJ, Hay KA, Hanafi LA, et al. Durable molecular remissions in chronic lymphocytic leukemia treated with CD19-Specific chimeric antigen Receptor-modified T cells after failure of ibrutinib. *J Clin Oncol.* 2017;35(26):3010—3020.
9. Lee DW, Gardner R, Porter DL, et al. Current concepts in the diagnosis and management of cytokine release syndrome. *Blood.* 2014;124(2).
10. Hay KA, Hanafi LA, Li D, et al. Kinetics and biomarkers of severe cytokine release syndrome after CD19 chimeric antigen receptor—modified T-cell therapy. *Blood.* 2017; 130(21):2295—2306.
11. Varadarajan I, Lee DW. Management of T-cell engaging immunotherapy complications. *Cancer J.* 2019;25(3):223—230.
12. Grigor EJM, Fergusson D, Kekre N, et al. Risks and benefits of chimeric antigen receptor T-cell (CAR-T) therapy in cancer: a systematic review and meta-analysis. *Transfus Med Rev.* 2019;33(2):98—110.
13. Turtle CJ, Hanafi LA, Berger C, et al. CD19 CAR-T cells of defined CD4+:CD8+ composition in adult B cell ALL patients. *J Clin Invest.* 2016;126(6):2123—2138.
14. Lee DW, Santomasso BD, Locke FL, et al. ASTCT consensus grading for cytokine release syndrome and neurologic toxicity associated with immune effector cells. *Biol Blood Marrow Transplant.* 2019;25(4).
15. von Stackelberg A, Locatelli F, Zugmaier G, et al. Phase I/Phase II study of blinatumomab in pediatric patients with relapsed/refractory acute lymphoblastic leukemia. *J Clin Oncol.* 2016;34(36):4381—4389.

16. Zucca E, Conconi A, Martinelli G, et al. Final results of the IELSG-19 randomized trial of mucosa-associated lymphoid tissue lymphoma: improved event-free and progression-free survival with rituximab plus chlorambucil versus either chlorambucil or rituximab monotherapy. *J Clin Oncol.* 2017;35(17):1905–1912.

17. Suntharalingam G, Perry MR, Ward S, et al. Cytokine storm in a phase 1 trial of the anti-CD28 monoclonal antibody TGN1412. *N Engl J Med.* 2006;355(10):1018–1028.

18. Norelli M, Camisa B, Barbiera G, et al. Monocyte-derived IL-1 and IL-6 are differentially required for cytokine-release syndrome and neurotoxicity due to CAR T cells. *Nat Med.* 2018;24(6):739–748.

19. Giavridis T, Van Der Stegen SJC, Eyquem J, Hamieh M, Piersigilli A, Sadelain M. CAR T cell-induced cytokine release syndrome is mediated by macrophages and abated by IL-1 blockade letter. *Nat Med.* 2018;24(6):731–738.

20. Orentas RJ, Lee DW, Mackall C. Immunotherapy targets in pediatric cancer. *Front Oncol.* 2012;2(JAN).

21. Berger C, Sommermeyer D, Hudecek M, et al. Safety of targeting ROR1 in primates with chimeric antigen receptor-modified T cells. *Cancer Immunol Res.* 2015;3(2):206–216.

22. Taraseviciute A, Tkachev V, Ponce R, et al. Chimeric antigen receptor T cell–mediated neurotoxicity in nonhuman primates. *Cancer Discov.* 2018;8(6):750–763.

23. Lee DW, Wayne AS. Chimeric Antigen Receptor (CAR) T Cells. In: Ascierto P, Stroncek D, Wang E, eds. Developments in T Cell Based Cancer Immunotherapies. Cancer Drug Discovery and Development. Cham: Humana Press; 2015.

24. Teachey DT, Lacey SF, Shaw PA, et al. Identification of predictive biomarkers for cytokine release syndrome after chimeric antigen receptor T-cell therapy for acute lymphoblastic leukemia. *Cancer Discov.* 2016;6(6):664–679.

25. Gust J, Hay KA, Hanafi LA, et al. Endothelial activation and blood–brain barrier disruption in neurotoxicity after adoptive immunotherapy with CD19 CAR-T cells. *Cancer Discov.* 2017;7(12):1404–1419.

26. Jones SA, Novick D, Horiuchi S, Yamamoto N, Szalai AJ, Fuller GM. C-reactive protein: a physiological activator of interleukin 6 receptor shedding. *J Exp Med.* 1999;189(3):599–604.

27. Turtle CJ, Hanafi LA, Berger C, et al. Immunotherapy of non-Hodgkin's lymphoma with a defined ratio of CD8+ and CD4+ CD19-specific chimeric antigen receptor-modified T cells. *Sci Transl Med.* 2016;8(355):355ra116.

28. National Cancer Institute. Common Terminology criteria for adverse events (CTCAE) version 4.0. *NIH Publ.* 2009.

29. National Cancer Institute. Common Terminology criteria for adverse events (CTCAE).v.5.0. *NIH Publ.* 2017.

30. Porter D, Frey N, Wood PA, Weng Y, Grupp SA. Grading of cytokine release syndrome associated with the CAR T cell therapy tisagenlecleucel. *J Hematol Oncol.* 2018;11(1):35.

31. Neelapu SS, Tummala S, Kebriaei P, et al. Chimeric antigen receptor T-cell therapy-assessment and management of toxicities. *Nat Rev Clin Oncol.* 2018;15(1):47–62.

32. Brudno JN, Somerville RPT, Shi V, et al. Allogeneic T cells that express an anti-CD19 chimeric antigen receptor induce remissions of B-cell malignancies that progress after allogeneic hematopoietic stem-cell transplantation without causing graft-versus-host disease. *J Clin Oncol.* 2016;34(10):1112–1121.

33. Kochenderfer JN, Dudley ME, Kassim SH, et al. Chemotherapy-refractory diffuse large B-cell lymphoma and indolent B-cell malignancies can be effectively treated with autologous T cells expressing an anti-CD19 chimeric antigen receptor. *J Clin Oncol.* 2015;33(6):540–549.

34. Maude SL, Frey N, Shaw PA, et al. Chimeric antigen receptor T cells for sustained remissions in leukemia. *N Engl J Med.* 2014;371(16):1507–1517.

35. Burstein DS, Maude S, Grupp S, Griffis H, Rossano J, Lin K. Cardiac profile of chimeric antigen receptor T cell therapy in children: a single-institution experience. *Biol Blood Marrow Transplant.* 2018;24(8):1590–1595.

36. Kochenderfer JN, Dudley ME, Carpenter RO, et al. Donor-derived CD19-targeted T cells cause regression of malignancy persisting after allogeneic hematopoietic stem cell transplantation. *Blood.* 2013;122(25):4129–4139.

37. Kalos M, Levine BL, Porter DL, et al. T cells with chimeric antigen receptors have potent antitumor effects and can establish memory in patients with advanced leukemia. *Sci Transl Med.* 2011;3(95):95ra73.

38. Brentjens RJ, Rivière I, Park JH, et al. Safety and persistence of adoptively transferred autologous CD19-targeted T cells in patients with relapsed or chemotherapy refractory B-cell leukemias. *Blood.* 2011;118(18):4817–4828.

39. Le RQ, Li L, Yuan W, et al. FDA approval summary: tocilizumab for treatment of chimeric antigen receptor T cell-induced severe or life-threatening cytokine release syndrome. *Oncologist.* 2018;23(8):943–947.

40. Genetech I. *ACTEMRA® (tocilizumab). Prescribing Information.* 2013.

41. Singh N, Hofmann TJ, Gershenson Z, et al. Monocyte lineage–derived IL-6 does not affect chimeric antigen receptor T-cell function. *Cytotherapy.* 2017;19(7):867–880.

42. Nishimoto N, Kishimoto T. Interleukin 6: from bench to bedside. *Nat Clin Pract Rheumatol.* 2006;2(11):619–626.

43. Van Rhee F, Wong RS, Munshi N, et al. Siltuximab for multicentric Castleman's disease: a randomised, double-blind, placebo-controlled trial. *Lancet Oncol.* 2014;15(9):966–974.

44. Amgen, KINERET™ (anakinra). *Prescribing Information.* 2001.

45. Fox E, Jayaprakash N, Pham TH, et al. The serum and cerebrospinal fluid pharmacokinetics of anakinra after intravenous administration to non-human primates. *J Neuroimmunol.* 2010;233(1-2):138–140.

46. Huizinga TW, Kivitz AJ, Rell-Bakalarska M, et al. OP0023 Sarilumab for the treatment of moderate-to-severe rheumatoid arthritis: results of a phase 2, randomized, double-blind, placebo-controlled, international study. *Ann Rheum Dis.* 2013;67(6):1424–1437.

47. Sterner RM, Sakemura R, Cox MJ, et al. GM-CSF inhibition reduces cytokine release syndrome and neuroinflammation but enhances CAR-T cell function in xenografts. *Blood.* 2019;133(7):697–709.

48. Tey SK, Dotti G, Rooney CM, Heslop HE, Brenner MK. Inducible caspase 9 suicide gene to improve the safety of allodepleted T cells after haploidentical stem cell transplantation. *Biol Blood Marrow Transplant.* 2007; 13(8):913–924.

49. Paszkiewicz PJ, Fräßle SP, Srivastava S, et al. Targeted antibody-mediated depletion of murine CD19 CAR T cells permanently reverses B cell aplasia. *J Clin Invest.* 2016; 126(11):4262–4272.

50. Bonini C, Ferrari G, Verzeletti S, et al. HSV-TK gene transfer into donor lymphocytes for control of allogeneic graft-versus-leukemia. *Science.* 1997;276(5319):1719–1724.

CHAPTER 6

Special Considerations for ICU Management of Patients Receiving CAR Therapy

KRIS M. MAHADEO, MD, MPH • FRANCESCO PAOLO TAMBARO, MD, PHD • CRISTINA GUTIERREZ, MD

Cancer is among the leading causes of death worldwide. The number of new cancer cases per year is expected to rise to 23.6 million by 2030.[1] Advancements in oncology therapeutics and associated improvements in survival mean that more patients may require advanced life support for cancer-related complications, treatment-related toxicities, and severe infections.[2] Cancer-specific guidelines for admission to the intensive care unit (ICU) as well as protocols for care, which may be implemented in any ICU (general or cancer specific), may be important to ensure advancements in cancer therapeutics are matched by appropriate critical care interventions when they are indicated.[2]

Chimeric antigen receptor (CAR) T-cells belong to the class of immune effector cell (IEC) therapies, which have been associated with striking outcomes in terms of overall and disease-free survival rates, particularly among patients with relapsed/refractory hematologic malignancies.[3,4] Yet, they have also been associated with unique toxicities, which may lead to very rapid and life-threatening cardiorespiratory, neurological, and multiorgan dysfunction.[4–7] Up to 40% of patients who receive CAR therapy may require ICU admission.[3,8,9] Cytokine release syndrome (CRS) and immune effector cell–associated neurotoxicity syndrome (ICANS) (previously referred to as CAR T-related encephalopathy syndrome or CRES) are well-described complications associated with CAR therapy and other immunotherapeutic agents (bispecific T-cell engager monoclonal antibodies (mAbs), e.g., blinatumomab, natural killer (NK) cells therapy, and CAR NK cells).[4,10–14] The pathophysiology, diagnosis, grading, and specific management of these complications are described elsewhere in this book.

The constellation of signs and symptoms of CAR-associated toxicities may require critical care recognition and intervention that is independent of CRS- and ICANS-specific treatment. Prompt recognition and supportive management by trained critical care staff of CAR-associated toxicities, including, but not limited to, hypotension and shock, acute respiratory distress syndrome (ARDS and pediatric ARDS [P-ARDS]), acute kidney injury (AKI), arrhythmias, coagulopathy, status epilepticus, and intracranial hypertension, may be lifesaving and/or preserve long-term organ function.

While CAR therapies may be limited to administration at tertiary care centers, emergency medical services, community hospitals, and local triage facilities require high vigilance to recognize and promptly escalate care in the event that a patient treated with CAR T-cell therapy presents to their facility in an emergency.[4] With this in mind, it is important for the ICU clinician to be knowledgeable and actively involved in the care and monitoring of patients receiving CAR therapy. In this chapter, we will discuss in detail considerations specific to the critically ill CAR patient.

OUTREACH, MONITORING, AND ICU ADMISSION CRITERIA

A successful CAR T-cell program requires multidisciplinary and interprofessional collaboration.[4] At inception of a program, ICU collaboration is imperative to develop ICU admission criteria, assist with monitoring of high-risk patients, and create guidelines for the management and care of severe toxicities. ICU admission criteria may vary among institutions and even within institutions based upon staffing and bed availability. In general, patients with > grade 3 CRS or neurological toxicity

Chimeric Antigen Receptor T-Cell Therapies for Cancer. https://doi.org/10.1016/B978-0-323-66181-2.00006-8

(ICANS) should be admitted to the ICU.[15] Other considerations for ICU admission include patients with rapid progression of pulmonary infiltrates on imaging and/or rapid progression of hypoxemia, hypotension especially when associated with elevated lactate levels, and signs of hypoperfusion (such as organ dysfunction and poor mental status) or rapidly progressing neurotoxicity.[16] Risk factors for severe CRS and ICANS such as high tumor burden, higher CAR T-cell dose administration, high number of comorbidities, and early onset of symptoms have been described.[6,8,11,12,17−19] The presence of one or more risk factors may prompt consideration of either close monitoring by the ICU team on the floors or early ICU admission.[16] Variability in the frequency and severity of toxicity seen based on product used and patient characteristics make close and regular communication between the cell therapy and ICU teams imperative to mitigate the impact to ICU staffing and bed availability.

For CAR T-cell patients admitted to the ICU, close and frequent communication is needed between the ICU team, consultants, and the cell therapy team. Evaluation and treatment of patients with CRS and ICANS should not be static, especially among those with grade 3 and grade 4 toxicities. Frequent reevaluation of response to treatment should occur, with a timely response and escalation of care if no response is observed.[16] Management algorithms and call escalation trees should be clearly delineated for staff.[4] Different products may be associated with specific toxicity management protocols. For example, while agents directed at interleukin-6 (IL-6), such as tocilizumab, and corticosteroids are commonly used for severe toxicities associated with CAR T-cells, other products may use first-line administration of drugs that trigger specific off-switch receptors. In recent clinical trials, an inducible caspase 9 (iCasp9) "safety switch" allows for the removal of inappropriately activated CAR T-cells by administration of the small molecule drug AP1903, which causes dimerization and activation of iCasp9, leading to rapid induction of apoptosis in transduced cells.[20−22] Coexpression on the CAR T-cell of a truncated protein recognized by clinically approved mAbs may also allow transduced T-cells to be eliminated by antibody-dependent cellular cytotoxicity or complement-dependent cytotoxicity after the administration of the relevant mAb, such as rituximab.[23,24]

Aggressive support in this patient population is important. Despite the advanced stage of malignancy, severe toxicities are usually reversible, and patients achieve long-term survival and durable cancer remission.[6,7] Considerations for ICU admission of CAR T-cell patients are summarized in Table 6.1.

SHOCK AND OTHER CARDIOVASCULAR MANIFESTATIONS

Vasodilation and secondary hypotension may occur as a consequence of the exaggerated inflammatory process observed in CRS. Hypotension and shock are pillars of CRS, varying from grade 2 (hypotension that responds to fluid resuscitation) and grade 3−4 that is shock (hypotension requiring one to multiple vasopressors).[15,25] Reports suggest that as many as 42% of patients with CRS will require vasopressors and ICU admission.[25] Hypotension might not initially present with overt shock; more subtle clinical signs such as a need to decrease the dose of antihypertensives could serve as an early indicator. Knowing the patient's baseline blood pressure is important. A drop in a patient's blood pressure from baseline may be a better indicator, rather than choosing a specific value for a systolic blood pressure to define hypotension (e.g.,: <90 mmHg).

Guidelines recommend 20−30 mL/kg of fluid resuscitation for patients in vasodilatory shock secondary to sepsis.[26] Shock due to CRS occurs as a vasodilatory response to cytokines and is associated with significant endothelial dysfunction and capillary leak.[8,15] In this setting, careful resuscitation is paramount, as fluid overload can worsen the inflammatory response and lead to secondary organ damage and increased mortality (in particular, among younger children and infants).[27−29] Assessment of intravascular fluid status using minimally invasive monitoring or targeted ultrasound should be considered to help guide fluid therapy in these patients.[5,16]

If a patient continues to be hypotensive after two fluid boluses, use of vasopressors should not be delayed.[15] While no specific vasopressors are recommended for this patient population, considerations such as ongoing arrhythmias and evidence of a cardiomyopathy with low cardiac output can help with the specific agents used. Data from other causes of vasodilatory shock, such as sepsis, could be extrapolated to this patient population. Norepinephrine can be considered as the vasopressor of choice, as it has shown to reduce the incidence of arrhythmias and mortality when compared with dopamine.[30] Epinephrine could be useful in patients with low cardiac output from new onset cardiomyopathy, as it has inotropic effects; however, it is important to note that supraventricular tachycardia can be increased with its use.[31] Adding noncatecholamine vasopressors such as vasopressin or angiotensin-2 agonists, especially in patients with refractory shock, can be considered.[26,32] Signs of end-organ hypoperfusion, increasing lactate, poor lactate clearance, or rapid increase in vasopressor requirement should lead to

TABLE 6.1
Indications for Admission to the Intensive Care Unit.

Considerations for ICU Admission	Clinical Conditions
Strong	- Shock requiring multiple/high-dose vasopressors - Hypoxemia requiring HFNC or BiPAP—mechanical ventilation - Need for continuous RRT - Refractory arrhythmias - Concern for HLH - Signs of impending shock in the pediatric patient - Decreased arousability concerning for poor airway protection - Nonconvulsive/convulsive/repetitive seizures or status epilepticus - Focal cerebral edema on imaging (will require monitoring for signs of elevated ICP) - Diffuse cerebral edema - Stupor or coma (need for endotracheal intubation for airway protection) - Motor deficits - Severe hyponatremia in patients presenting with neurotoxicity - Development of ischemic stroke or intracranial hemorrhage - Early onset of CRS or rapidly progressive symptoms - Grade 3 ICANS (ICE score 0–2 due to aphasia or seizures that resolve rapidly) in high-risk products
Equivocal	- Grade 2 CRS with more than two organ failure and/or a patient with significant comorbidities[a] - Hypotension without vasopressors with signs of hypoperfusion - Patients with a difficult airway at high risk for decompensation - Early onset of ICANS or rapidly progressive symptoms - Patients with underlying neurological deficits that could make evaluation or treatment challenging[b] - Moderate hyponatremia associated with grade 2 ICANS
Requires closer monitoring and early ICU consideration	- High-risk patients: Product known to cause high-grade toxicities or diffuse cerebral edema, multiple comorbidities, high risk of TLS or signs of TLS prior to infusion, high disease burden, baseline elevated CRP, and/or ferritin

HFNC, High-flow nasal cannula; BiPAP, Bilevel positive airway pressure; RRT, Renal replacement therapy; HLH, Hemophagocytic lymphohistiocytosis; ICP, Intracranial pressure; TLS, Tumor lysis syndrome; CRP, C-reactive protein.
[a] For example, patients with advanced heart failure, significant coronary artery disease, or baseline difficult to control arrhythmias; pediatric patients with significant cardiomyopathies or baseline neurocognitive defects that could pose difficult evaluation.
[b] For example, underlying history of seizures that are difficult to control; CNS involved with disease.

consideration of early use of both tocilizumab and corticosteroids[16] as the latter has been shown to be beneficial in patients with vasodilatory shock.[26,32]

Cardiomyopathy with a depressed ejection fraction can be observed in patients with CRS, and up to 5% of them can develop cardiogenic shock.[25] For patients with new onset cardiomyopathy, electrocardiographic changes and elevated troponins have been associated with increased mortality; therefore, early monitoring is recommended.[11,33,34] Moreover, an electrocardiogram, echocardiogram and serum troponins can help rule out other causes of shock and decreased cardiac output such as cardiac tamponade, acute coronary syndrome, and myocarditis or pericarditis. Treatment with inotropes such as dobutamine and milrinone can be considered in patients with low cardiac output. In these cases, minimally invasive monitoring devices can be beneficial to evaluate response to inotropes and guide treatment. Arrhythmias have also been described during CRS, most commonly sinus tachycardia and atrial fibrillation, but QT prolongation and fatal arrhythmias have also been observed.[11,18,33–35] Treatment for these arrhythmias should be supportive and no different than for any other critically ill patient. It is important to note that patients with significant cardiac risk could benefit from closer monitoring and telemetry postinfusion. Patients with Down syndrome, for example, should have an appropriate baseline cardiac evaluation to stratify their risk prior to CAR therapy, given their predisposition to cardiac abnormalities.

Lastly, CAR T-cell patients are at high risk of sepsis; therefore, following guidelines for neutropenic sepsis and septic shock is recommended while treating concomitantly for CRS.[36] A careful physical examination, cultures, imaging, and initiation of broad-spectrum antibiotics should not be delayed in this patient population.

Besides the supportive care described above, specific treatment for CRS with therapies such as anti-IL-6 and anti-IL-1 agents and steroids should be initiated without delay in patients with hypotension and shock.[4,12,16] In this patient population, the ICU clinician should monitor closely the patient's response to therapy, so treatment decisions and interventions are made in a timely manner.

RESPIRATORY FAILURE

In some series, as much as 45% of patients with CAR T-cell–related complications will require mechanical ventilation, although the data are unclear if this is all related to pulmonary complications versus a need for endotracheal intubation in patients with severe neurotoxicity and altered mentation.[25] Careful attribution of the need for intubation is important for delineating between true respiratory failure and the need for airway protection due to ICANS, with the latter not contributing to the grading of CRS as put forth by the recent ASTCT consensus manuscript.[25]

In regard to respiratory complications, the ASTCT consensus grading has defined grade 2 CRS as requiring low-flow nasal canula or blow by oxygen supplementation; grade 3 CRS as hypoxemia that requires oxygen supplementation with high flow devices; and grade 4 as the need for noninvasive ventilation (such as bilevel positive airway pressure [BiPAP]) or invasive mechanical ventilation.[25] When concurrent hypotension is present, thoughtful balance of fluid resuscitation with initiation of vasopressor support may avoid respiratory failure. We caution that for small infants, increasing oxygen supplementation even below a 2L threshold may signal worsening acuity. The overall trend in the need for oxygen supplementation should be considered carefully. The need for noninvasive ventilation (e.g., high-flow nasal cannula, bilevel positive airway pressure, continuous positive airway pressure) and invasive mechanical ventilation suggests very severe disease.

Respiratory failure in the patient post-CAR T-cell therapy may present with pleural effusions, noncardiogenic pulmonary edema, and cardiogenic pulmonary edema. When evaluating patients with hypoxemia, it is of great importance to consider if the hypoxemia is acute and related to CRS or if there are underlying chronic processes (e.g., malignant pleural effusions, progression of disease, pulmonary embolism, underlying chronic obstructive pulmonary disease) that require the patient to use oxygen supplementation. Therefore, as with hypotension, knowing the patients and their underlying comorbidities is of extreme importance. In patients requiring invasive mechanical ventilation, careful assessment of their airway prior to endotracheal intubation is important (Table 6.2). For example, patients with Down syndrome have a 20-fold increased likelihood of developing childhood leukemia.[37]

Respiratory illness is a significant cause of hospitalization for children with Down syndrome.[38] The upper airway in these patients is narrow, with smaller midface and lower face skeleton, macroglossia, narrow nasopharynx, relatively larger tonsils and adenoids, and short palate; laryngomalacia is a common cause of airway obstruction in Down syndrome patients.[39–41] These patients also have smaller trachea, with subglottic stenosis and dysfunctional cilia.[40,42–44] Hypotonia and obesity are also often present in these patients. Altogether, these patients may have difficult airways for intubation. Furthermore, they have a smaller functional residual capacity and may be prone to hypoxia during intubation[44] so preoxygenation may be helpful. Reverse Trendelenburg position (feet lower than head) may help displace the obese abdomen off the chest and may improve alignment of the external auditory meatus with the sternal notch. Techniques to minimize cervical manipulation are recommended given the potential for cervical spine instability. Using an endotracheal tube that is two times smaller than expected for age may account for the smaller trachea in these patients and facilitate successful intubation.[44–46]

Patients that present with noncardiogenic pulmonary edema due to CRS can progress quickly to ARDS or P-ARDS (definitions vary). The overall inflammatory state underlying CRS leads to endothelial dysfunction, capillary leak, and acute lung injury and ARDS. High-flow nasal cannula and BiPAP can be considered in these patients; however, intubation should not be delayed when indicated.[12] Patients requiring high-flow nasal cannula or noninvasive ventilatory support should be managed in the ICU.[18,47]

Once on mechanical ventilation due to ARDS, a lung-protective strategy with low tidal volumes (4–6 mL/kg) to avoid further lung injury is important.[48] Daily awakenings and minimizing sedation or oversedation to avoid delirium can have a positive impact on mortality in the critically ill.[18] Sedation choice can be complex in the CAR T-cell population and should be carefully considered. Sedatives such as

TABLE 6.2
Clinical Factors for Airway Evaluation in CAR T-Cell Patients.

Clinical Factors	Considerations during Endotracheal Intubation
Mucositis	- High risk of bleeding, can have difficulty visualizing the airway during direct laryngoscopy - Airway edema can cause difficulty during ventilation and endotracheal tube placement
Bulky disease compromising upper airway (head and neck)	- Assessment with imaging or by direct laryngoscopy can be helpful to evaluate airway patency prior to infusion - Bulky disease can limit mouth opening, thereby limiting the utility of direct laryngoscopy. Consider fiber optic intubation - Early evaluation by interventional pulmonary for airway stenting when possible (e.g., tracheal stents, main bronchus)
Bulky mediastinal disease	- Significant decrease in preload can occur when lying flat, particularly with sedation and paralytics - Consider awake fiber optic intubation
Shock and cardiomyopathy	- Consider etomidate for induction to avoid significant effects on hemodynamics and preload - Ketamine can be considered for induction; however, it requires careful consideration due to its risk of myocardial depression. In patients with ICANS, it should be avoided as it can elevate intracranial pressure
Radiation to the head and neck	- Can limit mouth opening, therefore limiting the use of direct laryngoscopy. Consider fiber optic intubation

dexmedetomidine and propofol can decrease the incidence of delirium when compared with benzodiazepines.[49] Moreover, their shorter time from discontinuation to light sedation or arousability could help with daily evaluation of ICANS. Despite these obvious benefits, concurrent cardiovascular toxicities from CRS (e.g., shock, baseline bradycardia, or high-grade heart blocks) may limit their use as both drugs are known to cause decreased systemic vascular resistance, hypotension, and bradycardia.

Careful fluid resuscitation and early diuresis should be paramount in patients with CRS-related respiratory failure. Available data in the critically ill show that patients with respiratory failure have increased mortality when there is evidence of fluid overload and overall positive fluid balance during their ICU stay.[50–52] Increased fluid balance has not been studied in the CAR T-cell patients with CRS; however, one may extrapolate data from the general ICU population in this setting; fluid overload leads to worsening inflammatory response, secondary organ damage, and increased mortality. Therefore, close monitoring of intake and output, diuresis when possible, and early consideration of renal replacement therapy (RRT) to avoid further complications are recommended.[12]

Treatment for grade 3 and 4 CRS with hypoxemia includes not only ICU support but also specific treatment such as steroids and anti-IL-6 or other anticytokine therapy if not already initiated.[50–52] Moreover, ruling out additional causes of respiratory failure while treating concomitantly for CRS is imperative. Other causes of respiratory failure to consider include viral, fungal, and bacterial pneumonia and disease progression involving the lungs. Diffuse alveolar hemorrhage can also occur as these patients may have disseminated intravascular coagulation (DIC) and thrombocytopenia. Studies such as computerized tomography (CT) of the chest, bronchoscopy with bronchioalveolar lavage, and microscopic studies are helpful to rule out other concomitant causes of respiratory failure.

NEUROLOGICAL COMPLICATIONS AND NEUROTOXICITY (ICANS)

The precise pathophysiology of ICANS remains unclear but may be related to a combination of endothelial activation in the central nervous system (CNS), elevated cytokine levels in the cerebrospinal fluid (CSF), and cerebral T-cell infiltration.[12,53–57,4] Risk factors, diagnosis, grading, and specific management of ICANS are discussed elsewhere in this book. Here, we focus on critical care management considerations of patients receiving CAR therapy who experience neurotoxicity.

ICANS may manifest as delirium, encephalopathy, aphasia, lethargy, impaired concentration, agitation, tremor, seizures, and, rarely, cerebral edema.[15] The onset can be biphasic, occurring concurrently with CRS and/or after CRS has resolved.[4,12] When corticosteroids and/or other definitive therapies are used, patients should be monitored closely for recurrence of neurotoxicity symptoms posttreatment or during tapering.[12] Patients with an ICANS grade of 3 or 4 require ICU monitoring for airway protection, management of possible seizures, status epilepticus, and signs of elevated intracranial pressure (ICP).[4,5,15] We will discuss in detail some specific considerations of patients with neurotoxicity while in the ICU.

Delirium

Delirium is a serious complication associated with critical illness and has been linked to increased mortality, prolongation and complication of hospitalization, and long-term disability.[57a,65] Manifestations include inattention, disturbance of consciousness within short periods, and sudden change in psychotic features from baseline. If a CAR therapy patient is admitted to the ICU for CRS, cognitive changes such as memory loss, confusion, language, or emotional disturbance may not be easily detected if there is severely reduced level of consciousness. Delirium represents the most frequent manifestation of acute brain dysfunction in the ICU. To minimize the incidence, severity, and duration of delirium, early diagnosis and management of ICU patients with delirium are crucial.[57a,58,65] When CAR patients are admitted to the ICU, interventions known to mitigate risk of delirium, such as reorientation, promoting sleep, pain management, and early ambulation, should be implemented.[49]

Among adult CAR therapy patients, an immune effector cell encephalopathy (ICE) score < 10 may indicate the presence of delirium and/or ICANS.[12,15] This tool is recommended by the ASTCT consensus grading as a screening assessment for neurological complications in adult patients treated with IEC therapies.[49] Among pediatric patients, the Cornell Assessment of Pediatric Delirium (CAPD) is used for delirium assessment.[4,12,15,59,60] CAPD is a validated screening tool for recognition of delirium among children and adolescents (from birth to 21 years old); the sensitivity and specificity of this tool are highest in patients aged <12 years. Use of CAPD with appropriate developmental anchor points enables developmentally appropriate delirium screening by nurses and other members of the healthcare team at the bedside.[4,12,15,59,60] A CAPD score >8 is indicative of delirium.[4,12,15,59,60]

While delirium may represent one of the earliest indications of ICANS, it is important to recognize that aside from CAR therapy, other risk factors, such as sepsis, pain, hypoperfusion, high fever, medications, withdrawal (alcohol and/or illicit drug use), and electrolyte imbalance, may also be present.[61] Administration of corticosteroids is the principle therapy for ICANS, but it has also been associated with delirium in the critically ill, especially in geriatric patients.[4,12,62-65] Thus, disparate etiologies may trigger a final common pathway, leading to delirium.[62-65] Hence, identifying the etiology of delirium is paramount in determining the best course of treatment.[4,12,65-68]

There are few evidence-based treatment strategies for management of delirium. For patients who have received CAR therapy, we suggest that they be evaluated for likelihood of ICANS. If the patient's risk factors, product type, and temporal relationship are consistent with ICANS, definitive treatment should be initiated per ICANS management guidelines. However, patients should be simultaneously evaluated for other underlying illness, iatrogenic causes, and abnormal environment. This may be particularly important for CAR patients admitted to the ICU. Environmental causes such as immobilization, pain, and poor sleep hygiene should be recognized and modified as possible.[65,69-71] If optimal ICANS management and addressing modifiable risk factors fail to improve symptoms, pharmacologic treatment with atypical antipsychotics (in particular, quetiapine) may be considered for delirium with a hyperactive component.[65] The use of antipsychotics in the ICU for patients with active delirium is common; however, data supporting improved outcomes with their use vary significantly.[49] With this in mind, the use of quetiapine or haloperidol is recommended for patients with distressing symptoms that could cause harm to themselves or others.[49] Special considerations of these medications among CAR T patients include close monitoring of QT on electrocardiogram, especially in patients with ongoing arrhythmias associated with CRS. Dexmedetomidine has been shown to reduce delirium in postoperative, intubated and nonintubated patients.[65,72,73] The use of dexmedetomidine can be beneficial in the CAR T patient population when the agitation precludes close evaluation and further testing (such as MRI of the brain, EEG, or lumbar puncture), and can be used without suppressing the patient's respiratory status.[49]

It is important to note that dexmedetomidine is known to cause hypotension and bradycardia; therefore, careful titration should be done in patients with hypotension associated with CRS.

Seizures

Seizures represent paroxysmal cortical discharges with either motor, sensory, and/or cognitive dysfunction and may be a manifestation of local or systemic factors exciting normal brain or may reflect a structural cerebral insult.[74] While the etiology of seizures may differ, the approach to the problem is similar.[74] An accurate diagnosis, prompt therapeutic intervention, and prevention of recurrence are imperative. Among CAR therapy patients, ICANS should be immediately suspected as the cause of observed seizure activity, and such patients should receive ICANS-specific management. However, other common causes of seizure activity must be considered, including but not limited to sepsis, metabolic abnormalities, intracranial hemorrhage (ICH), central nervous system (CNS) malignancy, and acute drug toxicity or withdrawal.[74-76] These factors may represent the etiology of seizures in a patient who has received CAR therapy and/or may result in a lower seizure threshold in a patient with ICANS.

Sepsis and CNS infections should be suspected in a patient with seizures, in particular among patients who are immunocompromised. Patients with refractory malignancies and those who have received lymphodepleting chemotherapy prior to CAR administration may be predisposed to infection. A sepsis evaluation should be conducted for CAR therapy patients who develop seizures with empiric antimicrobial coverage as indicated. Consideration of bacterial, viral, and fungal causes should be guided by the patient's specific risk profile and in conjunction with an interdisciplinary management team. For example, rare cases of prolonged grade 3 or 4 neutropenia before and after tisagenlecleucel infusion was associated with severe infections affecting the CNS (grade 3 human herpesvirus 6 [HHV-6] encephalitis) or were fatal (encephalitis and systemic mycosis).[3]

Patients receiving CAR therapy may be at risk for coagulopathy and CNS manifestations of their primary malignancy. Seizures that occur among these patients may also be related to ischemic stroke, intracerebral hemorrhage, and/or disease progression. Metabolic abnormalities including hyponatremia, hypocalcemia, hypophosphatemia, uremia, hypoglycemia, and alterations of serum osmolarity are also associated with lower seizure thresholds.[74] Fever, acidosis, or acute hyperventilation of ICU patients (leading to an increased pH by decreasing pCO2) may also contribute to lowering of seizure thresholds.[74-77] Alcohol ingestion and/or withdrawal and iatrogenic complications such as precipitous benzodiazepine and opiate withdrawal have also been associated with increased risk of seizures.

The large Boston Collaborative Drug Surveillance Program found drug-induced seizures to occur infrequently among admitted patients.[78] Antibiotics have been frequently cited as a class of medications associated with seizures in the ICU. Penicillin, cephalosporins, aztreonam, carbapenems, fluoroquinolones, isoniazid, and metronidazole all antagonize gamma-aminobutyric acid (GABA) activity through different proconvulsant mechanisms of action.[79] Therapeutic drug monitoring and dose adjustments in the setting of renal failure, congestive heart failure, and liver disease may mitigate some of the drug-associated risks of seizures.[74,79] Antidepressants have also been associated with variable risk of seizure activity. The serotonin selective reuptake inhibitors, trazodone, and the monoamine oxidase inhibitors have very low potential for causing seizures; the tricyclic antidepressants and bupropion have an intermediate risk profile; maprotiline and amoxapine are considered high risk.[74,80] Bupivacaine and lidocaine have also been associated with convulsions when used at therapeutic levels for arrhythmias.[74,81] Convulsions are usually a result of high-dose intravenous injection, but seizures have been reported following intratracheal instillation for bronchoscopy or even after topical application or when used for anesthesia during procedures.[74,81-86] Pain medications, such as fentanyl, have also been associated with proconvulsant risk profiles[74,87]

Patients who develop seizures after receiving CAR therapy should be comprehensively evaluated to ascertain the etiology. High vigilance for ICANS should alert interdisciplinary teams for definitive treatment (with, for example, corticosteroid administration). Patients should be immediately assessed for airway and breathing; a blood glucose check should quickly determine whether hypoglycemia is present. Nonconvulsive and convulsive status epilepticus, among CAR therapy patients, should be managed with benzodiazepines and additional antiepileptics (preferably with levetiracetam), as needed.[4,12] Intravenous administration of lorazepam may attain a rapid response with improvements in both EEG findings and mental status. Levetiracetam is generally well tolerated and is not thought to affect cytokine levels; it has minimal risk of adverse drug interactions, although dose adjustments might be necessary in the setting of renal dysfunction.[4,12,88,89] Loading doses with levetiracetam and then maintenance should be used until seizures have resolved and the patient is clinically stable. Phenobarbital is the preferred second antiepileptic for the management of seizures occurring among CAR recipients (a loading dose may be administered in the setting of refractory seizures).[5] Phenytoin and lacosamide can be considered but are associated with higher risks of cardiovascular adverse events, and this may be a concern among patients with concurrent CRS at risk for arrhythmias and hypotension. If seizures continue to be refractory, burst suppression with benzodiazepines, phenobarbital, or propofol might be necessary. While the choice of any of these might vary depending on availability and preference within institution, careful considerations should be taken with each of these medications in the CAR patient population. Benzodiazepines, while efficient for management of status epilepticus, are associated with higher prevalence of delirium and withdrawal when utilized at high doses and for prolonged periods of time.[49,90] Phenobarbital and propofol are known to cause hypotension and bradycardia; therefore, careful monitoring in patients with concomitant CRS is recommended. While rare, propofol infusion syndrome can occur and should be considered as a differential diagnosis in a CAR T-cell patient with shock and multiorgan failure. Patients with persistent seizures require ICU management with continuous electroencephalogram monitoring and neurology consultation.

Cerebral Edema

Among patients receiving CAR therapy, and in particular, those with or at risk for ICANS, there should be high vigilance for development of cerebral edema, as life-threatening cerebral edema can develop suddenly and without warning. Increased ICP (CSF opening pressure $\geq$20 mmHg or clinical signs of increased ICP) requires intensive care management and, in severe cases, osmotherapy. Institutional guidelines should be used for management of cerebral edema. "Cushing's triad," which is the presence of hypertension, bradycardia, and irregular respirations, is usually present when herniation is imminent. Careful monitoring and interventions should be instituted in CAR patients with cerebral edema prior to its presentation on exam.

Papilledema assessment according to the Frisén scale may guide severity stratification and management.[4,12,91] Stage 1 or 2 papilledema with CSF opening pressure of <20 mmHg without cerebral edema may be managed with intravenous administration of acetazolamide (with dose adjustments if indicated for renal function). Stages 3–5 papilledema, and or patients with any sign of cerebral edema on imaging studies,

or a CSF opening pressure of $\geq$20 mmHg may be managed with (1) high-dose corticosteroids, (2) elevation of the head of the patient's bed to an angle of 30 degrees, (3) avoiding repeat stimuli that could increase ICP (fevers, seizures, coughing or Valsalva, repeated suctioning), and/or (4) hyperosmolar therapy with either mannitol (20 g/dL solution) or hypertonic saline (3% or 23.4%).[12,16] Hyperventilation to achieve target partial pressure of arterial carbon dioxide ($PaCO_2$) of 28–30 mmHg should be reserved for patients with diffuse cerebral edema and with concerns of herniation. This, however, should be performed for no longer than 24 hours, as it can cause rebound vasodilation and elevated ICP.[92] It is important to note that funduscopic exam can be difficult to perform in patients with ICANS, especially those who are agitated; therefore, other modes of monitoring can be considered. Noninvasive methods such as transcranial Doppler or ocular ultrasound to measure optic nerve sheath diameter can be used; however, their role in patients with ICANS has not been studied. Careful monitoring of serum sodium levels and avoiding hyponatremia (which is common in this patient population) are of extreme importance in patients with cerebral edema.[93]

A neurosurgery consultation is recommended for patients with cerebral edema. The role of external ventricular devices in this patient population is limited, as many of these patients present with concomitant thrombocytopenia and coagulopathy.[92] If the patient has an Ommaya reservoir, CSF should be drained to target opening pressure of <20 mmHg. Metabolic profiling should be performed frequently with adjustments of medications as indicated to prevent rebound cerebral edema, renal failure, electrolyte abnormalities, hypovolemia, and hypotension.[4,12] Frequent imaging, perhaps daily, may guide response to management. While computed topography (CT) scan is useful to rule out other causes of altered mentation in this patient population, its sensitivity for early signs of edema is lower than that of MRI of the brain. Findings on MRI are more common in patients with severe neurotoxicity, and these include global or focal edema (such as in thalamus, brainstem, and basal ganglia).[8,94] When performing endotracheal intubation in CAR patients with suspected elevated ICP, use of lidocaine may be beneficial, and induction agents that cause hypotension (such as propofol) should be used cautiously.[8,94]

Intracranial Hemorrhage

ICH in patients with cancer commonly occurs due to intratumoral hemorrhage or related to coagulopathy, hypertensive hemorrhage, leukostasis and hyperviscosity, hemorrhagic conversion of ischemic stroke, venous sinus thrombosis, or posterior reversible encephalopathy syndrome.[95]

Among patients receiving CAR therapy, ICH has been reported, albeit rarely. In the phase 2, single-cohort, 25-center, global study of tisagenlecleucel in pediatric and young adult patients with CD19+ relapsed or refractory B-cell acute lymphoblastic leukemia (ALL), one patient died from cerebral hemorrhage in the context of coagulopathy and resolving CRS.[3] In a phase 1 study of EGFRvIII-targeted CAR T-cells in patients with EGFRvIII-expressing recurrent glioblastoma multiforme, one patient developed an ICH, but it occurred postoperatively.[96] Aside from CAR therapies, patients with relapsed/refractory hematologic malignancies may have baseline hyperleukocytosis, and patients with CNS malignancies may be predisposed to develop ICH. Patients with ICH typically present with focal neurological deficits, headache, and encephalopathy. Recognition of ICH as a distinct occurrence among patients who may concurrently have ICANS requires a high index of suspicion.

If a CAR therapy patient is suspected of developing ICH, radiologic imaging with a noncontrast CT scan of the head should be obtained. Postcontrast sequences (when feasible) may be helpful in identification of active sites of bleeding and prediction of hematoma expansion.[95] Once the patient is stable, brain magnetic resonance imaging (MRI) with contrast may identify ischemic stroke with hemorrhagic conversion and venous sinus thrombosis[95]

Management of ICH involves steroids to decrease mass effect from vasogenic edema, reversal of coagulopathy as it may be associated with CRS and aggressive management of thrombocytopenia. Patients at risk for ICANS and/or ICH should receive platelet transfusions per institutional guidelines to minimize risks of catastrophic bleeding (consider maintaining platelets > 30–50,000/mm^3). However, patients with ICH should be transfused to a target platelet value of ≥70–100,000/mm^3. Coagulation cascade impairment may result from liver failure, vitamin K deficiency due to poor nutrition and/or antibiotic use, and/or DIC. Repletion of vitamin K and/or correction of the underlying cause of DIC (e.g., CRS) and replacement of coagulation factors (cryoprecipitate, fresh frozen plasma, factor concentrates) are of vital importance.[95]

RENAL FAILURE

Nephrotoxic medications, postrenal obstruction, compression and infiltration by malignancy, tumor lysis

syndrome (TLS), sepsis, and contrast agent nephropathy may all contribute to AKI among patients with cancer.[97] Among patients receiving CAR therapy, increased cytokine production (as part of CRS) can also have direct actions and cause injury to glomerular cells.[54]

AKI is defined as an abrupt (within 2 weeks) reduction in kidney function based on an elevation in serum creatinine level, a reduction in urine output, the need for RRT (dialysis), or a combination of these factors.[98] AKI may be classified as prerenal (low blood flow into kidney), renal (kidney damage), and postrenal causes (ureteral or bladder outflow obstruction).[99] Elevations in creatinine are helpful in the classification of AKI in adult patients (>1.5 upper limit normal, 1.5–3× upper limit normal/baseline, 3–6× upper limit normal/baseline, or >6× upper limit normal/baseline).[99] Among pediatric patients, elevations in baseline creatinine and/or a drop in urine output below 0.5 mL/kg/hour for >6 hours or <0.3 mL/kg/hour for >24 hours is concerning for AKI.[100]

Positive fluid balance in the first 24 hours of ICU admission is associated with a significant risk of AKI in a mixed critically ill population.[101] Fluid administration and resuscitation may be used in CAR therapy patients during lymphodepleting chemotherapy, in response to tumor lysis prevention or management, for poor oral intake and/or hypotension related to CRS. Additionally, patients may receive intravenous medications and blood products that add to their total fluid intake. Patients receiving CAR therapy may be predisposed to clinical deterioration in the setting of acute fluid overload. Respiratory decompensation is frequently preceded by fluid resuscitation.[16,102] Fluid management is important in the setting of capillary leak, leading to nonpulmonary cardiogenic edema, CRS-related cardiomyopathy, and/or oliguric renal failure.[16,102] Therefore, early dialysis among oliguric patients with renal failure and CRS is recommended to avoid further complications associated with acute fluid overload.

TLS is characterized by hyperkalemia, hypocalcemia, hyperphosphatemia, hyperuricemia, and azotemia with high blood urea nitrogen. This potentially fatal complication may occur in particular, among CAR therapy patients with leukemia and lymphomas, as tumor cells are lysed in response to treatment. The metabolic abnormalities seen in TLS can ultimately result in acute uric acid nephropathy, AKI, seizures, cardiac arrhythmias, and death.[103] Patients at risk for TLS should receive prophylaxis with oral or intravenous allopurinol (a xanthine oxidase inhibitor that inhibits uric acid production); rasburicase, a synthetic urate oxidase enzyme, acts by degrading uric acid and can be used in lieu of allopurinol among higher-risk patients.[104] Patients ideally should also receive intravenous hydration to maintain high urine output (>2.5 L/day or 2 mL/kg/day)[105] though a careful balance between TLS management and risk of fluid-associated respiratory compromise is necessary. For patients that develop TLS, rasburicase is used as treatment to eliminate uric acid crystal accumulation, along with loop diuretics and intravenous hydration. Close and frequent monitoring of urine output and fluid balance is key for patients at risk and those with TLS. Cardiac monitoring and measurement of electrolytes, creatinine, and uric acid every 4−6 hours is indicated among patients at high risk for TLS. RRT may be indicated for patients who do not respond. Life-threatening dysrhythmias may occur with TLS that is associated with hyperkalemia and/or hypocalcemia. When RRT is indicated for hyperkalemia, glucose plus insulin or beta-agonists can be used as a temporizing measure. Symptomatic hypocalcemia should be treated with calcium at the lowest dose required to relieve symptoms; excessive calcium increases the calcium-phosphate product and the rate of calcium phosphate crystallization.[105]

Indications to commence RRT include intractable hyperkalemia, acidosis, uremic symptoms (nausea, pruritus, malaise), fluid overload (refractory to medical management), and chronic kidney disease.[105] The indications for RRT among patients receiving CAR therapy are the same among others with AKI. Among patients with TLS, lower thresholds may be considered for initiation of RRT; the potential for rapid potassium release and accumulation, particularly in patients with oliguria and hyperphosphatemia-induced symptomatic hypocalcemia, are valid reasons for early consideration of RRT.[106] Continuous RRT (CRRT) may better facilitate phosphate removal, as this increases with longer treatment duration[107]

APPROACH TO RENAL FUNCTION AMONG CAR THERAPY PATIENTS

Patients receiving CAR therapy may be predisposed to renal dysfunction based on underlying malignancy, prior medication/toxin exposures, CRS with vascular leak, fluid overload, and sepsis. A baseline assessment of renal function may be helpful for early detection of AKI among these patients. Patients at risk for development of AKI should have frequent assessment of serum electrolytes with creatinine and be monitored for adequate urine output. Patients at risk for TLS should be managed per TLS management guidelines. Where possible, avoidance of acute fluid overload and nephrotoxic medications (with dose adjustments based on

therapeutic drug monitoring and renal function) may be helpful. Early consideration of RRT should prompt attention for the need of vascular access for initiation of this procedure. For patients at risk of bleeding due to coagulopathy, avoidance of systemic anticoagulation by using citrate may be preferred over heparin with RRT. CRRT may be the preferred mode among patients with CRS, hypotension, hyperphosphatemia, and potential for cardiac dysfunction. Patients with cancer receiving RRT may not mount fevers with infections; high vigilance for sepsis is recommended.

OTHER CONSIDERATIONS
Complications Associated with Autologous Leukapheresis for CAR T-Cell Production
Generation of autologous CAR T-cells requires the collection of $CD3^+$ lymphocytes from the patient via leukapheresis. Pediatric patients often require a central venous catheter rather than a peripheral venous cannula for collection, which frequently requires sedation. Packed red blood cells (irradiated) and/or albumin may be needed to prime the collection in children weighing <30 kg, which adds an additional risk to this procedure. Candidates for CAR therapies may be refractory to standard treatments, making timing of apheresis challenging given the need for appropriate washout periods. In addition, comprehensive assessment of organ function may be important to guide whether patients undergoing autologous collection are hemodynamically stable and able to tolerate fluid shifts. Close monitoring for hypotension, hypocalcemia, and catheter-related pain is imperative during leukapheresis. Recognition of symptomatic hypocalcemia among infants and younger children who may not verbalize symptoms requires careful vigilance.[4,108−112]

Complications Associated With Infusion of CAR T-Cells
Infusion of cellular therapy products is generally safe, although serious adverse infusion reactions can occur. At the time of infusion, oxygen, suction, and emergency medications should be easily accessible. Adverse reactions include nausea, vomiting, abdominal pain, chills, fever, and, rarely, severe respiratory depression, neurotoxicity, and cardiac arrhythmias.[113−120] While these are mostly related to the cryoprotectant in the frozen cell product, anaphylactic reactions may occur when products manufactured with antibiotics are given to patients with an allergy to that antimicrobial.

General management principles for infusion reactions associated with adoptive cell therapy include slowing or halting the infusion, while severe reactions should prompt ICU evaluation. If a reaction does occur, the product identity should be verified again for accuracy. Bacterial infusion reactions may occur from infusion of contaminated products, typically with gram-negative organisms. Prompt initiation of empiric antimicrobial treatment and symptomatic management of fever, hypotension, and other unexpected signs and symptoms may be lifesaving.[4]

COAGULOPATHY

The risk of bleeding among patients receiving CAR therapy who develop CRS can be exacerbated by hypofibrinogenemia and/or thrombocytopenia, especially in those receiving anticoagulation therapy (including through continuous venovenous hemofiltration).[3,4,34,121] Prompt management of bleeding or hypofibrinogenemia and/or thrombocytopenia with the use of platelet transfusions, cryoprecipitate, or fresh frozen plasma infusions is recommended to avoid lethal hemorrhage. When possible, avoidance of anticoagulation or prioritization of citrate over heparin with RRT circuits may be helpful.

INFECTIOUS DISEASE

Patients receiving CAR therapy should be monitored closely for sepsis. Patients with CRS who receive anti-IL six therapies and/or corticosteroids may not mount fevers in response to infection. Other hemodynamic parameters such as persistent tachycardia and hypotension may be indicative of sepsis. Any patient with a suspicion of sepsis should be promptly cultured and initiated on broad-spectrum antimicrobial therapy, with continuation of other infectious disease prophylaxis against viral, bacterial, and/or fungal pathogens as appropriate.[4,12,34,122] Administration of growth factors (filgrastim/biosimilar) should be considered.

HEMOPHAGOCYTIC LYMPHOHISTIOCYTOSIS

Hemophagocytic lymphohistiocytosis (HLH) is a potentially life-threatening syndrome resulting from dysregulation of the immune response, leading to a hyperinflammatory status with increased cytokine release and organ infiltration.[122a-c,123,127] It is characterized by impaired cytotoxic activity of natural killer (NK) and cytotoxic T lymphocytes (CTLs), with continued capacity for activation and cytokine secretion. The result is mobilization, infiltration, and

overactivation of other IECs, mostly macrophages, which in turn try to stimulate the ineffective NK cells and CTLs, creating a vicious cycle and exaggerated secretion of cytokines responsible of the hyperinflammatory status.[124]

Malignancy-associated HLH (M-HLH) refers to HLH that occurs in the setting of cancer treatment and has an incidence of 1% with a median survival of 2.5–3.5 months.[125] Infection-associated HLH (I-AHS) is mostly associated with viral infections, most notably EBV,[126] but fungal and bacterial infections are also associated with I-AHS.[127,128] HLH associated with autoimmune or autoinflammatory diseases is also known as macrophage-activating syndrome (MAS) and requires immediate recognition and intervention.[126] The recent introduction and increased use of immunotherapies, such as checkpoint inhibitor mAbs, bispecific mAb T-cell engagers (BiTEs), CAR T-cell therapy, dendritic cell vaccines, and immunomodulatory drugs for a variety of malignancies may increase dysregulation of immune homeostasis created by cancer, leading to immune-related adverse events such as dermatitis, myocarditis, pericarditis, vasculitis, or HLH/MAS.[12] The occurrence of HLH/MAS in the course of CAR T-cell therapy may be underdiagnosed since it may be an overlapping syndrome with CRS and therefore difficult to differentiate.

The HLH 2004 diagnostic criteria requires the presence of five of the following eight criteria to make the diagnosis: fever, splenomegaly, cytopenias (affecting ≥ 2 of 3 lineages in blood), hypertriglyceridemia and/or hypofibrinogenemia, hemophagocytosis in bone marrow or spleen or lymph nodes, low or absent NK cell activity, ferritin ≥ 500 ng/mL, and soluble CD25 ≥ 2400 U/mL.[129] HLH shares other clinical and laboratory features with CRS, including multiorgan dysfunction, CNS disturbances, and high lactate dehydrogenase levels. Some practitioners tend to refer to them as part of a spectrum of systemic inflammatory disorders, even though patients with CRS may or may not have hepatosplenomegaly, lymphadenopathy, or overt evidence of hemophagocytosis.[15] Based on emerging clinical understanding, diagnostic criteria for CAR T-related HLH/MAS have been proposed based on the presence of elevated ferritin ($>10,000$ ng/mL) during the CRS phase and two of the following: grade ≥ 3 organ toxicities involving liver, lung and kidney, or hemophagocytosis in bone marrow.[12] CAR T-related HLH/MAS typically responds to management for grade 3 CRS, for example, with anti-IL-6 therapy and use of corticosteroids. The role of etoposide and intrathecal cytarabine or methotrexate for fulminant

HLH/MAS, not responding to 48 hours of treatment, has been strongly debated.[12,130] Anti-IL-1 therapy with anakinra could represent a valuable weapon, although further studies are needed to assess this agent in the treatment of refractory HLH/MAS.[131]

PEDIATRIC CRITICAL CARE CONSIDERATIONS

The main difference in assessing CAR T-cell toxicities between adults and children is not only physiological but also primarily related to identifying and understanding the early signs and symptoms of associated toxicities. Infants and young children may not clearly verbalize or communicate their symptoms, which typically help identify toxicity. All members of the healthcare team and parents, guardians, and caregivers must be properly educated to promptly recognize potential toxicities.

A central venous catheter may be required for leukapheresis in children. Children must be hemodynamically stable to tolerate fluid shifts, and priming with packed red blood cells and/or albumin may be performed among low-weight children (<30 kg). High vigilance for hypotension, hypocalcemia, and catheter-related pain is important during the procedure, as young children may not be able to adequately describe symptoms such as tetany related to hypocalcemia. Similarly, monitoring of children for adverse reactions during CAR T-cell infusion requires careful attention to recognizing symptoms such as shortness of breath, chills, rash, and back pain, which may present as irritability without localizing signs. Knowing the child's baseline heart rate and respiratory rate are helpful in recognizing changes, though it is important to interpret discrepancies in the context of the child's anxiety level (e.g., tachycardia associated with crying).

Standard monitoring for toxicities and adverse events in pediatrics requires early detection of changes in baseline heart rate, blood pressure, temperature, and engagement with parents or staff. Hypotension in children is determined by age and systolic blood pressure (BP), measured in mmHg as follows[131]:

- Term neonates (0–28 days): systolic BP < 60 mmHg.
- Infants (1–12 months): systolic BP < 70 mmHg.
- Children 1–10 years (fifth BP percentile): systolic BP < 70 mmHg + (age in years × 2).
- Children >10 years: systolic BP < 90 mmHg.

Signs and symptoms of impending hemodynamic shock among younger children include malaise, lethargy, weakness, oliguria, irritability, and reduced appetite. When hypotension is present, care should be taken to avoid overly aggressive fluid resuscitation moving, rather, to early pressor support with definitive therapies to avoid respiratory compromise. P-ARDS diagnosis and management should be performed per Pediatric Acute Lung Injury Consensus Conference (PALICC) criteria.[132] AKI in children may be graded per the Kidney Disease: Improving Global Outcomes (KDIGO) grading, which requires attention to urine output and serum creatinine.[100]

Children with Down syndrome (DS) have an increased risk of B-cell precursor ALL, which may now be treated with CAR T-cells for relapsed/refractory disease. Children with DS have genetic anomalies, which may influence their response to critical illness.[133] They may present with greater disease severity and disproportionately require cardiovascular and renal support than suggested by disease severity at admission. They may also require longer stays in the ICU with higher mortality rates associated with increased length of ICU admission.[133]

Attention to pediatric specific dosing for definitive therapies such as the anti-IL-6 agent, tocilizumab, for the management of the CRS is important (12 and 8 mg/kg for patients weighing > and <30 kg, respectively).[4]

HANDOFF COMMUNICATION BETWEEN CRITICAL CARE AND CELL THERAPY TEAMS

Effective transfer of care between clinical teams is an important and potentially modifiable factor that may prevent adverse patient outcomes.[134–136] Standardized verbal and written handoffs with closed loop communication may allow for effective patient transfers. Key elements of handoff communication for CAR T-cell patients are summarized in Table 6.2.

FUTURE DIRECTIONS

Current management of the critically ill CAR patient is based on extrapolation of data available for the general ICU population. In view of this, a large area of investigational data is still to be discovered. Further investigation in understanding the role of specific vasopressors in vasodilatory shock observed in patients with CRS and their impact on patient outcomes might be beneficial in patient care. Moreover, data on the use of noninvasive ventilation in the oncological population suggest that they have lower mortality than patients who require mechanical ventilation; however, its role in the CAR patient (noninvasive ventilation vs. early intubation) is unclear.[100] Also, interventions to manage cerebral edema and elevated ICP in CAR patients are based on experience in the general population. The role of certain tools such as transcranial Doppler, funduscopic exam, and ocular ultrasound to guide management of patients with ICANS is unknown and needs further evaluation. Lastly, data suggest that early initiation of CRRT in critically ill patients shows no benefit.[137] However, due to the high risk of fluid overload, further studies on early versus late RRT in this specific patient population are necessary.

Moreover, while rare, severe refractory CRS and ICANS can and do occur, so additional treatment options are needed for these complex cases. Ongoing work with agents such as anakinra, anti-GM-CSF, and ruxolitinib in animal models suggest that they may play a role in preventing or decreasing the severity of CRS and ICANS. However, further studies are required to know how to optimally treat these patients.

REFERENCES

1. NCI. *Cancer Statistics*; 2018. https://www.cancer.gov/about-cancer/understanding/statistics.
2. Koch A, Checkley W. Do hospitals need oncological critical care units? *J Thorac Dis*. 2017;9:E304−E309.
3. Maude SL, Laetsch TW, Buechner J, et al. Tisagenlecleucel in children and young adults with B-cell lymphoblastic leukemia. *N Engl J Med*. 2018;378:439−448.
4. Mahadeo KM, Khazal SJ, Abdel-Azim H, et al. Management guidelines for paediatric patients receiving chimeric antigen receptor T cell therapy. *Nat Rev Clin Oncol*. 2019;16:45−63.
5. Neelapu SS, Locke FL, Bartlett NL, et al. Axicabtagene ciloleucel CAR T-cell therapy in refractory large B-cell lymphoma. *N Engl J Med*. 2017;377:2531−2544.
6. Park JH, Riviere I, Gonen M, et al. Long-term follow-up of CD19 CAR therapy in acute lymphoblastic leukemia. *N Engl J Med*. 2018;378:449−459.
7. Locke FL, Ghobadi A, Jacobson CA, et al. Long-term safety and activity of axicabtagene ciloleucel in refractory large B-cell lymphoma (ZUMA-1): a single-arm, multicentre, phase 1-2 trial. *Lancet Oncol*. 2019;20:31−42.
8. Gust J, Hay KA, Hanafi LA, et al. Endothelial activation and blood-brain barrier disruption in neurotoxicity after adoptive immunotherapy with CD19 CAR-T cells. *Cancer Discov*. 2017;7:1404−1419.
9. Hay KA, Hanafi LA, Li D, et al. Kinetics and biomarkers of severe cytokine release syndrome after CD19 chimeric antigen receptor-modified T-cell therapy. *Blood*. 2017;130:2295−2306.
10. Fitzgerald JC, Weiss SL, Maude SL, et al. Cytokine release syndrome after chimeric antigen receptor T cell therapy for acute lymphoblastic leukemia. *Crit Care Med*. 2017;45:e124−e131.
11. Kochenderfer JN, Dudley ME, Feldman SA, et al. B-cell depletion and remissions of malignancy along with cytokine-associated toxicity in a clinical trial of anti-CD19 chimeric-antigen-receptor-transduced T cells. *Blood*. 2012;119:2709−2720.
12. Neelapu SS, Tummala S, Kebriaei P, et al. Chimeric antigen receptor T-cell therapy - assessment and management of toxicities. *Nat Rev Clin Oncol*. 2018;15:47−62.
13. Rezvani K, Rouce R, Liu E, et al. Engineering natural killer cells for cancer immunotherapy. *Mol Ther*. 2017;25:1769−1781.
14. Teachey DT, Rheingold SR, Maude SL, et al. Cytokine release syndrome after blinatumomab treatment related to abnormal macrophage activation and ameliorated with cytokine-directed therapy. *Blood*. 2013;121:5154−5157.
15. Lee DW, Santomasso BD, Locke FL, et al. ASBMT consensus grading for cytokine release syndrome and neurologic toxicity associated with immune effector cells. *Biol Blood Marrow Transplant*. 2018.
16. Gutierrez C, McEvoy C, Mead E, et al. Management of the critically ill adult chimeric antigen receptor-T cell therapy patient: a critical care perspective. *Crit Care Med*. 2018;46:1402−1410.
17. Corrigan-Curay J, Kiem HP, Baltimore D, et al. T-cell immunotherapy: looking forward. *Mol Ther*. 2014;22:1564−1574.
18. Lee DW, Gardner R, Porter DL, et al. Current concepts in the diagnosis and management of cytokine release syndrome. *Blood*. 2014;124:188−195.
19. Xu XJ, Tang YM. Cytokine release syndrome in cancer immunotherapy with chimeric antigen receptor engineered T cells. *Cancer Lett*. 2014;343:172−178.
20. Diaconu I, Ballard B, Zhang M, et al. Inducible caspase-9 selectively modulates the toxicities of CD19-specific chimeric antigen receptor-modified T cells. *Mol Ther*. 2017;25:580−592.
21. Gargett T, Brown MP. The inducible caspase-9 suicide gene system as a "safety switch" to limit on-target, off-tumor toxicities of chimeric antigen receptor T cells. *Front Pharmacol*. 2014;5:235.
22. Li J, Li W, Huang K, et al. Chimeric antigen receptor T cell (CAR-T) immunotherapy for solid tumors: lessons learned and strategies for moving forward. *J Hematol Oncol*. 2018;11(22).
23. Li H, Zhao Y. Increasing the safety and efficacy of chimeric antigen receptor T cell therapy. *Protein Cell*. 2017;8:573−589.
24. Wang X, Chang WC, Wong CW, et al. A transgene-encoded cell surface polypeptide for selection, in vivo tracking, and ablation of engineered cells. *Blood*. 2011;118:1255−1263.
25. Teachey DT, Lacey SF, Shaw PA, et al. Identification of predictive biomarkers for cytokine release syndrome after chimeric antigen receptor T-cell therapy for acute lymphoblastic leukemia. *Cancer Discov*. 2016;6:664−679.

26. Rhodes A, Evans LE, Alhazzani W, et al. Surviving sepsis campaign: international guidelines for management of sepsis and septic shock: 2016. *Intensive Care Med.* 2017; 43:304–377.

27. Alsous F, Khamiees M, DeGirolamo A, et al. Negative fluid balance predicts survival in patients with septic shock: a retrospective pilot study. *Chest.* 2000;117: 1749–1754.

28. Boyd JH, Forbes J, Nakada TA, et al. Fluid resuscitation in septic shock: a positive fluid balance and elevated central venous pressure are associated with increased mortality. *Crit Care Med.* 2011;39:259–265.

29. Vincent JL, Sakr Y, Sprung CL, et al. Sepsis in European intensive care units: results of the SOAP study. *Crit Care Med.* 2006;34:344–353.

30. Avni T, Lador A, Lev S, et al. Vasopressors for the treatment of septic shock: systematic review and meta-analysis. *PLoS One.* 2015;10. e0129305.

31. Myburgh JA, Higgins A, Jovanovska A, et al. A comparison of epinephrine and norepinephrine in critically ill patients. *Intensive Care Med.* 2008;34: 2226–2234.

32. Khanna A, English SW, Wang XS, et al. Angiotensin II for the treatment of vasodilatory shock. *N Engl J Med.* 2017; 377:419–430.

33. Park JH, Geyer MB, Brentjens RJ. CD19-targeted CAR T-cell therapeutics for hematologic malignancies: interpreting clinical outcomes to date. *Blood.* 2016;127: 3312–3320.

34. Brudno JN, Kochenderfer JN. Toxicities of chimeric antigen receptor T cells: recognition and management. *Blood.* 2016;127:3321–3330.

35. Schuster SJ, Svoboda J, Chong EA, et al. Chimeric antigen receptor T cells in refractory B-cell lymphomas. *N Engl J Med.* 2017;377:2545–2554.

36. Freifeld AG, Bow EJ, Sepkowitz KA, et al. Clinical practice guideline for the use of antimicrobial agents in neutropenic patients with cancer: 2010 update by the infectious diseases society of America. *Clin Infect Dis.* 2011;52: e56–93.

37. Holland WW, Doll R, Carter CO. The mortality from leukaemia and other cancers among patients with Down's syndrome (mongols) and among their parents. *Br J Cancer.* 1962;16:177–186.

38. So SA, Urbano RC, Hodapp RM. Hospitalizations of infants and young children with Down syndrome: evidence from inpatient person-records from a statewide administrative database. *J Intellect Disabil Res.* 2007;51: 1030–1038.

39. Uong EC, McDonough JM, Tayag-Kier CE, et al. Magnetic resonance imaging of the upper airway in children with Down syndrome. *Am J Respir Crit Care Med.* 2001;163: 731–736.

40. Hamilton J, Yaneza MM, Clement WA, et al. The prevalence of airway problems in children with Down's syndrome. *Int J Pediatr Otorhinolaryngol.* 2016;81:1–4.

41. Mitchell RB, Call E, Kelly J. Diagnosis and therapy for airway obstruction in children with Down syndrome. *Arch Otolaryngol Head Neck Surg.* 2003;129:642–645.

42. Shott SR. Down syndrome: analysis of airway size and a guide for appropriate intubation. *The Laryngoscope.* 2000; 110:585–592.

43. Miller R, Gray SD, Cotton RT, et al. Subglottic stenosis and Down syndrome. *Am J Otolaryngol.* 1990;11: 274–277.

44. Fox S. *Down Syndrome Airway*; 2018. https:// pedemmorsels.com/down-syndrome-airway/.

45. Lewanda AF, Matisoff A, Revenis M, et al. Preoperative evaluation and comprehensive risk assessment for children with Down syndrome. *Paediatr Anaesth.* 2016;26: 356–362.

46. Watts R, Vyas H. An overview of respiratory problems in children with Down's syndrome. *Arch Dis Child.* 2013;98: 812–817.

47. Gutierrez CP, Pastores SM. Oncologic emergencies. In: Hall B, Schmidt G, Kress J, eds. *Hall, Schmidt and Wood's Principles of Critical Care.* 4th. Burlington, NC: McGraw-Hill Education; 2015:872–880.

48. Fan E, Del Sorbo L, Goligher EC, et al. An official American thoracic society/European society of intensive care medicine/society of critical care medicine clinical practice guideline: mechanical ventilation in adult patients with acute respiratory distress syndrome. *Am J Respir Crit Care Med.* 2017;195:1253–1263.

49. Devlin JW, Skrobik Y, Gelinas C, et al. Clinical practice guidelines for the prevention and management of pain, agitation/sedation, delirium, immobility, and sleep disruption in adult patients in the ICU. *Crit Care Med.* 2018;46:e825–e873.

50. Murphy CV, Schramm GE, Doherty JA, et al. The importance of fluid management in acute lung injury secondary to septic shock. *Chest.* 2009;136:102–109.

51. National Heart L, Blood Institute Acute Respiratory Distress Syndrome Clinical Trials N, Wiedemann HP, et al. Comparison of two fluid-management strategies in acute lung injury. *N Engl J Med.* 2006;354:2564–2575.

52. Rosenberg AL, Dechert RE, Park PK, et al. Review of a large clinical series: association of cumulative fluid balance on outcome in acute lung injury: a retrospective review of the ARDSnet tidal volume study cohort. *J Intensive Care Med.* 2009;24:35–46.

53. Grupp SA, Kalos M, Barrett D, et al. Chimeric antigen receptor-modified T cells for acute lymphoid leukemia. *N Engl J Med.* 2013;368:1509–1518.

54. Maude SL, Frey N, Shaw PA, et al. Chimeric antigen receptor T cells for sustained remissions in leukemia. *N Engl J Med.* 2014;371:1507–1517.

55. Lee DW, Kochenderfer JN, Stetler-Stevenson M, et al. T cells expressing CD19 chimeric antigen receptors for acute lymphoblastic leukaemia in children and young adults: a phase 1 dose-escalation trial. *Lancet.* 2015;385: 517–528.

56. Hu Y, Sun J, Wu Z, et al. Predominant cerebral cytokine release syndrome in CD19-directed chimeric antigen receptor-modified T cell therapy. *J Hematol Oncol.* 2016;9:70.

57. Gust J, Taraseviciute A, Turtle CJ. Neurotoxicity associated with CD19-targeted CAR-T cell therapies. *CNS Drugs.* 2018;32:1091−1101.

57a. Barr J, Fraser GL, Puntillo K, Ely EW, Gélinas C, Dasta JF, Davidson JE, Devlin JW, Kress JP, Joffe AM, Coursin DB, Herr DL, Tung A, Robinson BR, Fontaine DK, Ramsay MA, Riker RR, Sessler CN, Pun B, Skrobik Y, Jaeschke R. American College of Critical Care Medicine. Clinical practice guidelines for the management of pain, agitation, and delirium in adult patients in the intensive care unit. *Crit Care Med.* 2013 Jan;41(1):263−306. https://doi.org/10.1097/CCM.0b013e3182783b72.

58. Arumugam S, El-Menyar A, Al-Hassani A, et al. Delirium in the intensive care unit. *J Emerg Trauma Shock.* 2017;10:37−46.

59. Traube C, Silver G, Kearney J, et al. Cornell Assessment of Pediatric Delirium: a valid, rapid, observational tool for screening delirium in the PICU*. *Crit Care Med.* 2014; 42:656−663.

60. Silver G, Kearney J, Traube C, et al. Delirium screening anchored in child development: the Cornell assessment for pediatric delirium. *Palliat Support Care.* 2015;13: 1005−1011.

61. Pandharipande PP, Ely EW, Arora RC, et al. The intensive care delirium research agenda: a multinational, interprofessional perspective. *Intensive Care Med.* 2017;43: 1329−1339.

62. Schreiber MP, Colantuoni E, Bienvenu OJ, et al. Corticosteroids and transition to delirium in patients with acute lung injury. *Crit Care Med.* 2014;42:1480−1486.

63. Mu JL, Lee A, Joynt GM. Pharmacologic agents for the prevention and treatment of delirium in patients undergoing cardiac surgery: systematic review and metaanalysis. *Crit Care Med.* 2015;43:194−204.

64. Wolters AE, Veldhuijzen DS, Zaal IJ, et al. Systemic corticosteroids and transition to delirium in critically ill patients. *Crit Care Med.* 2015;43:e585−e588.

65. Traube C, Silver G, Gerber LM, et al. Delirium and mortality in critically ill children: epidemiology and outcomes of pediatric delirium. *Crit Care Med.* 2017;45:891−898.

66. Karnik NS, Joshi SV, Paterno C, et al. Subtypes of pediatric delirium: a treatment algorithm. *Psychosomatics.* 2007; 48:253−257.

67. Schieveld JN, Leroy PL, van Os J, et al. Pediatric delirium in critical illness: phenomenology, clinical correlates and treatment response in 40 cases in the pediatric intensive care unit. *Intensive Care Med.* 2007;33:1033−1040.

68. Traube C, Augenstein J, Greenwald B, et al. Neuroblastoma and pediatric delirium: a case series. *Pediatr Blood Cancer.* 2014;61:1121−1123.

69. Smith HA, Brink E, Fuchs DC, et al. Pediatric delirium: monitoring and management in the pediatric intensive care unit. *Pediatr Clin North Am.* 2013;60:741−760.

70. Peritogiannis V, Bolosi M, Lixouriotis C, et al. Recent insights on prevalence and corelations of hypoactive delirium. *Behav Neurol.* 2015;2015:416792.

71. Silver G, Traube C, Gerber LM, et al. Pediatric delirium and associated risk factors: a single-center prospective observational study. *Pediatr Crit Care Med.* 2015;16:303−309.

72. Schieveld JN, Lousberg R, Berghmans E, et al. Pediatric illness severity measures predict delirium in a pediatric intensive care unit. *Crit Care Med.* 2008;36:1933−1936.

73. Stagno D, Gibson C, Breitbart W. The delirium subtypes: a review of prevalence, phenomenology, pathophysiology, and treatment response. *Palliat Support Care.* 2004;2:171−179.

74. Varelas PN, Mirski MA. Seizures in the adult intensive care unit. *J Neurosurg Anesthesiol.* 2001;13:163−175.

75. Bleck TP, Smith MC, Pierre-Louis SJ, et al. Neurologic complications of critical medical illnesses. *Crit Care Med.* 1993;21:98−103.

76. Wijdicks EF, Sharbrough FW. New-onset seizures in critically ill patients. *Neurology.* 1993;43:1042−1044.

77. Haltiner AM, Temkin NR, Dikmen SS. Risk of seizure recurrence after the first late posttraumatic seizure. *Arch Phys Med Rehabil.* 1997;78:835−840.

78. Miller R. *Comprehensive Drug Surveillance.* 1974:461−481.

79. Wallace KL. Antibiotic-induced convulsions. *Crit Care Clin.* 1997;13:741−762.

80. Rosenstein DL, Nelson JC, Jacobs SC. Seizures associated with antidepressants: a review. *J Clin Psychiatry.* 1993;54: 289−299.

81. Wu FL, Razzaghi A, Souney PF. Seizure after lidocaine for bronchoscopy: case report and review of the use of lidocaine in airway anesthesia. *Pharmacotherapy.* 1993;13:72−78.

82. Credle Jr WF, Smiddy JF, Elliott RC. Complications of fiberoptic bronchoscopy. *Am Rev Respir Dis.* 1974;109:67−72.

83. Giard MJ, Uden DL, Whitlock DJ, et al. Seizures induced by oral viscous lidocaine. *Clin Pharm.* 1983;2:110.

84. Mofenson HC, Caraccio TR, Miller H, et al. Lidocaine toxicity from topical mucosal application. With a review of the clinical pharmacology of lidocaine. *Clin Pediatr (Phila).* 1983;22:190−192.

85. Parish RC, Moore RT, Gotz VP. Seizures following oral lidocaine for esophageal anesthesia. *Drug Intell Clin Pharm.* 1985;19:199−201.

86. Rothstein P, Dornbusch J, Shaywitz BA. Prolonged seizures associated with the use of viscous lidocaine. *J Pediatr.* 1982;101:461−463.

87. Tempelhoff R, Modica PA, Bernardo KL, et al. Fentanyl-induced electrocorticographic seizures in patients with complex partial epilepsy. *J Neurosurg.* 1992;77:201−208.

88. Guenther S, Bauer S, Hagge M, et al. Chronic valproate or levetiracetam treatment does not influence cytokine levels in humans. *Seizure.* 2014;23:666−669.

89. Hovinga CA. Levetiracetam: a novel antiepileptic drug. *Pharmacotherapy.* 2001;21:1375−1388.

90. Girard TD, Pandharipande PP, Ely EW. Delirium in the intensive care unit. *Crit Care.* 2008;12(Suppl 3):S3.

91. Frisen L. Swelling of the optic nerve head: a staging scheme. *J Neurol Neurosurg Psychiatry.* 1982;45:13−18.

92. Godoy DA, Seifi A, Garza D, et al. Hyperventilation therapy for control of posttraumatic intracranial hypertension. *Front Neurol.* 2017;8:250.

93. Dixon B, Daley R, Horvat T, et al. Risk of hyponatremia and associated clinical characteristics in patients with acute lymphoblastic leukemia after CD19 targeted chimeric antigen receptor (CAR) T-cells. *Blood*. 2017; 130(Suppl 1):3584.

94. Santomasso BD, Park JH, Salloum D, et al. Clinical and biological correlates of neurotoxicity associated with CAR T-cell therapy in patients with B-cell acute lymphoblastic leukemia. *Cancer Discov*. 2018;8:958−971.

95. Velander AJ, DeAngelis LM, Navi BB. Intracranial hemorrhage in patients with cancer. *Curr Atheroscler Rep*. 2012; 14:373−381.

96. O'Rourke DM, Nasrallah MP, Desai A, et al. A single dose of peripherally infused EGFRvIII-directed CAR T cells mediates antigen loss and induces adaptive resistance in patients with recurrent glioblastoma. *Sci Transl Med*. 2017;9.

97. Darmon M, Ciroldi M, Thiery G, et al. Clinical review: specific aspects of acute renal failure in cancer patients. *Crit Care*. 2006;10:211.

98. Mehta RL, Kellum JA, Shah SV, et al. Acute Kidney Injury Network: report of an initiative to improve outcomes in acute kidney injury. *Crit Care*. 2007;11:R31.

99. NIH/NCI. *Common Terminology Criteria for Adverse Events (CTCAE)*; 2017. https://ctep.cancer.gov/protocoldevelopment/electronic_applications/docs/ctcae_v5_quick_reference_8.5x11.pdf.

100. Mizuno T, Sato W, Ishikawa K, et al. KDIGO (Kidney Disease: Improving Global Outcomes) criteria could be a useful outcome predictor of cisplatin-induced acute kidney injury. *Oncology*. 2012;82:354−359.

101. Salahuddin N, Sammani M, Hamdan A, et al. Fluid overload is an independent risk factor for acute kidney injury in critically ill patients: results of a cohort study. *BMC Nephrol*. 2017;18:45.

102. Hanidziar D, Bittner E. A growing problem of critical illness due to chimeric antigen receptor T-cell therapy. *Crit Care Med*. 2018;46:e1086−e1087.

103. Cheuk DK, Chiang AK, Chan GC, et al. Urate oxidase for the prevention and treatment of tumour lysis syndrome in children with cancer. *Cochrane Database Syst Rev*. 2014. CD006945.

104. Coiffier B, Mounier N, Bologna S, et al. Efficacy and safety of rasburicase (recombinant urate oxidase) for the prevention and treatment of hyperuricemia during induction chemotherapy of aggressive non-Hodgkin's lymphoma: results of the GRAAL1 (Groupe d'Etude des Lymphomes de l'Adulte Trial on Rasburicase Activity in Adult Lymphoma) study. *J Clin Oncol*. 2003;21: 4402−4406.

105. Howard SC, Jones DP, Pui CH. The tumor lysis syndrome. *N Engl J Med*. 2011;364:1844−1854.

106. Mirrakhimov AE, Voore P, Khan M, et al. Tumor lysis syndrome: a clinical review. *World J Crit Care Med*. 2015;4: 130−138.

107. Gutzwiller JP, Schneditz D, Huber AR, et al. Estimating phosphate removal in haemodialysis: an additional tool to quantify dialysis dose. *Nephrol Dial Transplant*. 2002;17:1037−1044.

108. Carausu L, Clapisson G, Philip I, et al. Use of totally implantable catheters for peripheral blood stem cell apheresis. *Bone Marrow Transplant*. 2007;40:417−422.

109. Gorlin JB, Humphreys D, Kent P, et al. Pediatric large volume peripheral blood progenitor cell collections from patients under 25 kg: a primer. *J Clin Apher*. 1996;11: 195−203.

110. Koristek Z, Sterba J, Havranova D, et al. Technique for PBSC harvesting in children of weight under 10 kg. *Bone Marrow Transplant*. 2002;29:57−61.

111. Michon B, Moghrabi A, Winikoff R, et al. Complications of apheresis in children. *Transfusion*. 2007;47: 1837−1842.

112. Ohara Y, Ohto H, Tasaki T, et al. Comprehensive technical and patient-care optimization in the management of pediatric apheresis for peripheral blood stem cell harvesting. *Transfus Apher Sci*. 2016;55:338−343.

113. Davis JM, Rowley SD, Braine HG, et al. Clinical toxicity of cryopreserved bone marrow graft infusion. *Blood*. 1990; 75:781−786.

114. Hoyt R, Szer J, Grigg A. Neurological events associated with the infusion of cryopreserved bone marrow and/or peripheral blood progenitor cells. *Bone Marrow Transplant*. 2000;25:1285−1287.

115. Miniero R, Vai S, Giacchino M, et al. Severe respiratory depression after autologous bone marrow infusion. *Haematologica*. 1992;77:98−99.

116. Otrock ZK, Beydoun A, Barada WM, et al. Transient global amnesia associated with the infusion of DMSO-cryopreserved autologous peripheral blood stem cells. *Haematologica*. 2008;93:e36−e37.

117. Stroncek DF, Fautsch SK, Lasky LC, et al. Adverse reactions in patients transfused with cryopreserved marrow. *Transfusion*. 1991;31:521−526.

118. Truong TH, Moorjani R, Dewey D, et al. Adverse reactions during stem cell infusion in children treated with autologous and allogeneic stem cell transplantation. *Bone Marrow Transplant*. 2016;51:680−686.

119. Zambelli A, Poggi G, Da Prada G, et al. Clinical toxicity of cryopreserved circulating progenitor cells infusion. *Anticancer Res*. 1998;18:4705−4708.

120. Zenhausern R, Tobler A, Leoncini L, et al. Fatal cardiac arrhythmia after infusion of dimethyl sulfoxide-cryopreserved hematopoietic stem cells in a patient with severe primary cardiac amyloidosis and end-stage renal failure. *Ann Hematol*. 2000;79:523−526.

121. Buechner J, Grupp S, Maude S, et al. Global registration trial of efficacy and safety of CTL019 in pediatric and young adult patients with relapsed/refractory (R/R) acute lymphoblastic leukemia (ALL): update to the interim analysis. *Clin Lymphoma Myeloma Leuk*. 2017;17: S263−S264.

122. Tomblyn M, Chiller T, Einsele H, et al. Guidelines for preventing infectious complications among hematopoietic cell transplantation recipients: a global perspective. *Biol Blood Marrow Transplant*. 2009;15:1143−1238.

122a Henter JI, Elinder G, Söder O, Ost A. Incidence in Sweden and clinical features of familial hemophagocytic lymphohistiocytosis. *Acta Paediatr Scand.* 1991 Apr; 80(4):428−435.

122b Wang Z, Wang Y, Huang W, et al. Hemophagocytic lymphohistiocytosis is not only a childhood disease: a multi-center study of 613 cases from Chinese HLH Workgroup. *Blood.* 2014;124(21):4146.

122c Stepp SE, Dufourcq-Lagelouse R, Le Deist F, Bhawan S, Certain S, Mathew PA, Henter JI, Bennett M, Fischer A, de Saint Basile G, Kumar V. Perforin gene defects in familial hemophagocytic lymphohistiocytosis. *Science.* 1999 Dec 3;286(5446):1957−1959.

123. Henter JI, Arico M, Elinder G, et al. Familial hemophagocytic lymphohistiocytosis. Primary hemophagocytic lymphohistiocytosis. *Hematol Oncol Clin North Am.* 1998;12:417−433.

124. Creput C, Galicier L, Buyse S, et al. Understanding organ dysfunction in hemophagocytic lymphohistiocytosis. *Intensive Care Med.* 2008;34:1177−1187.

125. Daver N, Kantarjian H. Malignancy-associated haemophagocytic lymphohistiocytosis in adults. *Lancet Oncol.* 2017;18:169−171.

126. Melek Oguz M, Sahin G, Altinel Acoglu E, et al. Secondary hemophagocytic lymphohistiocytosis in pediatric patients: a single center experience and factors that influenced patient prognosis. *Pediatr Hematol Oncol.* 2019;1−16.

127. Janka G, Imashuku S, Elinder G, et al. Infection- and malignancy-associated hemophagocytic syndromes. secondary hemophagocytic lymphohistiocytosis. *Hematol Oncol Clin North Am.* 1998;12:435−444.

128. Risdall RJ, McKenna RW, Nesbit ME, et al. Virus-associated hemophagocytic syndrome: a benign histiocytic proliferation distinct from malignant histiocytosis. *Cancer.* 1979;44:993−1002.

129. Henter JI, Horne A, Arico M, et al. HLH-2004: diagnostic and therapeutic guidelines for hemophagocytic lymphohistiocytosis. *Pediatr Blood Cancer.* 2007;48:124−131.

130. Teachey DT, Bishop MR, Maloney DG, et al. Toxicity management after chimeric antigen receptor T cell therapy: one size does not fit 'ALL'. *Nat Rev Clin Oncol.* 2018;15:218.

131. Maude SL, Barrett D, Teachey DT, et al. Managing cytokine release syndrome associated with novel T cell-engaging therapies. *Cancer J.* 2014;20:119−122.

132. Pediatric acute lung injury consensus conference G: pediatric acute respiratory distress syndrome: consensus recommendations from the pediatric acute lung injury consensus conference. *Pediatr Crit Care Med.* 2015;16: 428−439.

133. Tibby SM, Durward A, Goh CT, et al. Clinical course and outcome for critically ill children with Down syndrome: a retrospective cohort study. *Intensive Care Med.* 2012;38: 1365−1371.

134. Aylward MJ, Rogers T, Duane PG. Inaccuracy in patient handoffs: discrepancies between resident-generated reports and the medical record. *Minn Med.* 2011;94: 38−41.

135. Evans AS, Yee MS, Hogue CW. Often overlooked problems with handoffs: from the intensive care unit to the operating room. *Anesth Analg.* 2014;118:687−689.

136. Warrick D, Gonzalez-del-Rey J, Hall D, et al. Improving resident handoffs for children transitioning from the intensive care unit. *Hosp Pediatr.* 2015;5: 127−133.

137. Bhatt GC, Das RR. Early versus late initiation of renal replacement therapy in patients with acute kidney injury-a systematic review & meta-analysis of randomized controlled trials. *BMC Nephrol.* 2017;18:78.

CHAPTER 7

Neurotoxicities After CAR T-Cell Immunotherapy

JULIANE GUST, MD, PHD • FRANCESCO CEPPI, MD •
CAMERON J. TURTLE, MBBS, PHD, FRACP, FRCPA

INTRODUCTION

Chimeric antigen receptor (CAR)–modified T-cell immunotherapy can be a highly effective treatment for patients with relapsed and/or refractory hematologic malignancies, but significant adverse effects remain a concern. Systemic cytokine release syndrome (CRS) can occur in association with the inflammatory cytokine surge during in vivo CAR T-cell proliferation,[1–3] and neurologic adverse effects commonly occur in this context.[4,5] While most patients who experience neurotoxicity have mild and reversible symptoms and/or signs, fulminant cerebral edema and other serious events can occur in rare cases. Early studies considered neurotoxicity to be a component of CRS,[2] but it has become increasingly clear that it is a related but distinct entity. The close relationship between CRS and neurotoxicity is illustrated by the observation that neurotoxicity typically develops after the onset of CRS and may present after its resolution. In patients without CRS, neurotoxicity is uncommon, and if it does occur, manifestations are typically not severe. Most approaches to treat neurotoxicity have been adapted from the management of CRS, and in light of the natural history of neurotoxicity, it has been difficult to identify effective treatments for neurotoxicity. Consensus guidelines for diagnosis and grading of CAR T-cell treatment–associated CRS and neurotoxicity were developed by the American Society for Transplantation and Cellular Therapy (ASTCT) in 2018.[6] The group considered the diversity of signs and symptoms associated with CAR T-cell treatment–related neurologic dysfunction, as well as the fact that similar toxicities have been observed with other cancer therapies that engage immune effector cells (IECs) and arrived at the new designation of IEC-associated neurotoxicity syndrome (ICANS). For the purposes of this discussion, we will adopt the designation of ICANS, using "neurotoxicity" interchangeably when appropriate for discussing prior research that did not apply ICANS criteria for the diagnosis of neurotoxicity.

INCIDENCE OF NEUROLOGIC ADVERSE EVENTS IN PUBLISHED CLINICAL TRIALS OF CHIMERIC ANTIGEN RECEPTOR T-CELL THERAPY

Neurologic adverse events have been reported in all trials of CD19-directed CAR T-cells that showed significant anticancer efficacy and have also been noted with other CAR T-cell modalities (Table 7.1). However, prior to the development of consensus criteria for the diagnosis, identification and reporting of the severity of neurologic adverse events related to CAR T-cell immunotherapy (ICANS) was not standardized. Therefore, the reported incidence of neurotoxicity varies between individual studies at least in part due to differences in the specific cancers treated, prior treatment history, patient age, CAR design, CAR T-cell manufacturing approach, lymphodepletion regimen, CAR T-cell dose and infusion regimen, product potency and efficacy, toxicity grading schemas, and toxicity treatment strategies in each study.[2,7]

The role of the CAR costimulatory domain has been considered as a possible determinant of neurotoxicity risk. In studies using a CD19-targeting CAR with 4-1BB costimulation, neurotoxicity was reported in 40% −44% of children and young adults with acute lymphoblastic leukemia (ALL; 13%−21% severe, defined as Common Terminology Criteria for Adverse Events (CTCAE) grade 3 or greater)[8–10] and 47% of adults with ALL (30% severe).[11] 4-1BB CAR trials for adults with non-Hodgkin's lymphoma (NHL) reported neurotoxicity in 32%−39% of subjects (11%−13% severe),[12,13] and in adults with chronic lymphocytic leukemia (CLL), the incidence was 6%−33% (0% −29% severe).[14,15] Patients with ALL who underwent

TABLE 7.1
Neurotoxicity, CRS, and Immunomodulatory Treatment in Selected Clinical Trials of CAR T-Cells for Hematologic Malignancies.

Disease—CAR Antigen	Clinical Trial Registration	N	Age Range (years)	CAR Construct	Lymphodepletion (N)	CRR (%)	ORR (%)	NT (%)	sNT (%)	CRS[a] (%)	sCRS[a] (%)	Toci (%)	Steroids (%)
ALL—CD19													
Park 2018[17]	NCT01044069	53	23–74	28z (19-28z)	Cy (43) or Flu/Cy (10)	83#/67^	n/a	44	42	85[M]	26	42	38
Maude 2018[8]	NCT02435849	75	3–23	4-1BB (tisagenlecleucel)	Flu/Cy (71) or Cy/Etop (1)	81#/81^	n/a	40	13	77[P]	46	48	0
Gardner 2017[9]	NCT02028455	43	1–25	4-1BB	Cy (27) or Flu/Cy (14)	93#/93^	n/a	44	21[b]	93[C*]	23	42	25
Turtle 2016[11,c]	NCT01865617	30	20–73	4-1BB	Cy/Etop (2), Cy (11) or Flu/Cy (17)	100#/93^	n/a	50	50	83[C]	23	27	37
Lee 2015[16]	NCT01593696	20	5–27	28z	Flu/Cy	70#/60^	n/a	30	5	75[C*]	30	27	13
Maude 2014[10]	NCT01626495 NCT01029366	30	5–60	4-1BB (CTL019, tisagenlecleucel)	Cy/VP (5), AraC/Etop (1), Flu/Cy (15), Cy (3), Clo (1), CVAD-A (1) or CVAD-B (1)	90#/79^	n/a	43	–	88*	27	30	20
NHL—CD19													
Neelapu 2017[20]	NCT02348216	101	23–76	28z (axicabtagene ciloleucel)	Flu/Cy	54	82	64	28	93[L]	13	43	27
Schuster 2017[12]	NCT02030834	28	25–77	4-1BB (CTL019)	Cy (11), modEPOCH (3), bend (8), Cy/TBI (4), Cy/Etop (1), Flu/Cy (1), Carbo/Gem (10)	57	64	39	11	57[P]	18	20	6
Turtle 2016[13,c]	NCT01865617	32	36–70	4-1BB	Cy or Cy/Etop (12) or Flu/Cy (20)	33	63	28	28[d]	63[C*]	13	9	13
Kochenderfer 2015[19]	NCT00924326	11	30–68	28z	Flu/Cy	36	80	–	45	–	36[C]	25	0
CLL—CD19													
Fraietta 2018[14]	NCT01029366 NCT01747486 NCT02640209	41	61–66[e]	4-1BB	–	20	39	6[f]	0[f]	69[f]	38[f]	–	–

Study	NCT number	N	Age range	Costimulatory domain	Conditioning								
Turtle 2017[15,c]	NCT01865617	24	40–73	4-1BB	Cy (1), Flu (2) Flu/Cy (21)	29	71	33	25[d]	83[L]	8	25	25
ALL—CD22													
Fry 2018[26]	NCT02315612	21	7–30	4-1BB	Flu/Cy	57#43^	n/a	25	0	76[C*]	0	0	0
HL—CD30													
Ramos 2017[25]	NCT01316146	9[h]	20–65	28z	None	33	33	0	0	0[C]	0	n/a	n/a
Wang 2017[27]	NCT02259556	18	13–77	4-1BB	Flu/Cy (5), Gem/Cy+ (8), Pac/Cy+ (3), AraC/Cy+ (1), Etop/Cy+ (1)	0	39	0	0	0[C]	0	n/a	n/a
MM—BCMA													
Brudno 2018[32,g]	NCT02215967	14	–	28z	Flu/Cy	7[&]	81	–	14	93[C]	29	21	29
Zhao 2018[33]	NCT03090659	57	27–72	4-1BB	Cy	68[&]	88	2	0	90[L]	7	46	0
Ali 2016[28]	NCT02215967	12	–	28z	Flu/Cy	8[&]	33	25	8	50[C]	25	33	0
AML—LEY													
Ritchie 2013[29]	CTX 08-0002	4	–	28z	Ida/AraC (1), Flu/AraC/ AraC (1), Ida/AraC/ Gem (1), Ida/AraC/ Flu (1)	25	50	0	0	25[C]	0	0	0

#, morphologic remission; &, complete remission; ˟, complete response or stringent complete response; —, not reported; ˆ, MRD negative remission; 28z, CD28-CD3zeta costimulatory domain; 4-1BB, 4-1BB costimulatory domain; ALL, acute lymphoblastic leukemia; AML, acute myeloid leukemia; AraC, cytarabine; Bend, bendamustine; Carbo, carboplatin; CLL, chronic lymphocytic leukemia; Clo, clofarabine; CRR, complete remission rate; CRS, cytokine release syndrome (CTCAE grade 2 or less, or as defined in the publication); CVAD-A, cyclophosphamide+vincristine+adriamycin; CVAD-B, methotrexate+cytarabine; Cy, cyclophosphamide; Etop, etoposide; Flu, fludarabine; Gem, gemcitabine; HL, Hodgkin's lymphoma; Ida, idarubicin; MM, multiple myeloma; modEPOCH, modified EPOCH (doxorubicin, etoposide, cyclophosphamide); n/a, not applicable; NHL, non-Hodgkin's lymphoma; NT, neurotoxicity; ORR, overall response rate; Pac, nab-paclitaxel; sCRS, severe cytokine release syndrome (CTCAE grade 3 or greater, or as defined in the publication); sNT, severe neurotoxicity (CTCAE grade 3 or greater); steroids, corticosteroids; TBI, total body irradiation; Toci, tocilizumab.

a CRS grading is indicated by superscript: C = CTCAE criteria[2], L = Lee criteria[2], P = Penn/CHOP criteria[7], M = MSKCC criteria[17], *indicates modified criteria; please refer to the individual publication for details.

b CTCAE grade 3 or greater, and/or any seizures.

c Data on expanded cohort available in Ref. 5.

d CTCAE grade 3 or greater, and/or grade 2 delirium.

e Only median age reported.

f Toxicities only reported for the 16 patients who responded to CAR T-cells.

g Excluded two patients previously reported in Ref. 28.

h Two patients with anaplastic large cell lymphoma.

treatment with CD19-targeted CAR T-cells using a CD28 costimulatory domain experienced neurotoxicity rates of 30% in children and young adults (5% severe)[16] and 44% in adults (42% severe).[17] The same CAR construct, but a different manufacturing approach, was used in the ROCKET trial, which was closed due to a high incidence of fatal cerebral edema.[18] In adults with NHL who received a CD28-containing CD19 CAR, neurotoxicity developed in up to 64% (28% −45% severe).[19,20] Interestingly, no neurotoxicity was observed in patients who received CAR T-cells immediately following autologous hematopoietic cell transplant (HCT),[21,22] possibly due to a paucity of target antigen-expressing cells and consequently less robust CAR T-cell proliferation. Neurotoxicity was also absent in early clinical trials targeting CD19$^+$ malignancies, where CAR T-cells were given without preconditioning chemotherapy; however, response rates in these studies were low.[23,24]

ICANS is not exclusive to CD19-targeted CAR T-cell therapy and has been reported for a number of IEC-engaging treatments targeting B-cell malignancies and other hematologic or solid tumors.[25–30] CD22-directed CAR T-cells for children and young adults with ALL had a 25% rate of neurotoxicity but without any severe neurotoxicity or severe CRS.[26] 81% of the patients in the study had previously received CD19 CAR T-cells, and the morphologic complete remission rate (CRR) was 57%, which is lower than the 70%−100% morphologic CRR reported for ALL treated with CD19-directed CAR T-cells.[8–11,16,17,31] In trials of CAR T-cells directed against B-cell maturation antigen (BCMA) expressed on multiple myeloma, neurotoxicity was reported in 25% of patients (8%−14% severe) for a product using CD28 costimulation[28,32] and only 2% (none severe) in a trial using a 4-1BB containing CAR.[33] No neurotoxicity has been reported to date in CAR T-cell trials for non-CNS solid tumors,[30] which could be either related to different toxicity profiles, or due to the fact that robust antitumor responses have so far rarely been achieved in solid tumor treatment with CAR T-cells.[34] Transient neurologic adverse events, including seizures and focal weakness, occurred after systemic (EGFRvIII CAR)[35] or intra-CNS (IL13Rα2 CAR)[36] treatment with CAR T-cells for malignant glioma.

IEC-engaging therapies have also been implicated in similar neurologic syndromes. Blinatumomab, a bispecific CD3/CD19 T-cell engager for the treatment of ALL, can cause CRS and neurotoxicity.[37] Treatment of NHL with lymphodepletion followed by haploidentical natural killer cell−enriched donor cells and recombinant IL-15 was associated with neurotoxicity in 38% of patients, but neurotoxicity and CRS only occurred if the IL-15 was given subcutaneously instead of intravenously.[38,39]

With the rapid expansion of the CAR T-cell field, toxicity profiles may change as new epitopes are targeted, and combinatorial approaches are developed to target multiple antigens at once.

CLINICAL PRESENTATION OF NEUROTOXICITY ASSOCIATED WITH CHIMERIC ANTIGEN RECEPTOR T-CELL IMMUNOTHERAPY

Timing of Neurotoxicity

Neurologic signs and symptoms that are associated with CAR T-cell treatment typically follow a monophasic time course. Manifestations such as delirium, language disturbance, tremor, transient focal weakness, behavioral disturbances, ataxia, peripheral neuropathy, visual changes and generalized weakness, seizures, and acute cerebral edema[4,5,40−42] usually develop in the first 10 days after CAR T-cell infusion. Headache is often present in conjunction with neurotoxicity but may also be present in the absence of neurologic symptoms. In many cases, the findings worsen over the course of several days and usually take a similar amount of time to resolve (Fig. 7.1). In most patients, several different signs and symptoms occur at the same time, but confusion, language dysfunction, or delirium are often the first manifestations to appear and the last to resolve. In a study of neurotoxicity in 133 adults with ALL, NHL, or CLL who received T-cells expressing a CD19-targeting CAR with a 4-1BB costimulatory domain, neurotoxicity onset occurred a median of 4 days after CAR T-cell infusion, with a peak on day 7, and a duration of 5 days.[5] In a similar study of 53 adults who received CD28-costimulated CD19-targeted CAR T-cells for treatment of ALL, neurotoxicity started a median of 5 days after CAR T-cell infusion, the first severe neurotoxicity symptom occurred at a median 9 days postinfusion, and resolution occurred a median of 11 days after onset.[4]

The kinetics of presentation may differ between studies investigating different CAR T-cell therapies and studies where dedicated assessment tools are employed to identify early signs of subtle neurotoxicity.[5,8,12,26,41] Most signs and symptoms of neurotoxicity resolve within 21 days of CAR T-cell infusion, although in rare cases they can persist longer, either owing to irreversible neurologic injury, prolonged headaches, or cognitive and attentional

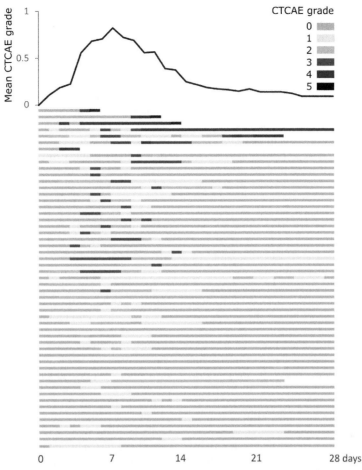

FIG. 7.1 **Kinetics of neurotoxicity in a cohort of 133 patients treated with CD19-directed chimeric antigen receptor (CAR) T-cells.** The graph (top) shows the mean of the highest grade of neurotoxicity occurring in all patients on each day after CAR T-cell infusion. The swimmer plot (bottom) shows the kinetics of the severity of neurotoxicity in each patient who developed neurotoxicity through 28 days after CAR T-cell infusion (n = 53). Each row represents one patient, and the colors indicate the highest grade of neurotoxicity recorded on each day. (Adapted with permission from Gust J, Hay K.A., Hanafi L.-A, et al., Endothelial activation and blood-brain barrier disruption in neurotoxicity after adoptive immunotherapy with CD19 CAR T-cells, Cancer Discov 7, 2017, 1404–1419.)

complaints.[4,5,8] Rarely, neurotoxicity onset has occurred after 14 days due to delayed CAR T-cell expansion and CRS.[43] One-month outcomes on neurocognitive screening tests were overall stable or improved in a cohort of 22 pediatric patients treated with CD22-targeting CAR T-cells.[43] However, long-term cognitive and neurodevelopmental outcomes have not yet been reported in the CAR T-cell–treated patient population. Comprehensive long-term follow-up as well as prospective neurocognitive testing would be required to determine whether acute neurotoxicity causes chronic changes that affect brain health.

Signs and Symptoms

The most common manifestation of neurotoxicity is a transient impairment of attention and cognitive processing, typically described as delirium or confusion.[5,8,12,26,41] Language disturbance is also frequent and is one of the more characteristic signs of ICANS.[4–6] This can easily be missed in subtle cases or when patients are systemically very ill. Impaired language production can be a manifestation of true aphasia, which is due to dysfunction of cortical and subcortical language modules, but abnormal language output can also occur related to impaired attention or arousal, as occurs in delirium and depressed level of consciousness. Validated mental status exam tools are required to make the distinction.[44,45] Of note, no imaging abnormalities have been reported in neurotoxicity patients that specifically localize to language centers of the brain such as Broca's or Wernicke's areas without affecting other brain regions.

Headache is very common and often an early sign of neurotoxicity. Although this temporal association suggests that headache can be a symptom of neurotoxicity, it is nonspecific and can be seen without other associated neurologic symptoms. Therefore, headache does not contribute to the criteria for diagnosis and grading of ICANS.[6]

Seizures have primarily been reported in patients with ALL who received CD19-directed CAR T-cells,[4,5,8–10,41,46] with incidences ranging from 0% to 30% after CD28-costimulated and 3%–14% after 4-1BB CAR treatment. Only isolated cases of seizure have been reported from other CAR T-cell trials (BCMA, 1 of 57 patients treated[33]; EGFRvIII for glioblastoma, 1 of 10 patients[35]), although there may be additional cases that are not reported here because not all authors have provided comprehensive listings of toxicities. The reason for the higher seizure risk in ALL patients is unknown but could be related to younger patient age (which appears less likely, since both pediatric and adult ALL trials report similar seizure incidences), more severe CRS, or higher rates of preexisting CNS comorbidities.

Other frequently reported signs and symptoms include tremor, visual hallucinations, behavioral disturbances, ataxia, peripheral neuropathy, visual changes, and generalized weakness. The overall pattern is that of a global, toxic-metabolic encephalopathy.

Focal pathology leading to focal neurologic dysfunction, such as unilateral limb weakness or cranial neuropathy, is unusual, and other etiologies should be considered. These include CNS infection, hemorrhagic or ischemic stroke, and malignant CNS involvement. Since patients with relapsed/refractory hematologic malignancies are at overall increased risk of such neurologic complications, further study will be needed to determine whether their incidence is affected by CAR T-cell therapy.

Pediatric CAR T-cell patients appear to have similar neurotoxicity profiles as adults. However, subtle cognitive dysfunction and language disturbance may be more difficult to detect in young children, requiring specific pediatric assessment tools. Proposed pediatric-specific measures include a neurologic symptom checklist that can be filled out by caregivers[43] or an observational tool for mental status assessment that can be used instead of language-based instruments that require patient cooperation (see ICANS Diagnostic Criteria section).[6]

Acute cerebral edema is a life-threatening complication that to date has only been described after treatment with CD19-directed CAR T-cells. In one clinical trial for adults with ALL, fatal cerebral edema occurred in five patients.[47] This forced the termination of the trial. Deaths due to cerebral edema have been reported in clinical trials using CAR constructs containing either 4-1BB or CD28 costimulatory domains, in children and adults with ALL, and in adults with NHL and CLL.[5,12,47–50] All published cases have been associated with CRS. Cerebral edema typically develops in the first week after CAR T-cell infusion and often at a time when CRS-associated signs such as fever and hypotension are abating after treatment with tocilizumab and/or steroids. The first signs of impending cerebral edema can occur with no preceding neurotoxicity, or as a worsening of existing neurologic signs and symptoms, occasionally after initial improvement. Within hours, symptoms can evolve from mild somnolence and confusion to those associated with increased intracranial pressure such as headache, nausea, vomiting, and decreasing level of consciousness. Blood pressure may rise due to autoregulatory responses to preserve cerebral perfusion. Patients then become comatose and require invasive ventilation and may develop seizures. Bradycardia is a late sign of impending herniation. Even if treated aggressively with measures directed toward CRS management and neuroprotection, edema can quickly become irreversible to the point of herniation and brain death.

Other fatal neurologic events after CD19 CAR T-cell therapy have included cortical necrosis, acute cerebral hemorrhage during resolving CRS, edema and hemorrhage of the brainstem and deep brain structures, and multifocal thrombotic microangiopathy.[5,8,47] One case of chronic, progressive neurologic decline was reported in a patient with preexisting optic atrophy, and pathologic examination revealed severe diffuse white matter degeneration and neuronal loss.[12] Since this case did not have the typical acute presentation of neurotoxicity, a distinct underlying pathophysiology may have contributed to the clinical findings.

Findings on Standard Clinical Blood Tests

Abnormalities in several standard clinically available markers have been identified in patients with neurotoxicity. However, many of these patients have concurrent CRS, and it is difficult to ascertain whether any of these abnormalities are specifically associated with neurotoxicity. We assessed clinical laboratory markers for CRS and neurotoxicity in a cohort of 133 adult patients after 4-1BB-costimulated CAR T-cell treatment.[1,5] The most pronounced abnormalities were seen in patients with grade ≥ 4 CRS as well as in patients with grade ≥ 3 neurotoxicity. For example, the acute phase reactants CRP and ferritin were significantly higher in patients with grade ≥ 3 neurotoxicity during the first week after CAR T-cell infusion compared with patients with grade 0–2 neurotoxicity,[5] and the increase in CRS was seen as early as 0–36 h after CAR T-cell infusion. The pattern of ferritin and CRP increases was the same when comparing patients with grade ≥ 4 CRS with those with grade 3 CRS.[1] In a different study, day 3 and peak CRP levels, as well as day 3 but not peak ferritin levels, correlated with the severity of neurotoxicity.[4] Other markers that were abnormal in patients with neurotoxicity and/or CRS in our cohort during the acute toxicity phase in the first 14 days after CAR T-cell infusion include decreased serum total protein and albumin levels, and derangements of coagulation assays (including elevated PT, PTT, and D-dimer, and decreased fibrinogen and platelet counts).

Findings on Standard Clinical Cerebrospinal Fluid Examination

Neurotoxicity is associated with increased cerebrospinal fluid (CSF) protein concentration and leukocyte counts,[4,5,41] consistent with increased trafficking of cells and serum proteins across the blood-CSF barrier. The protein concentration in the CSF can be very high, occasionally above 1 g/dL, but the increase is transient and normalizes soon after resolution of neurologic symptoms.[5,41] CSF cell counts are typically modestly elevated and rarely above 100 cells/μL.[5,41] The cellular composition of the CSF is typically lymphocyte predominant, and presence of significant numbers of neutrophils should prompt investigation for other causes of neurologic dysfunction, such as infection.[5,41] Although infectious workup is usually negative in patients with a typical course of neurotoxicity, empiric antibacterial and antiviral coverage, as well as CSF culture and viral PCRs, should be strongly considered.

CNS Imaging

Head imaging should be considered in all cases of neurotoxicity, but the clinical utility of normal or abnormal imaging results is not well studied. Magnetic resonance imaging (MRI) is preferred if the patient is stable enough to undergo the study, and contrast administration may be helpful for detecting evidence of inflammatory infiltrates by leptomeningeal enhancement and blood-brain barrier breakdown by enhancement of lesions in the brain parenchyma (Fig. 7.2). Head CT is useful to rule out acute abnormalities such as hemorrhage but is not sensitive to most of the changes that are seen with neurotoxicity. In patients with mild acute neurotoxicity, imaging is frequently normal.[5,10,16] The incidence of MRI abnormalities is higher in patients with severe neurotoxicity,[4,5] and head imaging may be considered in such cases both to rule out other etiologies such as stroke and to monitor response to treatment.

The most common and characteristic MRI pattern during neurotoxicity is one of symmetric T2 hyperintensities and swelling of the thalami and other deep gray matter structures, which is indicative of interstitial edema.[4,5,41] These lesions were noted to be reversible in patients who underwent repeat imaging after resolution of neurologic symptoms.[41] The deep gray matter lesions are typically nonenhancing and without restricted diffusion, but there may be associated microhemorrhages. This pattern is often seen in patients with decreased level of consciousness but can also occur in patients with mild, nonspecific symptoms.[41] Similar symmetric deep gray matter edema, with or without diffusion restriction, may be seen in many other neurologic disorders, such as hypoxic-ischemic brain injury, a number of toxic-metabolic etiologies, central posterior reversible encephalopathy syndrome (PRES), acute disseminated encephalomyelitis, and acute necrotizing encephalopathy.[51–53]

Patchy reversible T2 hyperintensities can also be seen in the cerebral white matter and can be associated with patchy enhancement that resolves over time.[5] This can affect the supratentorial or the cerebellar white matter, similar to what is seen in inflammatory disorders of the white matter, such as multiple sclerosis or CNS vasculitis. An unusual involvement of the extreme and external capsule white matter has been reported by several groups.[4,41] Acute T2 hyperintensities, with or without patchy enhancement, have also been described in areas of known CNS injury from other causes such as catheter placement or hemorrhage that were present prior to CAR T-cell treatment.[5,41]

Diffuse leptomeningeal enhancement can occur during neurotoxicity, indicating meningeal inflammation that is likely associated with increased cell and protein trafficking across the blood-CSF barrier.[54] Diffusion restriction, which is associated with cytotoxic edema, has been seen in regions of cortical gray matter and can be reminiscent of PRES. This can evolve into cortical laminar necrosis, which is irreversible and leads to

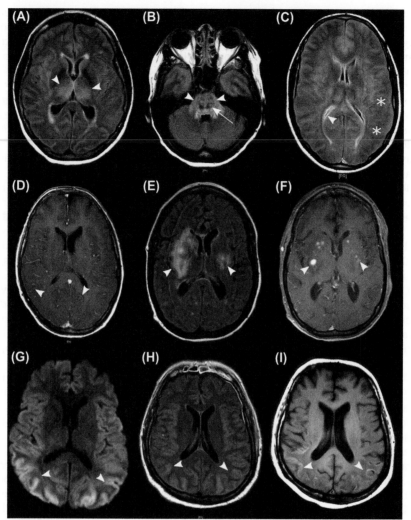

FIG. 7.2 Brain magnetic resonance imaging (MRI) findings in patients with severe neurotoxicity after CD19 chimeric antigen receptor (CAR) T-cell immunotherapy. **(A–B)** Symmetric edema of deep structures in a patient with grade 5 neurotoxicity. FLAIR hyperintensities were seen in the bilateral thalami **(A**, *arrowheads***)** and the pons **(B**, *arrowheads***)**, consistent with vasogenic edema. Punctate hemorrhages in the most affected areas are seen as T2 dark lesions **(B**, *arrow***)**. **(C)** Global edema with blurring of the gray-white junction (*stars*) and slit-like ventricles (*arrowhead*) on FLAIR imaging in a patient with grade 5 neurotoxicity. **(D)** Diffuse leptomeningeal enhancement (*arrowheads*) in a patient with grade 5 neurotoxicity. **(E–F)** White matter FLAIR hyperintensities **(E**, *arrowheads***)** that in some cases were contrast enhancing **(F**, *arrowheads*; T1 + gadolinium) in a patient with grade 3 neurotoxicity without focal neurologic deficits on exam. **(G–I)** Cytotoxic edema of the cortical ribbon is seen on diffusion weighted imaging **(G**, *arrowheads***)** and concomitant cortical swelling on FLAIR **(H**, *arrowheads***)**. In the same patient, injury progressed to irreversible cortical laminar necrosis indicated by T1 hyperintensities within the cortical ribbon 10 days later **(I**, *arrowheads***)**. (Reproduced with permission from Gust J, Hay K.A., Hanafi L.-A, et al., Endothelial activation and blood-brain barrier disruption in neurotoxicity after adoptive immunotherapy with CD19 CAR T-cells, Cancer Discov 7, 2017, 1404–1419.)

chronic neurologic deficits that refer to the cortical location of the lesion.[5,41] Finally, global cerebral edema can be identified on imaging and is associated with devastating neurologic injury.[5]

It is not known whether the different imaging patterns are all indicative of the same underlying pathophysiology or whether separate processes contribute. Individual patients frequently manifest multiple of the findings listed above, often without a clear clinical correlate of specific symptomatology or severity of symptoms. This supports the conclusion that they may all be part of the same process, which may manifest differently based on individual patient characteristics.

Since neurotoxicity is a clinical diagnosis, imaging typically plays a supportive role in management of CAR T-cell patients, both to rule out alternative diagnoses and to monitor the evolution of known abnormalities. Preexisting head imaging abnormalities such as diffuse T2 hyperintensities in the supratentorial white matter are common in patients who have undergone chemotherapy and/or radiation, and comparison with prior or follow-up imaging is needed to distinguish these chronic changes from acute toxicities. Consideration can be given to obtaining head imaging prior to CAR T-cell treatment in all patients; however, it is unclear whether this would change management. Since no studies have defined criteria for obtaining head imaging, either before, during, or after treatment, the true incidence of MRI abnormalities in neurotoxicity is unknown. It is also not known whether the presence or absence of abnormalities on head imaging correlates with neurologic and overall outcomes after CAR T-cell therapy and whether treatment decisions should be made based on imaging findings. To clarify these issues, prospective imaging studies using standardized neurologic assessment criteria will be needed.

Electroencephalography

The role of electroencephalography (EEG) monitoring in neurotoxicity is not yet well defined, although its routine use for risk assessment has been advocated.[55] EEG can either be useful for detecting subtle trends in background patterns, which may be an early warning sign for deterioration, or to rule out subclinical seizures. In neurotoxicity patients who underwent EEG, the most common finding was diffuse slowing, a nonspecific indicator of encephalopathy that is common in critically ill patients.[4,5,55] Causes of diffuse slowing can include medication effects, toxic metabolites, or hypoxia/ischemia.[56] The presence of interictal epileptiform discharges is associated with a higher risk of seizures, although their absence does not rule out the possibility of seizures. Nonconvulsive seizures or subclinical status

epilepticus have been reported in CAR T-cell patients, although this is typically only seen after clinical seizures are treated with antiseizure medications, and EEG monitoring is started to assess treatment response.[4] Only rarely, subclinical seizures are found to be the cause of depressed mental status without other clinical indicators of seizure activity.[55] To compare the true incidence of epileptiform abnormalities and seizures between different CAR T modalities and patient populations, defined EEG monitoring criteria will be needed. Ideally, prospective studies should use standardized criteria for neurotoxicity grading to trigger initiation of EEG monitoring and develop protocols to guide its duration.

DEVELOPMENT OF A CONSENSUS SYSTEM FOR DIAGNOSIS AND GRADING OF ICANS
Background

A unified system for detecting and grading neurotoxicity is a crucial component for advancing research into neurotoxicity pathogenesis, prevention, and management. Neurotoxicity signs and symptoms in clinical trials were initially graded by CTCAE, with grades 1 through 5 representing mild, moderate, severe, life-threatening, and fatal toxicity, respectively. As awareness increased of CAR T-cell–associated neurotoxicity as a novel clinical syndrome that is distinctive from CRS, modified grading systems were proposed to better reflect the clinical significance of certain findings, such as new-onset seizures, which are nearly always treated as an emergency.

In our report of neurotoxicity in 133 adults treated with CD19 CAR T-cells incorporating 4-1BB costimulation, the presence of delirium or seizures resulted in a designation of grade $\geq$3 neurotoxicity because of the requirement for hospitalization. Gardner et al. used CTCAE grading, with the exception that seizures were designated as grade $\geq$3 neurotoxicity.[9] The CARTOX group also assigned grade $\geq$3 neurotoxicity for any seizures and added grade $\geq$4 for any motor weakness.[55] This group also proposed a new name for the emergent syndrome. Based on the predominance of encephalopathy, it was termed CAR T-cell–related encephalopathy syndrome (CRES). For early detection of neurologic decline, this group devised the CARTOX-10 assessment tool that uses a modified minimental status exam for daily screening of patients.[55]

Pediatric-specific consensus criteria were proposed in 2018 by a group comprised by the MD Anderson CARTOX program and the Pediatric Acute Lung Injury and Sepsis Investigators (PALISI) network.[57] This group also adopted the designation of CRES for

CAR-T-cell–associated neurotoxicity and proposed the use of the Cornell Assessment of Pediatric Delirium (CAPD)[58] in children age ≤12, with a score ≥9 indicating grade 3 CRES. For children older than 12 years, the CARTOX-10 score is used. CTCAE criteria are applied for somnolence, confusion, encephalopathy, dysphasia, seizure, and tremor. Additional criteria include papilledema, opening pressure on lumbar puncture, as well as requirement for mechanical ventilation. A lumbar puncture opening pressure of ≥20 mm Hg alone could qualify for grade 4 CRES.

Shalabi et al.[43] prospectively monitored pediatric CD22-CAR patients with a brief cognitive assessment that was performed by a psychologist at baseline and 21–28 days after CAR T-cell infusion, and also provided a caregiver checklist, which reported additional neurologic symptoms that were not captured by standard clinical monitoring. No grading systems have yet been shown to correlate with long-term clinical outcomes in prospectively validated studies.

Given the diversity of proposed systems that largely reflect investigators' local experience with neurotoxicity, the need became apparent for a unified approach. Ideally, a neurotoxicity grading system would have consistent and predictive value for the patient's subsequent clinical course and thus could serve as a tool to support the treating clinician in decision-making regarding location of care (outpatient, inpatient, or ICU), workup, and interventions.

ICANS Diagnostic Criteria

To unify adverse event reporting in the field, the ASTCT developed a consensus approach to grading of CRS and neurotoxicity after IEC-engaging therapies.[6] The ASTCT ICANS grading criteria are based on a substantial body of research that was reviewed at a 2018 ASTCT meeting by a group of 49 experts from academia, industry, and the NIH. A writing group was then convened to develop consensus criteria that are based on standardized bedside exams and easily verifiable clinical data. The term ICANS was chosen to reflect the fact that a similar neurotoxicity syndrome has been observed with other effector cell engaging immunotherapies such as bispecific antibodies and to encompass the broad array of neurologic signs and symptoms that go beyond encephalopathy. The group's definition of ICANS is as follows: "a disorder characterized by a pathologic process involving the central nervous system, following any immune therapy that results in activation or engagement of endogenous or infused T-cells or other immune effector cells. Symptoms or signs can be progressive and may include aphasia, altered level of consciousness, impairment of cognitive skills, motor weakness,

seizures, and cerebral edema." Several signs and symptoms that have previously been considered to be included in the diagnosis of neurotoxicity, including headache, tremor, myoclonus, asterixis, hallucinations, weakness, balance problems, and intracranial hemorrhage, were excluded from the diagnostic criteria. These were felt to be not specific to ICANS, as they can be seen with other interventions, including chemotherapy and transplant. Patients who do not meet criteria for neurotoxicity (see ICANS Diagnosis and Grading for Adults and ICANS Diagnosis and Grading for Children sections) but who display signs and symptoms attributable to the nervous system should continue to be graded by CTCAE.

ICANS Diagnosis and Grading for Adults

For adults and children older than age 12 years, the ICANS grade is based on a score from a standardized bedside mental status exam as well as criteria in the domains of level of consciousness, seizure, motor findings, and intracranial pressure (Table 7.2). The mental status exam was developed specifically for the assessment of ICANS and is termed the IEC-associated encephalopathy (ICE) exam (Table 7.3). The exam replaces more subjective assessments of confusion or delirium and is designed to efficiently detect the type of impairments that are most typical of ICANS. It was adapted from the CARTOX-10[55] and minimental state[59] exams to test orientation, naming, comprehension, writing, and attention. Patients unable to participate in the exam due to decreased alertness are assigned ICANS grade 4, unless the altered mental status can be ascribed to sedating medications.

Level-of-consciousness assessments form the other main axis of ICANS grading. Level of consciousness is scored according to routine neurologic practice as the degree of stimulation that is required to obtain a response from the patient, thus avoiding ill-defined terms such as drowsiness or obtundation. Patients with grade 1 ICANS must have normal alertness, and grade 4 is assigned for patients who only respond to vigorous or repetitive stimuli or do not respond at all. Additional refinements include a special category for seizures, where the presence of any seizures qualifies as grade 3, and any seizures lasting 5 minutes or more, or repeated seizures without return to normal mental status, qualify for grade 4. No modification to this scheme is made for patients with preexisting epilepsy. The final contributor to ICANS grading is evidence of increased intracranial pressure. Findings of localized or focal edema on imaging are considered grade 3 ICANS, although no recommendations are made on when to obtain imaging and what imaging

TABLE 7.2
ASTCT ICANS Consensus Grading.

Neurotoxicity Domain	Grade 1	Grade 2	Grade 3	Grade 4
ICE score[a] (for adults and children >12 years) OR	7–9	3–6	0–2	0 (patient is unarousable and unable to perform ICE)
CAPD (for Children ≤12 years)	<9	<9	≥9	Unable to perform CAPD
Depressed level of consciousness[b]	Awakens spontaneously	Awakens to voice	Awakens only to tactile stimuli	Patient unarousable or requires vigorous or repetitive tactile stimuli to arouse. Stupor or coma
Seizure			Any clinical seizure (focal or generalized) that resolves rapidly, or nonconvulsive seizures on EEG that resolve with intervention	Life-threatening prolonged seizure (>5 minutes), or repetitive clinical or electrographic seizures without return to baseline in between
Motor findings[c]				Deep focal motor weakness such as hemiparesis or paraparesis
Raised ICP/cerebral edema			Focal/local edema on neuroimaging[d]	Diffuse cerebral edema on neuroimaging, decerebrate or decorticate posturing, or cranial nerve VI palsy, or papilledema, or Cushing's triad

ICANS grade is determined by the most severe event (ICE score, level of consciousness, seizure, motor findings, raised ICP/cerebral edema) not attributable to any other cause. For example, a patient with an ICE score of 3 who has a generalized seizure is classified as having grade 3 ICANS. *CAPD*, Cornell Assessment of Pediatric Delirium; *EEG*, electroencephalogram; *ICE*, immune effector cell–associated encephalopathy; *ICP*, intracranial pressure. Empty boxes indicate grade is not applicable.
[a] A patient with an ICE score of 0 may be classified as having grade 3 ICANS if the patient is awake with global aphasia. But a patient with an ICE score of 0 may be classified as having grade 4 ICANS if the patient is unarousable.
[b] Depressed level of consciousness should be attributable to no other cause (e.g., no sedating medication).
[c] Tremors and myoclonus associated with immune effector cell therapies may be graded according to CTCAE v5.0, but they do not influence ICANS grading.
[d] Intracranial hemorrhage with or without associated edema is not considered a neurotoxicity feature and is excluded from ICANS grading. It may be graded according to CTCAE v5.0.
Adapted with permission from Lee DW, Santomasso BD, Locke FL, et al. ASTCT Consensus Grading for Cytokine Release Syndrome and Neurological Toxicity Associated with Immune Effector Cells. *Biol Blood Marrow Transplant*. 2019;25(4):625–638. Available from: https://www.bbmt.org/article/S1083-8791(18)31691-4/abstract.

protocols should be used. The clinical significance of focal edema varies and can range from small, nonspecific FLAIR hyperintensities to massive hemispheric swelling with midline shift. Therefore, this criterion may need to be refined in future iterations of the grading scale. Grade 4 ICANS is assigned for several alarm signs that can be seen with impending herniation, such as diffuse cerebral edema on imaging, extensor or flexor posturing, cranial nerve VI palsy, or Cushing's triad. Papilledema is also considered grade

4 neurotoxicity, although this is more often seen with chronic intracranial pressure elevation.

ICANS Diagnosis and Grading for Children

Children as young as age 1 are eligible for treatment with CD19-directed CAR T-cells, which necessitates pediatric-specific approaches for detecting and managing ICANS. The prevalence of language disturbance may be underestimated in children, who may respond to language difficulty simply with a decrease in

TABLE 7.3
Immune Effector Cell—Associated Encephalopathy (ICE) Scoring Tool.

Exam Item	Task	Points
Orientation	Orientation to year, month, city, hospital	4
Naming	Name 3 objects (e.g., point to clock, pen, button)	3
Commands	Show me 2 fingers, or close your eyes and stick out your tongue	1
Writing	Write standard sentence (e.g., our national bird is the bald eagle)	1
Attention	Count backward from 100 by tens	1
Total		10

Score 10: No impairment; Score 7—9: Grade 1 ICANS; Score 3—6: Grade 2 ICANS; Score 0—2: Grade 3 ICANS; Score 0 due to patient unarousable or unable to perform ICE assessment: grade 4 ICANS.
Adapted with permission from Lee DW, Santomasso BD, Locke FL, et al. ASTCT Consensus Grading for Cytokine Release Syndrome and Neurological Toxicity Associated with Immune Effector Cells. *Biol Blood Marrow Transplant*. 2019;25(4):625—638. Available from: https://www. bbmt.org/article/S1083-8791(18)31691-4/abstract.

language output, or a regression of previously acquired language skills. Acute assessment of neurologic function can be made more difficult by a paucity of information on the child's premorbid function, which in adults can typically be assumed to be normal. In addition, young children are often not cooperative with structured exams. Given these concerns, for children age 12 years or younger, the ICE exam is replaced by the Cornell Assessment of Pediatric Delirium (CAPD), which is a validated clinical tool that is widely used in pediatric critical care.[58] This is a purely observational measure that can be completed by bedside nurses, does not require patient cooperation, and has been validated in children with developmental delay. CAPD scores ≥9 are consistent with delirium, and grade 3 ICANS is assigned in that case. Grade 4 is assigned when CAPD cannot be performed, although the CAPD can also be done in comatose patients (Table 7.2). The other ICANS criteria remain unchanged from the adult version. In the interest of uniformity in the field, we advocate for the use of the pediatric ICANS criteria in children, which differ from the adult criteria only in the use of the CAPD instead of the language-based ICE bedside assessment.

Patient Risk Factors

CRS is a clear risk factor for neurotoxicity and typically precedes the first neurologic symptoms. In fact, no cases of severe neurotoxicity without CRS have been described, although mild neurologic symptoms can occur even in patients who do not meet criteria for CRS. Multiple studies have confirmed that the severity of CRS is strongly associated with the severity of neurotoxicity.[3—5,8,9,20,46] Consequently, CRS risk factors such as higher in vivo CAR T-cell numbers, higher CAR T-cell dose, greater tumor burden, and use of fludarabine for lymphodepletion can also be associated with a higher risk of ICANS.[5] Other risk factors that have been identified include higher preinfusion tumor burden in ALL,[4,5] greater peak blood CAR T-cell counts,[4,5,20] and preexisting neurologic comorbidities, such as peripheral neuropathy or history of seizures.[5,46] Since many of the above variables may not be independent of each other (such as higher CAR T-cell dose and higher in vivo CAR T-cell numbers), we conducted additional multivariable analysis and found that preexisting neurologic comorbidities, percentage of disease in marrow, lymphodepletion with cyclophosphamide plus fludarabine, and CAR T-cell dose were associated with neurotoxicity risk.[5] CAR-specific features such as the type of costimulatory domain and CAR T-cell manufacturing processes may also contribute to differences in the risk of neurotoxicity, although no specific manufacturing approach or CAR design feature has been clearly shown to be responsible.[60]

PATHOGENESIS OF NEUROTOXICITY

Serum and CSF Cytokine Profiles During Acute Neurotoxicity

Cytokine release accompanies the in vivo expansion of CAR T-cells and is hypothesized to be the inciting event for the development of neurotoxicity, since severe neurotoxicity does not occur in isolation without preceding CRS. The task of identifying neurotoxicity-specific cytokines is made more difficult by the simultaneous presence of CRS. Certainly, serum concentrations of several inflammatory mediators are higher after CAR T-cell infusion in patients with severe or life-threatening neurotoxicity compared with those with grade ≤2 neurotoxicity. Consistently identified cytokines that are elevated during acute neurotoxicity include IL-6,[4,5,20,41] IL-10,[4,20,41] and IFNγ.[4,5,41] Associations of neurotoxicity with higher serum concentrations of GM-CSF, granzyme B, IL-15, IL-2, IL-2Rα, IL-5, and TNFα[4,5,20,41,46] have been reported, although many of these markers have also been noted to be elevated during CRS alone.[1,3] In one study that reported separate analyses for neurotoxicity and CRS, serum IL-2, sIL-4R, and hepatocyte growth factor elevations were associated only with neurotoxicity, but not with CRS.[46]

In the CSF, cytokine elevations during acute neurotoxicity often mirror those in the serum, likely due to both increased blood brain barrier (BBB) permeability and local production within the CNS.[4,5,41] However, enrichment of IL-8, IP10, and MCP-1 was seen in the CSF compared with the blood in some patients with severe neurotoxicity.[4] One may hypothesize that production of specific cytokines within the CNS may be present during neurotoxicity, but such an association has not been proven to date.

The source of cytokines in blood and CSF has not been well characterized, although animal studies suggest a key role for monocytes in producing IL-6 and IL-1 during CRS.[61] Macrophage inflammatory responses are amplified by autocrine-positive feedback loops using catecholamine signaling, whose role has been shown for CRS but not yet in neurotoxicity.[62,63] Endothelial cells are likely involved in cytokine production as well, as indicated in an autopsy study of a patient with fatal CRS that was accompanied by mental status changes. Here, IL-6 was expressed by brain endothelial cells but not infiltrating T-cells.[64] This is similar to endothelial responses seen with other inflammatory stimuli such as lipopolysaccharide challenge.[65,66]

Endothelial Dysfunction

A role for vascular dysfunction and endothelial activation is suggested by a correlation of neurotoxicity with elevated D-dimer, prothrombin (PT) and activated partial thromboplastin times (aPTT), decreased fibrinogen and platelet counts, and high red cell and platelet transfusion requirements.[4,5] Consumptive coagulopathy can be pronounced in patients with severe neurotoxicity.[5,67] Endothelial activation during neurotoxicity may be initially induced by systemic cytokine signaling. IL-6, IFNγ, and TNFα can be selectively transported across

the BBB but can also act on endothelial cells to open the tight junctions.[68–70] Endothelial activation then leads to increased permeability of the BBB to proteins and cells. For example, IFNγ and TNFα are able to transit across a leaky BBB, which may induce pericyte stress, thereby amplifying endothelial permeability and alteration of the neurovascular unit.[68,71]

The role of the angiopoietin (ANG)-TIE2 axis has been extensively investigated in sepsis and cerebral malaria,[72,73] and we hypothesized that similar signaling mechanisms are active in CRS and neurotoxicity. ANG1 is constitutively produced by pericytes and smooth muscle cells. In the quiescent state, it is the predominant binding partner of TIE2 receptor on endothelial cells, which inhibits proinflammatory pathways. Endothelial activation leads to a switch to a procoagulant state and release of ANG2 from Weibel-Palade bodies, which raises the ANG2:ANG1 ratio and increases binding of ANG2 to the TIE2 receptor to promote proinflammatory and prothrombotic pathways.[73] Additionally, von Willebrand factor (VWF) is released from endothelial cells when they are activated, which promotes stabilization of platelet aggregates.[74]

In patient samples, the presence of endothelial activation was corroborated by higher ANG2, ANG2:ANG1 ratio, and VWF serum concentrations in adult patients with grade ≥4 neurotoxicity after 4-1BB-costimulated CAR T-cell treatment. Interestingly, the elevated ANG2:ANG1 ratio was already present prior to lymphodepletion chemotherapy in some patients who then went on to develop grade ≥4 neurotoxicity, suggesting that preexisting endothelial activation may have predisposed them to dysfunction of the endothelium and BBB during the inflammatory state that accompanies in vivo CAR T-cell expansion.[4,64] An elevated ANG2:ANG1 ratio was also seen in adult patients who developed grade 3–4 neurotoxicity after receiving CD28-costimulated CAR T-cells.[4] Evidence of endothelial and vascular disruption was also noted on pathologic examination of the brain of a patient with fatal neurotoxicity, where endothelial activation was indicated by VWF aggregation, and a thrombotic microangiopathy with multifocal vascular disruption and microhemorrhages.[5]

The Role of Astrocytes and Microglia

On autopsy, acute cerebral edema has been associated with proteinaceous exudates in the perivascular spaces and evidence of astrocyte injury.[49] CSF levels of the astrocyte marker GFAP increased significantly during neurotoxicity in children and young adults treated with CD19-CAR T-cells.[41] Astrocyte endfeet are a key component of the BBB,[75] and astrocytes are crucial in the handling of extracellular space volume in the brain via the aquaporin-4 channel, as well as regulating endothelial permeability in response to inflammatory stimuli via VEGF and nitric oxide signaling.[71,76] Dysregulation of water handling by the astrocytes is associated with neurologic injury in epilepsy[77,78] and could conceivably play a role in development of fulminant cerebral edema. Indeed, perivascular edema with extravasation of perivascular fluid into the brain parenchyma was noted in an autopsy study of a patient with fatal cerebral edema.[49]

Microglial activation has been noted on brain pathology in patients who died from CAR T-cell–related neurotoxicity.[12,18,49] Microglia are brain-resident macrophages that respond to peripheral inflammatory stimuli, such as sepsis, by switching from a surveillance resting state toward an effector state, in which they release proinflammatory mediators.[79] This can lead to neuronal dysfunction with behavioral manifestations such as delirium and, if unchecked, can lead to irreversible neuronal injury.[80,81] It is unclear if this mechanism is active during neurotoxicity after CAR T-cell immunotherapy.

Inflammatory Cellular Infiltrates in the Brain
The role of inflammatory cellular infiltrates in the development of neurotoxicity is not well understood. Although CAR T-cells are detected in the CSF of most patients who undergo sampling during neurotoxicity, they can also be detected in the CSF of patients without neurotoxicity and after resolution of neurotoxicity.[4,5,82] This suggests that their presence in CSF alone is not sufficient to induce neurologic dysfunction.

CD4[+] CAR T-cells were slightly enriched in CSF compared with blood in patients with neurotoxicity, suggesting that CNS migration may differ between CAR T-cell subsets.[5] Neuropathologic studies at autopsy after fatal neurotoxicity have not yet shown definitive evidence of intraparenchymal invasion of CAR T-cells. Flow cytometry of fresh autopsy brain tissue demonstrated that 93% of the T-cells present were indeed CAR T-cells, half of which expressed CD4 and the other half expressed CD8, findings similar to those in CSF obtained at autopsy.[5] Although this technique could not distinguish between intravascular or intraparenchymal location of the T-cells, histology showed predominantly perivascular infiltration of CD8[+] T-cells in this[5] and other[12] cases, with few intraparenchymal inflammatory cells.

Perivascular macrophage infiltration has been reported by multiple autopsy studies.[12,18,49] In some patients with severe CRS and neurotoxicity, serum ferritin concentrations are markedly elevated, similar to those in macrophage activation syndrome (MAS) and

hemophagocytic lymphohistiocytosis (HLH), suggesting a role for macrophage activation in the pathophysiology.[83] We observed profound monocytopenia during severe neurotoxicity and CRS, which could be consistent with monocyte activation and extravasation into tissues.

Excitotoxicity
During systemic inflammation, such as sepsis, cognitive dysfunction has been shown to be mediated by IL-1β signaling, which may induce excitotoxicity via dysregulation of glial glutamate handling.[84–86] During CAR T-cell neurotoxicity, affected patients had increased CSF levels of glutamate and the excitotoxin quinolinic acid, compared with pre- and posttreatment levels.[4] It is not yet known how these measurements compare with those in CAR T-cell patients with active CRS but no neurotoxicity. Quinolinic acid is an NMDA receptor agonist that is part of the kynurene signaling pathway and is produced in the brain by infiltrating macrophages and activated microglia. Its production is stimulated by cytokines, most importantly IFNγ, and it has been implicated as an excitotoxin in neurodegenerative disorders such as Alzheimer's and Parkinson's disease.[87] Clinical trials of NMDA receptor blockade to prevent excitotoxicity in stroke and traumatic brain injury failed to show any efficacy.[88]

ANIMAL MODELS OF NEUROTOXICITY
Nonhuman Primate Model
A nonhuman primate model of CAR T-cell–induced neurotoxicity has been established by treating rhesus macaques with autologous, CD20-targeted CAR T-cells.[89] CAR T-cells were infused into healthy animals after lymphodepletion with cyclophosphamide and showed robust expansion in the blood, leading to B-cell aplasia as expected. Two animals later received T-cells engineered to express CD20 (T-APCs) to boost CAR T-cell proliferation. All animals developed CRS and neurotoxicity, which peaked between 7 and 14 days after CAR T-cell infusion, and clinically manifested as lethargy, tremor, and ataxia. This was accompanied by elevation of IL-6, IL-8, IL-1RA, MIG (CXCL9), and I-TAC (CXCL11) in serum. In CSF obtained via lumbar or foramen magnum puncture, there was disproportionate elevation of IL-6, IL-2, GM-CSF, VEGF, IL-1β, IL-1RA, MCP-1 (CCL2), and IP-10 (CXCL10), with levels of these cytokines and chemokines exceeding those found in serum. Neurotoxicity was associated with accumulation of both CAR and non-CAR T-cells in the CSF and in the brain parenchyma. Rare focal perivascular edema, as well as foci of perivascular T-cell cuffing, was seen during active

neurotoxicity. In the T-cells infiltrating the brain parenchyma, the fraction of CAR T-cells among total T-cells was similar to that in blood. Overall, the nonhuman primate model appears to recapitulate aspects of the human phenotype and may be a useful tool to study prophylactic or therapeutic strategies in future.

Mouse Models

Preclinical trials of in vivo CAR T-cell efficacy typically rely on xenograft modeling in immunodeficient mice treated with human CAR T-cells. However, given their limited ability to mount immune responses, these mice are not expected to develop CAR T-cell or cytokine-related side effects. Surprisingly, one group did find evidence of neurologic dysfunction and CRS in NSG mice implanted with primary ALL blasts that were treated with human CD19-directed CAR T-cells.[90] The mice developed weight loss, motor problems, and hunched posture and had increased contrast enhancement on brain MRI, which was ameliorated by concurrent treatment with the GM-CSF neutralizing antibody lenzilumab. Mice did not develop toxicity when they were engrafted with the NALM6 leukemia cell line.

To better understand the interaction between CAR T-cells and other components of the immune system, complex chimera and transgenic mouse models have been increasingly employed to investigate toxicity mechanisms. Norelli et al. developed a xenograft mouse model that allows for human hematopoiesis by engrafting human cord blood hematopoietic stem and progenitor cells (HSPCs) into irradiated newborn NSG mice transgenic for human hematopoietic signaling factors (stem cell factor, GM-CSF, and IL-3) (nHuSGM3 mice).[61] These mice then generate human T-cells that can be engineered to express a CAR. These CAR T-cells, when directed against CD19 or the myeloid antigen CD44v6, successfully eradicated ALL xenografts in adult SGM3 triple transgenic mice without causing CRS. However, when the adult SGM3 mice were transplanted with human HSPCs to provide a full human myeloid and monocyte complement, CAR T-cell expansion was accompanied by robust CRS with fever, weight loss, and elevated human IL-6. The IL-6 was chiefly produced by monocytes, which were also the main source of IL-1. CRS was prevented by depleting monocytes with liposomal clodronate prior to CAR T-cell infusion, but this also negatively impacted CAR T-cell expansion. In contrast, both the IL-1 receptor antagonist, anakinra, and IL-6 receptor blocking antibody, tocilizumab, prevented CRS when given at the time of CAR T-cell infusion and aborted CRS when they were given immediately after the onset of fever, without impairing

antitumor efficacy of the CAR T-cells. At a median of 30 days after CAR T-cell infusion, approximately 30% of mice developed lethal generalized paralysis and seizures. This occurred well after resolution of CRS and was accompanied by macrophage infiltration into the subarachnoid space. The lethal neurotoxicity phenotype was prevented by anakinra, either when given prophylactically or after development of fever, whereas tocilizumab did not prevent the neurotoxicity.

The same triple transgenic (human stem cell factor, GM-CSF, and IL-3) HuSGM3 mice were used to investigate the role of myeloid autocrine catecholamine signaling in the release of key cytokines implicated in CRS and neurotoxicity.[62] Pharmacologic blockade of catecholamine signaling with atrial natriuretic peptide or α-methyltyrosine abrogated cytokine release in tumor-bearing SGM3 mice that received human CAR T-cells, without impairing tumor killing by the CAR T-cells. In addition, the same treatment also decreased cytokine release in a syngeneic mouse model bearing murine ALL and receiving murine CAR T-cells. However, this study only reported effects on cytokine release and did not make mention of any neurologic abnormalities in the animals.

The key role of macrophages in cytokine release was also shown by Giavridis et al. in a model of xenograft tumor-bearing SCID-beige mice treated with human CD19-28z CAR T-cells.[91] These mice, which are more immunocompetent than standard NSG strains, developed a systemic inflammatory syndrome 2−3 days after CAR T-cell infusion. This was accompanied by increases of murine IL-6 and other proinflammatory cytokines. The source of the IL-6 were tumor-associated murine macrophages that interacted directly with the transfused human CAR T-cells via CD40 ligand, which induces upregulation of inducible nitric oxide synthase (iNOS). CRS was reduced via IL-1 inhibition by anakinra or overexpression of IL-1RA on the infused CAR-T-cells, without affecting antitumor efficacy. The investigators found no clinical or histopathologic evidence of neurotoxicity in the animals.

When human CD19-directed CAR T-cells were infused into mice who express human CD19 in their T-cells, there was a decrease in microglia on histology.[92] This finding is intriguing given the complex interaction of brain-resident microglia and systemic macrophages in CNS injury.[93]

To date, mouse models have not replicated the full phenotype and timing of human neurotoxicity, which typically occurs very soon after CRS develops. However, understanding the mechanism of CRS will provide important insights in how to prevent CRS without affecting antitumor efficacy of the CAR T-cells. Given the strong association of CRS and neurotoxicity, one might hypothesize that eliminating or greatly decreasing the incidence of CRS could also decrease the risk of neurotoxicity. Certainly, it is possible that the two are truly mechanistically different, but then one would expect the frequency of neurotoxicity to be unchanged even if there is much less CRS.

CANDIDATE BIOMARKERS TO PREDICT NEUROTOXICITY RISK

Early recognition of at-risk patients provides the best chance for prevention and timely treatment of ICANS. There has been intense interest in the development of predictive tools, which may include clinical measures such as specific vital sign changes or neurotoxicity scoring systems, or the use of standard clinical and novel laboratory biomarkers.

Early fever was found by several investigators to be predictive of subsequent higher neurotoxicity risk. All patients who developed grade ≥4 neurotoxicity had a fever ≥38.9°C within 36 hours of CAR T-cell infusion in one study.[5] Fever ≥38.0°C within the first 3 days, combined with a platelet count of ≤50,000 cells/μL, identified 74% of patients who went on to develop grade ≥3 neurotoxicity in another study.[4]

Algorithms have been developed to predict the development of severe CRS and neurotoxicity[1,94,95] and may add sensitivity and specificity to clinical parameters. Different biomarkers have been identified to predict different grades of neurotoxicity in patients of different ages who were treated with different CAR T-cell products, and no prospective validation studies have been performed to date. Adult patients who received 4-1BB-costimulated CAR T-cells were more likely to develop grade ≥4 neurotoxicity if they had higher serum levels of MCP-1, IL-15, IL-10, and IL-2 in the first 36 hours after infusion. This group of patients also had an earlier peak of serum IL-6 levels compared with patients with grade ≤3 neurotoxicity. Intriguingly, the ANG2:ANG1 ratio prior to lymphodepleting chemotherapy was also higher in patients who subsequently developed grade ≥4 neurotoxicity.[5] In a trial of a different 4-1BB-costimulated CAR T-cell product for pediatric patients, higher peak serum levels of sTNFR-1 identified patients who went on to develop any degree of neurotoxicity. In multivariable regression analysis, later development of neurotoxicity was best predicted by elevated ≤3 day serum levels of IL-12, sVEGFR-1 and sVEGFR-2, sgp130, STNFR-1, and sCD30. Patients who developed grade ≥3 neurotoxicity after receiving a CAR T-cell product with CD28

costimulation were found to have elevated IL-10, IL-15, and low EGF by day 3 after infusion.[4] The interpretation of all current predictive models is tempered by the fact that each study showed a robust association neurotoxicity risk with CRS. This raises the possibility of a confounding effect of CRS on these models.

In summary, biomarker-based neurotoxicity risk stratification is a promising approach, whose generalizability remains limited by the heterogeneity of time points, biomarkers assessed, serum concentration cutoff levels, and definition of neurotoxicity. With new ICANS consensus criteria available, the stage is now set for trials of prospective validation of early recognition and intervention strategies.

MANAGEMENT OF CHIMERIC ANTIGEN RECEPTOR T-CELL—ASSOCIATED NEUROTOXICITY

The role of disease-modifying interventions for neurotoxicity is debated, given the fact that neurologic symptoms are typically reversible, with little data available on possible adverse long-term sequelae. It is also unknown whether there are distinct pathogenic mechanisms for different clinical manifestations of ICANS. This has to be weighed against the risk of adverse effects from experimental treatments and possible decreased efficacy of CAR T-cells when exposed to immunomodulating interventions. Since most patients with neurotoxicity also experience CRS, many will be treated with CRS-targeted therapies such as tocilizumab and/or steroids,[2,3,96] further complicating the assessment of treatment effects on neurotoxicity. Given these uncertainties, some investigators advocate use of supportive care only.[5,8] Others advocate aggressive and early treatment with immunomodulators to decrease the risk of life-threatening complications.[55,97]

Tocilizumab

After recognition of the role of IL-6 in the pathogenesis of CRS, tocilizumab quickly gained acceptance as a first-line intervention strategy for CRS, while its role in the treatment of neurotoxicity remains debated.[2,98] This humanized monoclonal antibody targets the cell-associated and soluble IL-6 receptor (IL-6R), thereby blocking the binding of IL-6.[99–101] Its use in rheumatologic disorders is well established, and it is FDA approved for multiple rheumatologic indications.[102–105] Although no randomized controlled clinical trials of tocilizumab for CRS treatment have been reported to date, its impressive clinical efficacy has made it a mainstay for the treatment of severe CRS. Retrospective analyses showed sufficient likelihood of efficacy and safety to warrant FDA approval of tocilizumab for the treatment of CRS in 2017.[106] When used in patients who develop CRS in the setting of robust CAR T-cell proliferation, tocilizumab does not appear to impair the antitumor response.[9] However, when CAR T-cell proliferation is weaker, there remains a theoretical risk that it could impair antitumor response.

Tocilizumab may reduce neurotoxicity indirectly by decreasing the severity of CRS or by directly blocking IL-6-initiated cerebral dysfunction. However, neurotoxicity can still develop when CRS has already resolved after tocilizumab administration, which led to concerns that IL-6R blockade with tocilizumab may actually worsen the risk of neurotoxicity. Since tocilizumab is a large molecule that may be unable to cross the BBB, increased circulating IL-6 after IL-6R blockade would lead to an increase of free IL-6 that can then act unopposed on the CNS.[107,108] Indeed, in a recent study in healthy nonhuman primates, systemic administration of tocilizumab was associated with very low penetration into the CSF, whereas intraventricular delivery established therapeutic CSF concentrations without adverse effects.[109]

No randomized controlled studies of tocilizumab for the treatment of neurotoxicity have been reported to date. In phase 1 and 2 clinical trials, tocilizumab was used to treat CRS and/or neurotoxicity in 23% −48% of affected patients with ALL,[8–11,16,17] 6−43% with NHL,[12,13,19,20] and 0%−25% with CLL[15,19] (Table 7.1). However, the precise indication for treatment (CRS vs. neurotoxicity) and outcomes after the intervention have not been consistently reported. The guidelines for tocilizumab use differ between institutions, in some cases being recommended as a first-line therapy for neurotoxicity,[55] whereas in others, it is not used at all for this indication.[60]

In one study, the rate of severe CRS decreased after the guidelines for tocilizumab administration were altered to allow for treatment at first fever instead of giving tocilizumab only for dose-limiting toxicities.[110] However, there was no change in the incidences of any grade of neurotoxicity or of grade ≥3 neurotoxicity. This suggests that more aggressive treatment with tocilizumab, while not effective for preventing neurotoxicity, may not increase the risk of neurotoxicity, either. In contrast, in the expansion cohort of another trial, prophylactic tocilizumab was administered to all patients on day 2 after CAR T-cell infusion. With this intervention, the incidence of grade ≥3 CRS decreased from 13% to 3%, whereas grade ≥3 neurotoxicity was seen in 39% (including one death from cerebral edema), compared with 28% in historical controls in the phase 2 trial.[20,48] Thus, based on current evidence, we cannot yet make a recommendation regarding the use of tocilizumab in prevention and treatment of neurotoxicity.

Corticosteroids

Immunomodulation with corticosteroids is a mainstay in the treatment of acute inflammatory CNS conditions, making dexamethasone and other corticosteroids a logical choice for first-line therapy for neurotoxicity.[3,110] The excellent CNS penetration of dexamethasone has made it standard of care in the treatment of cerebral edema and inflammation in the setting of brain tumors and neurotrauma,[111,112] while high-dose methylprednisolone has well-established effectiveness and safety in neuroinflammatory disorders such as multiple sclerosis and acute demyelinating encephalomyelitis.[113,114] Glucocorticoids can affect T-cell function,[115] raising concern that they may decrease the efficacy of CAR T-cell immunotherapy. However, patients who develop toxicity in the setting of robust CAR T-cell expansion appear to tolerate short courses of low- to moderate-dose corticosteroids (e.g., dexamethasone 10 mg twice daily for two to four doses or equivalent) without clearly impacting response rates.[110] High-dose corticosteroids (e.g., methylprednisolone 1 g/day) may impart a higher risk of severe lymphopenia with reduced circulating CAR T-cell counts that could compromise efficacy, but this has not been proven.[116] Therefore, the use of corticosteroids for the prevention and treatment of neurotoxicity is a plausible approach based on their efficacy in other neuroinflammatory disorders and interstitial cerebral edema, but dedicated trials will be required to establish their safety, efficacy, and effect on CAR T-cell efficacy.

Based on the above considerations, we currently prefer to use dexamethasone for treatment of neurotoxicity alone. When CRS and neurotoxicity occur together, we give tocilizumab in conjunction with steroids, given the well-established efficacy of tocilizumab for CRS and the concern that tocilizumab alone is not sufficient to abrogate neuroinflammation.

Other Rational Therapies

The great need for targeted interventions for immunotherapy-associated toxicities has pushed forward research efforts to improve our mechanistic understanding. Out of initial findings, several rational therapies have been proposed, although human clinical data are not yet established.

Since IL-6 is a key cytokine implicated in both CRS and neurotoxicity, the use of siltuximab has been proposed as an alternative to tocilizumab. Siltuximab is a chimeric monoclonal antibody that binds IL-6 and prevents it from binding with soluble and membrane-bound IL-6R, which circumvents the concern for paradoxically increased availability of soluble IL-6 in the CNS after tocilizumab administration.[107,117] It has been administered in the setting of CRS and/or neurotoxicity and to manage neurologic adverse events during CAR T-cell treatment of glioblastoma.[35,118]

The role of IL-1 signaling in CRS and ICANS has been established in several animal models,[61,91] prompting consideration of IL-1 blockade for treatment of these toxicities. Anakinra is a recombinant IL-1 receptor antagonist (IL-1RA), which is FDA approved for the treatment of multiple rheumatologic disorders,[119] but safety and efficacy in CAR T-cell patients have not been established.

Other mechanism-based therapeutic approaches may include plasma exchange, angiopoietin-1 augmentation, or platelet hypertransfusion to counteract endothelial activation and coagulopathy.[5,120] GM-CSF blockade with lenzilumab has shown promise for abrogating CRS and neurotoxicity in a xenograft mouse model.[90] There are no data yet in humans to support the efficacy of targeting any of these pathways.

Seizure Prophylaxis

New-onset seizures are a frequent complication in ICANS, and the additional metabolic stress from seizures may further exacerbate CNS injury and edema. Therefore, prophylactic administration of antiseizure medications is an attractive risk-reduction strategy, but high-quality data are not yet available to show whether this is effective. Some CAR T-cell investigators start all patients on seizure prophylaxis, some use it only for patients with CRS, and others do not use seizure prophylaxis at all.[4,5,55,97] Seizures may still occur despite prophylaxis.[4,5,41] Levetiracetam is the medication of choice for seizure prophylaxis given its benign side effect profile with low risk of cognitive, hematologic, or metabolic disturbances. Levetiracetam does not significantly affect the metabolism of other drugs and has equivalent i.v. and p.o. dosing with consistent bioavailability.[121]

Acute Management of Life-Threatening Neurotoxicity

Fulminant cerebral edema and other life-threatening manifestations of neurotoxicity are rare, which makes optimization of neurocritical care strategies challenging. It is reasonable to offer standard neuroprotective interventions that are applied in other situations where increased intracranial pressure is suspected. This includes aggressive prevention of fever, normocarbia or short-term mild hyperventilation, and optimization of cerebral perfusion by preventing hypotension, treating hypertension with caution and keeping the head of bed midline.[122,123]

In patients with unexplained altered mental status, continuous EEG (cEEG) monitoring should be considered to rule out subclinical seizures. Electrographic-only seizures are also commonly seen in patients who have received treatment for clinically apparent seizures, and cEEG is an important modality for monitoring treatment response. cEEG can also be used to watch for changes in background patterns, which may be an earlier indicator of changes in cerebral function, which can be especially useful in critically ill patients with limited ability to participate in the exam.[56] It is reasonable to treat seizures aggressively, since they pose additional metabolic demand on the brain, but this has to be weighed against potential adverse effects from treatment.

The role of head imaging in guiding treatment of neurotoxicity has not been studied systematically, but urgent imaging should be considered in all patients with sudden neurologic deterioration to rule out potentially treatable etiologies such as intracranial hemorrhage. Imaging findings of cerebral edema can be subtle even when clinical symptoms are well established, and a normal head CT should not be used alone for reassurance. MRI is more sensitive for subtle abnormalities but is often not feasible in emergent situations.

When cerebral edema is suspected, hyperosmolar therapy with mannitol or hypertonic saline, high-dose corticosteroids, sedation, and optimization of cerebral perfusion are reasonable interventions but are without definite evidence of benefit in this setting. There is no evidence that invasive neuromonitoring is helpful, and it is associated with significant risk as patients are frequently coagulopathic. The role of surgical management of increased intracranial pressure is likely limited, since ventriculostomy is often not possible due to effacement of the ventricles from edema. Decompressive craniectomy for cerebral edema from diffuse inflammatory or metabolic causes is rarely attempted and carries an extremely high risk of complications.[124,125] Early detection of risk for deterioration is most likely the best way to prevent fulminant cerebral edema, since once established, it progresses rapidly and may not be reversible.

CONCLUSION AND AREAS OF FUTURE INVESTIGATION

Optimal diagnosis and management of ICANS will require a great deal of further investigation in both its clinical phenotype and mechanistic underpinnings. The heterogeneity of clinical adverse event reporting has hampered conclusions, and efforts have started to harmonize toxicity criteria across institutions.[6] These criteria will need to undergo prospective validation and iterative refinement. As CD19-directed CAR T-cell therapy moves rapidly from small academic trials to multicenter industry-sponsored investigations and postmarketing surveillance, it will be imperative to collect standardized clinical data. Of special interest to neurotoxicity investigators will be validation of early detection algorithms that can be based on bedside exam and/or biomarkers, defining the utility of ancillary studies, including CSF studies, imaging and electroencephalography, and long-term cognitive outcome monitoring.

The first trials of toxicity treatment are underway (i.e., NCT02906371). At this point, priority may be given to validating approaches with established track records of safety and mechanistic plausibility, including corticosteroids and blockade of IL-1 and IL-6 signaling. Careful a priori definition of outcome measures is crucial to ensure that data from different trials are comparable, and the value of collaborative efforts cannot be overstated.

REFERENCES

1. Hay KA, Hanafi L-A, Li D, et al. Kinetics and biomarkers of severe cytokine release syndrome after CD19 chimeric antigen receptor-modified T-cell therapy. *Blood.* 2017; 130:2295−2306.
2. Lee DW, Gardner R, Porter DL, et al. Current concepts in the diagnosis and management of cytokine release syndrome. *Blood.* 2014;124:188−195.
3. Brudno JN, Kochenderfer JN. Toxicities of chimeric antigen receptor T cells: recognition and management. *Blood.* 2016;127:3321−3330.
4. Santomasso BD, Park JH, Salloum D, et al. Clinical and biologic correlates of neurotoxicity associated with CAR T-cell therapy in patients with B-cell acute lymphoblastic leukemia. *Cancer Discov.* 2018;8:958−971.
5. Gust J, Hay KA, Hanafi L-A, et al. Endothelial activation and blood-brain barrier disruption in neurotoxicity after adoptive immunotherapy with CD19 CAR-T cells. *Cancer Discov.* 2017;7:1404−1419.
6. Lee DW, Santomasso BD, Locke FL, et al. ASTCT consensus grading for cytokine release syndrome and neurologic toxicity associated with immune effector cells. *Biol Blood Marrow Transplant.* 2019;25(4):625−638.
7. Porter D, Frey N, Wood PA, Weng Y, Grupp SA. Grading of cytokine release syndrome associated with the CAR T cell therapy tisagenlecleucel. *J Hematol Oncol;* 2018: 11. Available from: https://www.ncbi.nlm.nih.gov/pmc/articles/PMC5833070/.
8. Maude SL, Laetsch TW, Buechner J, et al. Tisagenlecleucel in children and young adults with B-cell lymphoblastic leukemia. *N Engl J Med.* 2018;378:439−448.
9. Gardner RA, Finney O, Annesley C, et al. Intent-to-treat leukemia remission by CD19 CAR T cells of defined formulation and dose in children and young adults. *Blood.* 2017;129(25):3322−3331.
10. Maude SL, Frey N, Shaw PA, et al. Chimeric antigen receptor T cells for sustained remissions in leukemia. *N Engl J Med.* 2014;371:1507−1517.
11. Turtle CJ, Hanafi L-A, Berger C, et al. CD19 CAR-T cells of defined CD4+:CD8+ composition in adult B cell ALL patients. *J Clin Invest.* 2016;126:2123−2138.
12. Schuster SJ, Svoboda J, Chong EA, et al. Chimeric antigen receptor T cells in refractory B-cell lymphomas. *N Engl J Med.* 2017;377:2545−2554.
13. Turtle CJ, Hanafi L-A, Berger C, et al. Immunotherapy of non-Hodgkin's lymphoma with a defined ratio of CD8+ and CD4+ CD19-specific chimeric antigen receptor-modified T cells. *Sci Transl Med.* 2016;8:355ra116.
14. Fraietta JA, Lacey SF, Orlando EJ, et al. Determinants of response and resistance to CD19 chimeric antigen receptor (CAR) T cell therapy of chronic lymphocytic leukemia. *Nat Med.* 2018;1.
15. Turtle CJ, Hay KA, Hanafi L-A, et al. Durable molecular remissions in chronic lymphocytic leukemia treated with CD19-specific chimeric antigen receptor-modified T cells after failure of Ibrutinib. *J Clin Oncol.* 2017;35: 3010−3020.
16. Lee DW, Kochenderfer JN, Stetler-Stevenson M, et al. T cells expressing CD19 chimeric antigen receptors for acute lymphoblastic leukaemia in children and young adults: a phase 1 dose-escalation trial. *The Lancet.* 2015; 385:517−528.
17. Park JH, Rivière I, Gonen M, et al. Long-term follow-up of CD19 CAR therapy in acute lymphoblastic leukemia. *N Engl J Med.* 2018;378:449−459.
18. DeAngelo DJ, Ghobadi A, Park JH, et al. Abstract P217. Clinical outcomes for the phase 2, single-arm, multicenter trial of JCAR015 in adult B-ALL (ROCKET Study). *J Immunother Cancer.* 2017;5:86.
19. Kochenderfer JN, Dudley ME, Kassim SH, et al. Chemotherapy-refractory diffuse large B-cell lymphoma and indolent B-cell malignancies can be effectively treated with autologous T cells expressing an anti-CD19 chimeric antigen receptor. *J Clin Oncol.* 2015;33: 540−549.
20. Neelapu SS, Locke FL, Bartlett NL, et al. Axicabtagene Ciloleucel CAR T-cell therapy in refractory large B-cell lymphoma. *N Engl J Med.* 2017;377:2531−2544.
21. Kebriaei P, Singh H, Huls MH, et al. Phase I trials using Sleeping Beauty to generate CD19-specific CAR T cells. *J Clin Invest.* 2016;126:3363−3376.

22. Wang X, Popplewell LL, Wagner JR, et al. Phase 1 studies of central memory-derived CD19 CAR T-cell therapy following autologous HSCT in patients with B-cell NHL. *Blood*. 2016;127:2980−2990.

23. Cruz CRY, Micklethwaite KP, Savoldo B, et al. Infusion of donor-derived CD19-redirected virus-specific T cells for B-cell malignancies relapsed after allogeneic stem cell transplant: a phase 1 study. *Blood*. 2013;122:2965−2973.

24. Kochenderfer JN, Dudley ME, Carpenter RO, et al. Donor-derived CD19-targeted T cells cause regression of malignancy persisting after allogeneic hematopoietic stem cell transplantation. *Blood*. 2013;122:4129−4139.

25. Ramos CA, Ballard B, Zhang H, et al. Clinical and immunological responses after CD30-specific chimeric antigen receptor-redirected lymphocytes. *J Clin Invest*. 2017;127:3462−3471.

26. Fry TJ, Shah NN, Orentas RJ, et al. CD22-targeted CAR T cells induce remission in B-ALL that is naive or resistant to CD19-targeted CAR immunotherapy. *Nat Med*. 2018;24:20.

27. Wang C-M, Wu Z-Q, Wang Y, et al. Autologous T cells expressing CD30 chimeric antigen receptors for relapsed or refractory Hodgkin lymphoma: an open-label phase I trial. *Clin Cancer Res*. 2017;23:1156−1166.

28. Ali SA, Shi V, Maric I, et al. T cells expressing an anti-B-cell maturation antigen chimeric antigen receptor cause remissions of multiple myeloma. *Blood*. 2016;128:1688−1700.

29. Ritchie DS, Neeson PJ, Khot A, et al. Persistence and efficacy of second generation CAR T cell against the LeY antigen in acute myeloid leukemia. *Mol Ther*. 2013;21:2122−2129.

30. Gust J, Taraseviciute A, Turtle CJ. Neurotoxicity associated with CD19-targeted CAR-T cell therapies. *CNS Drugs*. 2018;32:1091−1101.

31. Annesley CE, Summers C, Ceppi F, Gardner RA. The evolution and future of CAR T cells for B-cell acute lymphoblastic leukemia. *Clin Pharmacol Ther*. 2018;103:591−598.

32. Brudno JN, Maric I, Hartman SD, et al. T cells genetically modified to express an anti-B-cell maturation antigen chimeric antigen receptor cause remissions of poor-prognosis relapsed multiple myeloma. *J Clin Oncol*. 2018;36:2267−2280.

33. Zhao W-H, Liu J, Wang B-Y, et al. A phase 1, open-label study of LCAR-B38M, a chimeric antigen receptor T cell therapy directed against B cell maturation antigen, in patients with relapsed or refractory multiple myeloma. *J Hematol Oncol*. 2018;11:141.

34. Chen N, Li X, Chintala NK, Tano ZE, Adusumilli PS. Driving CARs on the uneven road of antigen heterogeneity in solid tumors. *Curr Opin Immunol*. 2018;51:103−110.

35. O'Rourke DM, Nasrallah MP, Desai A, et al. A single dose of peripherally infused EGFRvIII-directed CAR T cells mediates antigen loss and induces adaptive resistance in patients with recurrent glioblastoma. *Sci Transl Med*. 2017;9.

36. Brown CE, Alizadeh D, Starr R, et al. Regression of glioblastoma after chimeric antigen receptor T-cell therapy. *N Engl J Med*. 2016;375:2561−2569.

37. Topp MS, Stelljes M, Zugmaier G, et al. Safety and activity of blinatumomab for adult patients with relapsed or refractory B-precursor acute lymphoblastic leukaemia: a multicentre, single-arm, phase 2 study. *Lancet Oncol*. 2015;16:57−66.

38. Cooley S, He F, Bachanova V, et al. Neurological consequences of cytokine release syndrome following subcutaneous recombinant IL-15 and haploidentical donor natural killer cell therapy for advanced acute myeloid leukemia. *Blood*. 2017;130:2649.

39. Bachanova V, Sarhan D, Defor T, et al. Haploidentical natural killer cells induce remissions in non-Hodgkin lymphoma patients with low levels of immune-suppressor cells. *Cancer Immunol Immunother*. 2018;67:483−494.

40. Prudent V, Breitbart WS. Chimeric antigen receptor T-cell neuropsychiatric toxicity in acute lymphoblastic leukemia. *Palliat Support Care*. 2017;15:499−503.

41. Gust J, Finney O, Gardner R, et al. Glial injury in neurotoxicity after pediatric CD19-directed chimeric antigen receptor T cell therapy. *Ann Neurol*. 2019;86:42−54.

42. Research C for BE and. Approved Products − KYMRIAH (tisagenlecleucel). [cited 2018 May 14]. Available from: https://www.fda.gov/BiologicsBloodVaccines/CellularGeneTherapyProducts/ApprovedProducts/ucm573706.htm.

43. Shalabi H, Wolters PL, Martin S, et al. Systematic evaluation of neurotoxicity in children and young adults undergoing CD22 chimeric antigen receptor T-cell therapy. *J Immunother*. 2018;41(7):350−358.

44. El Hachioui H, Visch-Brink EG, de Lau LML, et al. Screening tests for aphasia in patients with stroke: a systematic review. *J Neurol*. 2017;264:211−220.

45. Flamand-Roze C, Falissard B, Roze E, et al. Validation of a new language screening tool for patients with acute stroke: the Language Screening Test (LAST). *Stroke*. 2011;42:1224−1229.

46. Gofshteyn JS, Shaw PA, Teachey DT, et al. Neurotoxicity after CTL019 in a pediatric and young adult cohort. *Ann Neurol*. 2018;84:537−546.

47. DeAngelo DJ, Ghobadi A, Park JH, et al. Clinical outcomes for the phase 2, single-arm, multicenter trial of JCAR015 in adult B-ALL (ROCKET Study). 2017.

48. Locke FL, Neelapu SS, Bartlett NL, et al. Preliminary results of prophylactic tocilizumab after Axicabtagenecilo-leucel (axi-cel; KTE-C19) treatment for patients with Refractory,Aggressive non-Hodgkin lymphoma (NHL). *Blood*. 2017;130:1547.

49. Torre M, Solomon IH, Sutherland CL, et al. Neuropathology of a case with fatal CAR T-cell-associated cerebral edema. *J Neuropathol Exp Neurol*. 2018;77:877−882.

50. Gardner R, Ceppi F, Rivers J, et al. Preemptive Mitigation of CD19 CAR T Cell Cytokine Release Syndrome Without Attenuation of Anti-Leukemic Efficacy. *Blood*. 2019. https://doi.org/10.1182/blood.2019001463 [Epub ahead of print].

51. Neilson DE. The interplay of infection and genetics in acute necrotizing encephalopathy. *Curr Opin Pediatr.* 2010;22:751—757.

52. McKinney AM, Short J, Truwit CL, et al. Posterior reversible encephalopathy syndrome: incidence of atypical regions of involvement and imaging findings. *AJR Am J Roentgenol.* 2007;189:904—912.

53. Fugate JE, Rabinstein AA. Posterior reversible encephalopathy syndrome: clinical and radiological manifestations, pathophysiology, and outstanding questions. *Lancet Neurol.* 2015;14:914—925.

54. Engelhardt B, Vajkoczy P, Weller RO. The movers and shapers in immune privilege of the CNS. *Nat Immunol.* 2017;18:123—131.

55. Neelapu SS, Tummala S, Kebriaei P, et al. Chimeric antigen receptor T-cell therapy - assessment and management of toxicities. *Nat Rev Clin Oncol.* 2018;15:47—62.

56. Herman ST, Abend NS, Bleck TP, et al. Consensus statement on continuous EEG in critically ill adults and children, Part I: indications. *J Clin Neurophysiol.* 2015;32: 87—95.

57. Mahadeo KM, Khazal SJ, Abdel-Azim H, et al. Management guidelines for paediatric patients receiving chimeric antigen receptor T cell therapy. *Nat Rev Clin Oncol.* 2018;1.

58. Traube C, Silver G, Kearney J, et al. Cornell assessment of pediatric delirium: a valid, rapid, observational tool for screening delirium in the PICU. *Crit Care Med.* 2014;42: 656—663.

59. Folstein MF, Folstein SE, McHugh PR. "Mini-mental state": a practical method for grading the cognitive state of patients for the clinician. *J Psychiatr Res.* 1975;12: 189—198.

60. Grupp S. Beginning the CAR T cell therapy revolution in the US and EU. *Curr Res Transl Med.* 2018;66:62—64.

61. Norelli M, Camisa B, Barbiera G, et al. Monocyte-derived IL-1 and IL-6 are differentially required for cytokine-release syndrome and neurotoxicity due to CAR T cells. *Nat Med.* 2018;1.

62. Staedtke V, Bai R-Y, Kim K, et al. Disruption of a self-amplifying catecholamine loop reduces cytokine release syndrome. *Nature.* 2018;564:273.

63. Flierl MA, Rittirsch D, Nadeau BA, et al. Phagocyte-derived catecholamines enhance acute inflammatory injury. *Nature.* 2007;449:721—725.

64. Obstfeld AE, Frey NV, Mansfield K, et al. Cytokine release syndrome associated with chimeric-antigen receptor T-cell therapy: clinicopathological insights. *Blood.* 2017; 130:2569—2572.

65. Jirik FR, Podor TJ, Hirano T, et al. Bacterial lipopolysaccharide and inflammatory mediators augment IL-6 secretion by human endothelial cells. *J Immunol.* 1989;142: 144—147.

66. Reyes TM, Fabry Z, Coe CL. Brain endothelial cell production of a neuroprotective cytokine, interleukin-6, in response to noxious stimuli. *Brain Res.* 1999;851: 215—220.

67. Park JH, Santomasso B, Riviere I, et al. Baseline and early post-treatment clinical and laboratory factors associated with severe neurotoxicity following 19-28z CAR T cells in adult patients with relapsed B-ALL. *J Clin Oncol.* 2017;35:7024.

68. Rochfort KD, Collins LE, McLoughlin A, Cummins PM. Tumour necrosis factor-α-mediated disruption of cerebrovascular endothelial barrier integrity in vitro involves the production of proinflammatory interleukin-6. *J Neurochem.* 2016;136:564—572.

69. Pan W, Stone KP, Hsuchou H, Manda VK, Zhang Y, Kastin AJ. Cytokine signaling modulates blood-brain barrier function. *Curr Pharm Des.* 2011;17: 3729—3740.

70. Erickson MA, Banks WA. Cytokine and chemokine responses in serum and brain after single and repeated injections of lipopolysaccharide: multiplex quantification with path analysis. *Brain Behav Immun.* 2011;25: 1637—1648.

71. Argaw AT, Gurfein BT, Zhang Y, Zameer A, John GR. VEGF-mediated disruption of endothelial CLN-5 promotes blood-brain barrier breakdown. *Proc Natl Acad Sci.* 2009;106:1977—1982.

72. van Meurs M, Kümpers P, Ligtenberg JJ, Meertens JH, Molema G, Zijlstra JG. Bench-to-bedside review: angiopoietin signalling in critical illness — a future target? *Crit Care.* 2009;13:207.

73. Page AV, Liles WC. Biomarkers of endothelial activation/dysfunction in infectious diseases. *Virulence.* 2013;4: 507—516.

74. Savage B, Saldívar E, Ruggeri ZM. Initiation of platelet adhesion by arrest onto fibrinogen or translocation on von Willebrand factor. *Cell.* 1996;84:289—297.

75. Engelhardt B, Ransohoff RM. Capture, crawl, cross: the T cell code to breach the blood—brain barriers. *Trends Immunol.* 2012;33:579—589.

76. Potokar M, Jorgačevski J, Zorec R. Astrocyte aquaporin dynamics in health and disease. *Int J Mol Sci.* 2016;17.

77. Eid T, Lee T-SW, Thomas MJ, et al. Loss of perivascular aquaporin 4 may underlie deficient water and K+ homeostasis in the human epileptogenic hippocampus. *Proc Natl Acad Sci U S A.* 2005;102:1193—1198.

78. Sofroniew MV. Astrocyte barriers to neurotoxic inflammation. *Nat Rev Neurosci.* 2015;16:249—263.

79. Hoogland ICM, Houbolt C, van Westerloo DJ, van Gool WA, van de Beek D. Systemic inflammation and microglial activation: systematic review of animal experiments. *J Neuroinflammation;* 2015:12. Available from: https://www.ncbi.nlm.nih.gov/pmc/articles/PMC4470063/.

80. Das A, Arifuzzaman S, Yoon T, et al. RNA sequencing reveals resistance of TLR4 ligand-activated microglial cells to inflammation mediated by the selective jumonji H3K27 demethylase inhibitor. *Sci Rep.* 2017;7:6554.

81. Glass CK, Saijo K, Winner B, Marchetto MC, Gage FH. Mechanisms underlying inflammation in neurodegeneration. *Cell.* 2010;140:918—934.

82. Rheingold SR, Chen LN, Maude SL, et al. Efficient trafficking of chimeric antigen receptor (CAR)-Modified T cells to CSF and induction of durable CNS remissions

in children with CNS/combined relapsed/refractory ALL. *Blood*. 2015;126:3769.

83. Rosário C, Zandman-Goddard G, Meyron-Holtz EG, D'Cruz DP, Shoenfeld Y. The Hyperferritinemic Syndrome: macrophage activation syndrome, Still's disease, septic shock and catastrophic antiphospholipid syndrome. *BMC Med*. 2013;11:185.

84. Fogal B, Hewett SJ. Interleukin-1β: a bridge between inflammation and excitotoxicity? *J Neurochem*. 106: 1−23.

85. Tilleux S, Hermans E. Neuroinflammation and regulation of glial glutamate uptake in neurological disorders. *J Neurosci Res*. 85:2059−2070.

86. Skelly DT, Griffin ÉW, Murray CL, et al. Acute transient cognitive dysfunction and acute brain injury induced by systemic inflammation occur by dissociable IL-1-dependent mechanisms. *Mol Psychiatry*. 2018;1.

87. Guillemin GJ. Quinolinic acid, the inescapable neurotoxin. *FEBS J*. 2012;279:1356−1365.

88. Ikonomidou C, Turski L. Why did NMDA receptor antagonists fail clinical trials for stroke and traumatic brain injury? *Lancet Neurol*. 2002;1:383−386.

89. Taraseviciute A, Tkachev V, Ponce R, et al. Chimeric antigen receptor T cell-mediated neurotoxicity in nonhuman primates. *Cancer Discov*. 2018;8:750−763.

90. Sterner RM, Sakemura R, Cox MJ, et al. GM-CSF inhibition reduces cytokine release syndrome and neuroinflammation but enhances CAR-T cell function in xenografts. *Blood*. 2019;133:697−709.

91. Giavridis T, van der Stegen SJC, Eyquem J, Hamieh M, Piersigilli A, Sadelain M. CAR T cell−induced cytokine release syndrome is mediated by macrophages and abated by IL-1 blockade. *Nat Med*. 2018;1.

92. Pennell CA, Barnum JL, McDonald-Hyman CS, et al. Human CD19-targeted mouse T cells induce B cell aplasia and toxicity in human CD19 transgenic mice. *Mol Ther J Am Soc Gene Ther*. 2018;26:1423−1434.

93. Yin J, Valin KL, Dixon ML, Leavenworth JW. The role of microglia and macrophages in CNS homeostasis, autoimmunity, and cancer. *J Immunol Res*. 2017;2017: 5150678.

94. Davila ML, Riviere I, Wang X, et al. Efficacy and toxicity management of 19-28z CAR T cell therapy in B cell acute lymphoblastic leukemia. *Sci Transl Med*. 2014;6:224ra25.

95. Teachey DT, Lacey SF, Shaw PA, et al. Identification of predictive biomarkers for cytokine release syndrome after chimeric antigen receptor T cell therapy for acute lymphoblastic leukemia. *Cancer Discov*. 2016;6:664−679.

96. Gauthier J, Turtle CJ. Insights into cytokine release syndrome and neurotoxicity after CD19-specific CAR-T cell therapy. *Curr Res Transl Med*. 2018;66:50−52.

97. Teachey DT, Bishop MR, Maloney DG, Grupp SA. Toxicity management after chimeric antigen receptor T cell therapy: one size does not fit "ALL.". *Nat Rev Clin Oncol*. 2018;15:218.

98. Maude SL, Teachey DT, Porter DL, Grupp SA. CD19-targeted chimeric antigen receptor T-cell therapy for acute lymphoblastic leukemia. *Blood*. 2015;125:4017−4023.

99. Atreya R, Mudter J, Finotto S, et al. Blockade of interleukin 6 trans signaling suppresses T-cell resistance against apoptosis in chronic intestinal inflammation: evidence in crohn disease and experimental colitis in vivo. *Nat Med*. 2000;6:583−588.

100. Mihara M, Nishimoto N, Ohsugi Y. The therapy of autoimmune diseases by anti-interleukin-6 receptor antibody. *Expert Opin Biol Ther*. 2005;5:683−690.

101. Venkiteshwaran A. Tocilizumab. *mAbs*. 2009;1:432−438.

102. Rubbert-Roth A, Furst DE, Nebesky JM, Jin A, Berber E. A review of recent advances using tocilizumab in the treatment of rheumatic diseases. *Rheumatol Ther*. 2018; 1−22.

103. Curtis JR, Perez-Gutthann S, Suissa S, et al. Tocilizumab in rheumatoid arthritis: a case study of safety evaluations of a large postmarketing data set from multiple data sources. *Semin Arthritis Rheum*. 2015;44:381−388.

104. Stone JH, Tuckwell K, Dimonaco S, et al. Trial of tocilizumab in giant-cell arteritis. *N Engl J Med*. 2017;377:317−328.

105. Tarp S, Amarilyo G, Foeldvari I, et al. Efficacy and safety of biological agents for systemic juvenile idiopathic arthritis: a systematic review and meta-analysis of randomized trials. *Rheumatology*. 2016;55:669−679.

106. Le RQ, Li L, Yuan W, et al. FDA approval summary: tocilizumab for treatment of chimeric antigen receptor T cell-induced severe or life-threatening cytokine release syndrome. *The Oncologist*. 2018;23:943−947.

107. Chen F, Teachey DT, Pequignot E, et al. Measuring IL-6 and sIL-6R in serum from patients treated with tocilizumab and/or siltuximab following CAR T cell therapy. *J Immunol Methods*. 2016;434:1−8.

108. Nishimoto N, Terao K, Mima T, Nakahara H, Takagi N, Kakehi T. Mechanisms and pathologic significances in increase in serum interleukin-6 (IL-6) and soluble IL-6 receptor after administration of an anti-IL-6 receptor antibody, tocilizumab, in patients with rheumatoid arthritis and Castleman disease. *Blood*. 2008;112: 3959−3964.

109. Nellan A, McCully CML, Garcia RC, et al. Improved CNS exposure to tocilizumab after cerebrospinal fluid compared to intravenous administration in rhesus macaques. *Blood*. 2018;132:662−666.

110. Gardner R, Leger KJ, Annesley CE, et al. Decreased rates of severe CRS seen with early intervention strategies for CD19 CAR-T cell toxicity management. *Blood*. 2016; 128:586.

111. Koehler PJ. Use of corticosteroids in neuro-oncology. *Anticancer Drugs*. 1995;6:19−33.

112. Michinaga S, Koyama Y. Pathogenesis of brain edema and investigation into anti-edema drugs. *Int J Mol Sci*. 2015;16:9949−9975.

113. Berkovich RR. Acute multiple sclerosis relapse. *Continuum (Minneap Minn)*. 2016;22:799−814.

114. Wingerchuk DM, Weinshenker BG. Acute disseminated encephalomyelitis, transverse myelitis, and neuromyelitis optica. *Continuum (Minneap Minn)*. 2013;19:944−967.

115. Elenkov IJ. Glucocorticoids and the Th1/Th2 balance. *Ann N Y Acad Sci*. 2004;1024:138−146.

116. Martínez-Cáceres EM, Barrau MA, Brieva L, Espejo C, Barberà N, Montalban X. Treatment with methylprednisolone in relapses of multiple sclerosis patients: immunological evidence of immediate and short-term but not long-lasting effects. *Clin Exp Immunol.* 2002;127:165–171.

117. Kurzrock R, Voorhees PM, Casper C, et al. A phase I, open-label study of siltuximab, an anti–IL-6 monoclonal antibody, in patients with B-cell non-Hodgkin lymphoma, multiple myeloma, or Castleman disease. *Clin Cancer Res.* 2013;19:3659–3670.

118. Shah B, Huynh V, Sender LS, et al. High rates of minimal residual disease-negative (MRD−) complete responses (CR) in adult and pediatric and patients with relapsed/refractory acute lymphoblastic leukemia (R/R ALL) treated with KTE-C19 (Anti-CD19 chimeric antigen receptor [CAR] T cells): preliminary results of the ZUMA-3 and ZUMA-4 trials. *Blood.* 2016;128:2803.

119. Cavalli G, Dinarello CA. Anakinra therapy for non-cancer inflammatory diseases. *Front Pharmacol.* 2018;9:1157.

120. Saharinen P, Eklund L, Alitalo K. Therapeutic targeting of the angiopoietin-TIE pathway. *Nat Rev Drug Discov.* 2017; 16:635–661.

121. Ramael S, De Smedt F, Toublanc N, et al. Single-dose bioavailability of levetiracetam intravenous infusion relative to oral tablets and multiple-dose pharmacokinetics and tolerability of levetiracetam intravenous infusion compared with placebo in healthy subjects. *Clin Ther.* 2006;28:734–744.

122. Chesnut RM, Temkin N, Dikmen S, et al. A method of managing severe traumatic brain injury in the absence of intracranial pressure monitoring: the imaging and clinical examination protocol. *J Neurotrauma.* 2018;35: 54–63.

123. Kukreti V, Mohseni-Bod H, Drake J. Management of raised intracranial pressure in children with traumatic brain injury. *J Pediatr Neurosci.* 2014;9:207–215.

124. Wendell LC, Khan A, Raser J, et al. Successful management of refractory intracranial hypertension from acute hyperammonemic encephalopathy in a woman with ornithine transcarbamylase deficiency. *Neurocrit Care.* 2010;13:113–117.

125. Honeybul S, Ho KM, Gillett GR. Long-term outcome following decompressive craniectomy: an inconvenient truth? *Curr Opin Crit Care.* 2018;24:97–104.

CHAPTER 8

Hematologic and Non-CRS Toxicities

FRANCESCO CEPPI, MD • CORINNE SUMMERS, MD • REBECCA A. GARDNER, MD

INTRODUCTION

Chimeric antigen receptor (CAR)—modified T-cell immunotherapy is highly effective for patients with relapsed and/or refractory B-cell malignancies, but significant adverse effects remain a concern. Systemic cytokine release syndrome (CRS) can occur in association with the inflammatory cytokine surge during in vivo CAR T-cell proliferation,[1–3] and neurologic adverse effects commonly occur in this context.[4,5] Significant progress has been made in CRS management, leading to a reduction in its incidence and severity. But there are additional toxicities that require further research focus for management guidance.

HEMOPHAGOCYTIC LYMPHOHISTIOCYTOSIS AND MACROPHAGE ACTIVATION SYNDROME

Hemophagocytic lymphohistiocytosis (HLH) and macrophage activation syndrome (MAS) are potentially life-threatening syndromes brought on by excessive and unreserved immune activation.[6,7] Primary HLH is frequently observed in infants and toddlers due to underlying genetic mutations.[8,9] These mutations result in a lack of downregulation following immune activation, leading to a dysfunctional hyperinflammatory state. This is felt to involve macrophages, natural killer (NK) cells and cytotoxic T-cells. Macrophage activation leads to cytokine production which ultimately causes end organ destruction and organ failure.[7] In normal states, NK and T-cells function to eliminate macrophages that have been activated in a negative feedback loop. In the pathologic state, lack of negative feedback allows for continued activation and cytokine production from macrophages. While MAS is observed in patients with rheumatologic disorders such as systemic juvenile idiopathic arthritis, secondary HLH describes patients who develop HLH in response to an identified inciting trigger such as a neoplastic process or viral infection.[10] Diagnostic criteria include identification of a known genetic mutation or five of the following: fever >38.5C, splenomegaly, cytopenias involving two lines (hemoglobin <9 g/dL, platelets <100,000/uL or absolute neutrophil count <1000/uL), hypertriglyceridemia (fasting triglycerides >265 mg/dL) and/or hypofibrinogenemia (fibrinogen <150 mg/dL), hemophagocytosis in bone marrow, spleen, lymph node or liver, low or absent NK cell function, elevated ferritin (>500 ng/mL) and elevated soluble CD25 or IL-2 receptor alpha.[6]

There is significant overlap between HLH/MAS diagnostic criteria and the signs and symptoms of CRS that develop in response to CAR T-cell therapy. In many of the patients meeting criteria for grade 3 or greater CRS, they also meet criteria for HLH/MAS.[11,12] CAR T-cell—related HLH/MAS is currently considered to be secondary HLH/MAS, as it is felt to be due to the hyperinflammatory state initiated by CAR T-cell activation. The incidence of CRS-associated HLH/MAS is difficult to define, and there is controversy regarding the prevalence of CRS-associated HLH/MAS. Mahadeo et al. suggested considering the diagnosis of HLH/MAS if a patient's serum ferritin is greater than 10,000 ng/mL with concurrent hepatic, renal, or pulmonary toxicity (CTCAE grade 3 or higher) or hemophagocytosis noted on pathology.[13] Neelapu et al. suggest it is rare, approximately 1% of patients treated in their experience.[14] However, Teachey et al. report a different experience noting the significant overlap in CRS and HLH/MAS in patients with grade 3 or high CRS, suggesting a higher observed incidence.[11,12] Given that most patients receive lymphodepleting chemotherapy prior to the CAR T-cell infusion and are immunocompromised, they are also at risk for infections concurrently and other potential causes for secondary HLH/MAS must also be evaluated if patients do not improve following CRS-targeted therapy. Teachey et al.

Chimeric Antigen Receptor T-Cell Therapies for Cancer. https://doi.org/10.1016/B978-0-323-66181-2.00008-1

suggested elevated levels of IFN-γ (>75 pg/mL) and IL10 (>60 pg/mL) were more suggestive of potential CRS-associated HLH and less likely to be due to infection, though this has not been demonstrated in analysis of cytokines evaluated during periods of CRS and documented infection.[15,16] In addition, if a patient has a history suggestive of a previous HLH/MAS event or hyperinflammation is not improved with CRS-targeted therapies, one should consider investigating for primary HLH genetic mutations.

In line with general principles of secondary HLH/MAS treatment, therapy should be focused on the underlying cause, which is the CRS and the CAR T-cell activation. Some have recommended IL-6-directed therapy, which is also used for CRS and if there is lack of clinical response in 48−72 hours to consider HLH management per HLH-2004.[13] Additionally, some practitioners are trialing anakinra, an IL-1 blocking agent for severe HLH.[17] However, one must balance the need for additional therapy and the potential for eliminating the CAR T-cells with further cytotoxic therapy. These above issues highlight the difficulty in distinguishing the two entities, and further research is needed to guide management to intervene early if a patient is more likely to develop HLH/MAS and is in need of therapeutic interventions beyond IL-6-directed therapy and corticosteroids.

HEMATOLOGIC COMPLICATIONS
Cytopenias

Cytopenias are a common occurrence following CAR T-cell infusion. Grades 3−4 anemias, thrombocytopenia, leukopenia, neutropenia, and lymphopenia are frequently reported. There is often difficulty in determining the etiology of cytopenias occurring after CAR T-cell infusions. Cytopenias are seen following the chemotherapy that is often given before CAR T-cell infusions. Additionally, many patients have suboptimal marrow function prior to the receipt of the CAR T-cells and have preexisting transfusion requirements. However, patients not receiving conditioning chemotherapy have also experienced cytopenias following CAR T-cell infusion, demonstrating that the CAR T-cells cause myelosuppression by a cytokine-mediated mechanism or some other mechanism.[18−20]

In a phase I study targeting CD19, most patients had grade 3 or 4 cytopenias attributed to lymphodepleting chemotherapy.[3] Median duration of absolute neutrophil count less than 500 was 8 days (0−38 days in responding patients), but prolonged (≥14 days) grade 4 neutropenia was noted in 7 of 21 patients (33%). Anemia grade 3 was present in 63% of the patients, and thrombocytopenia grades 3 and 4 were 16% and 37%, respectively.[3]

In the tisagenlecleucel registration trial, a total of 31 of 75 patients (41%) had grade 3 or 4 thrombocytopenia that had not resolved by day 28.[2] Of those 31 patients, 22 had resolution to grade 2 or lower by the last assessment, and 9 did not. By month 3, the Kaplan-Meier estimate of the percentage of patients with resolution to grade 2 or lower was 73%. A grade 3 or 4 decreased neutrophil count that had not resolved by day 28 was reported in 40 of 75 patients (53%). Of those 40 patients, 32 had resolution to grade 2 or lower by the last assessment, and 8 did not; the Kaplan-Meier estimate of the percentage of patients who had resolution to grade 2 or lower by month 3 was 66%. Of these 40 patients, 18 (45%) had grade 3 or 4 infections. In rare cases, prolonged grade 3 or 4 neutropenia before and after tisagenlecleucel infusion was associated with infections that were severe (grade 3 human herpesvirus 6 [HHV-6] encephalitis) or fatal (encephalitis and systemic mycosis). The frequency of cytopenias not resolved by day 28 was 37% for any grade and 32% for grades 3 and 4.[2]

Hay et al. evaluated recovery of blood counts in 104 adult patients who had received lymphodepletion with cyclophosphamide/fludarabine chemotherapy followed by a CD19 CAR T-cell infusion.[21] They were able to demonstrate the association between hematological toxicity and severity of CRS providing evidence for cytokine-induced aplasia. The absolute neutrophil count, hematocrit, hemoglobin concentration, and platelet count declined after cyclophosphamide/fludarabine chemotherapy, reaching nadirs between days 2 and 5 after CAR T-cell infusion. The absolute neutrophil count, hematocrit, and platelet nadirs were lower in patients with more severe CRS, and patients with grade ≥4 CRS received more platelet and red cell transfusions than those with grade ≤3 CRS. Of 10 patients with grade ≥4 CRS, 5 became refractory to platelet transfusion. They also found an association of marrow tumor burden, the number of prior therapies, and the occurrence of CRS with longer hematologic recovery. The time to hematologic recovery was longer than expected in most patients with grade 4 CRS and was delayed in patients with grades 1 to 3 CRS (median, 13.5 days [IQR, 6.5−18.1 days]) compared with those without CRS (median, 4.1 days [IQR, 2.9−7.5 days]).

Coagulopathy

Findings of Turtle et al. were consistent with development of a consumptive coagulopathy in patients with severe CRS.[21] They examined the PT, aPTT, D-dimer, and fibrinogen in patients at intervals after CAR T-cell infusion. Patients receiving therapeutic anticoagulation were excluded from the analyses (n = 9). In the first week after CAR T-cell infusion, patients with grade ≤3 CRS had normal or mildly elevated PT, aPTT, D-dimer, and fibrinogen. In contrast, those with grade ≥4 CRS developed early prolongation of the PT and aPTT, which peaked approximately 2–5 days after CAR T-cell infusion. Increasing D-dimer and falling fibrinogen concentrations started on days 2–5, with hypofibrinogenemia occurring from days 9–12, consistent with disseminated intravascular coagulation (DIC).[22] Compared with patients with grades 1–3 CRS, those with grade ≥4 CRS received more cryoprecipitate transfusions to correct coagulopathy and had more severe and prolonged thrombocytopenia. Grade ≥3 bleeding occurred in only three patients (2%), all of whom had grade ≥4 CRS.

Similar results were also reported by Upenn/CHOP group in their pediatric cohort. Teachey et al. found a strong association with low fibrinogen and grade 4 CRS in the pediatric cohort but not in adults.[15,23] Children became mildly coagulopathic with more significant coagulopathy with severe CRS. Adults also developed hypofibrinogenemia and mild coagulopathy; however, this was seen across CRS grades. Although bleeding was rare, understanding the coagulopathy has direct clinical implications, as many of the patients required cryoprecipitate in addition to fresh frozen plasma to maintain hemostasis.

In conclusion, the coagulopathy, during CAR T-cell therapy, often presents with early prolongation of the prothrombin time (PT) and activated partial thromboplastin time (aPTT),[3,19,24] and increasing D-dimer[18] with low fibrinogen[18,24] occurring after CRS resolution, consistent with DIC.[24] Cryoprecipitate and plasma transfusions are the actual recommended supportive therapy along with close laboratory monitoring.

INFECTION

Patients who receive CAR T-cells are at increased risk for infection for a multitude of reasons. Malignancies along with the therapy used to treat them leave patients with poor immune function, which leads to increased infectious risk. CAR T-cell therapy's preceding lymphodepleting chemotherapy not only causes cytopenias but can also lead to destruction of the body's protective barriers, particularly mucosal barriers. Additionally,

therapies directed at CRS, aimed to dampen a hyperinflammatory state, are broadly targeting medications that can further increase one's infection risk. All patients should receive prophylaxis against *Pneumocystis jirovecii*. Trimethoprim-sulfamethoxazole is frequently used for this reason, but considering the potentially myelosuppressive effect, it is advised to instead use alternative agents such as pentamidine to avoid agents that may promote or prolong aplasia. Consideration for VZV prophylaxis should also strongly be considered in patients who are VZV seropositive to prevent reactivation during the period of lymphopenia and B-cell aplasia (BCA).

Researchers at Fred Hutchinson Cancer Research Center (FHCRC) evaluated the infectious complications in the first 90 days following CD19 CAR T-cell therapy in adult subjects.[25] Within the first 4 weeks following cell infusion, documented infections were observed in 23% of the subjects, with bacterial infections being the most common events, followed by viral infections. Only 3% of subjects developed invasive fungal infections, and all had developed severe CRS or neurotoxicity requiring therapy. The median time to first infection was 6 days with a majority occurring within the first 10 days. Most subjects that developed infection also developed CRS with CRS occurring prior to the infection. Following the initial 4 weeks, researchers noted a reduction in the infection density. Only 14% of subjects were diagnosed with an infection during this period, with viral infections being the most common, followed by bacterial infections. Fungal infections were relatively rare (2%). Of those who developed late infections, persistent malignant disease was noted in half of the subjects and persistent neutropenia in approximately 20%. Of all infections, less than half were considered severe, and only 6% of infectious events were life-threatening. Further analysis revealed that adult subjects with a history of four or more chemotherapeutic regimens, who received a CAR T-cell dose of 2×10^7 cells/kg (the maximum dose given) or who developed more severe CRS, were potentially at an increased infectious risk.[25]

The group at Memorial Sloan Kettering evaluated infectious events that occurred within the first 180 days following CD19 CAR T-cell infusion in 53 adult subjects.[16] Most patients were on antifungal, antiviral, and anti-*Pneumocystis* prophylaxis. None were on antibacterial prophylaxis at the time of T-cell infusion. During the first 30 days following cell infusion, 42% of subjects developed infections (26 infections in 22 patients), a majority occurred during a period of neutropenia. Bacterial infections were again the most common: eight episodes of bacteremia, four *Clostridium difficile* colitis, two pneumonias, one abdominal infection, one pyelonephritis, and one abscess. The researchers noted four invasive fungal infections in the patients on micafungin prophylaxis. There was one case of pulmonary mucormycosis, two probable invasive pulmonary aspergillosis infections, and one *Saccharomyces cerevisiae* fungemia. Five viral infections occurred during this period, one herpes simplex, one varicella zoster infection, and three viral upper respiratory tract infections. Following the first 30 days, 31% of subjects (that had continued remission) had 15 infections, which were predominantly viral infections (eight of the nine were respiratory tract viral infections). There were five bacterial infections (one *Clostridium difficile* colitis, two pneumonias, one cellulitis with potential associated osteomyelitis, and one urinary tract infection) and one fungal infection (probable pulmonary aspergillosis) noted between days 30 and 180. Again, the highest density period for infectious complications was during the first month following CAR T-cell infusion. Only three subjects died from infectious complications. Discrete from the finding of the FHCRC study, researchers evaluated for potential predictors of infection and did not observe increased risks associated with the number of prior chemotherapy cycles or CAR T-cell dose in their analysis. They did, however, corroborate the findings of an increased risk of infection, particularly blood stream infections, in patients who developed grade 3 or higher CRS.[16]

It is unclear if the relationship between severe CRS and infection is due to the pathophysiology of CRS or the therapies directed at treating CRS. Researchers have evaluated cytokine panels to assist in potentially delineating the cause (infection vs. CRS) of a patient's inflammatory state given severe infection and CRS have overlapping signs and symptoms.[15,21] Park et al. were not able to identify a distinct cytokine pattern that would be more suggestive of one over the other.[16] Therefore, practitioners must consider both entities during such a period. Additionally, as we gain more knowledge regarding the prevention of severe CRS, we may subsequently reduce potential infectious complications for patients who receive CAR T-cell therapy.

B-CELL APLASIA

Prolonged BCA, and resultant hypogammaglobulinemia, is an expected on-target toxicity of successful CD19- and CD22-directed CAR T-cell therapy.[1,3,19,20,24,26,27] CD19 and CD22 CAR therapies eliminate nonmalignant precursor and mature B-cells. However, BCA has the potential to be indefinite after B-cell targeting CAR T-cell therapy, as long as the CAR T-cells maintain functional persistence. BCA can serve as a surrogate measure of the pharmacodynamic persistence of CAR T-cells. BCA and hypogammaglobulinemia may last 2 months to over 2 years following CAR T-cell infusion and is longer in those patients who receive 4-1BB costimulatory domain products over CD28 costimulatory domain products.[2,18,24,28] However, BCA as a measure of functional persistence should be interpreted with caution, as patients may be B-cell deplete prior to receiving CAR T-cell therapy. In fact, Kochenderfer et al., in their NHL anti-CD19 CAR T (CD28 costimulatory domain) cell trial, had a median blood B-cell count at enrollment of 1/mL (range, 0−123/mL).[29]

Good clinical practice following B-cell−directed therapy includes monitoring of IgG levels, and repletion can be accomplished with either intravenous immunoglobulin (IVIG) or subcutaneous dosing of IgG according to institutional standards, and these may be different with adult and pediatric programs, with pediatric programs more frequently replacing for asymptomatic low levels. Although immunoglobulin replacement mitigates most infectious complications, longer follow-up is needed to assess late toxicity of BCA. This is not unique to CAR T-cell therapy, as IgG is also monitored and replaced following CD20-targeting therapy with rituximab, or during treatment with the CD19-targeting, bispecific T-cell engaging drug, blinatumomab.

Interestingly, it is possible that CD19-negative plasma cells (PCs) persist and contribute to sustained immunoglobulin production of antibodies against vaccine-related antigens.[30] Bhoj et al. found that while total serum immunoglobulin concentrations decline following CTL019-induced BCA, several vaccine/pathogen-specific serum immunoglobulin G and A titers remain relatively stable for at least 6 and 12 months posttreatment, respectively.[30] Analysis of bone marrow biopsies after CTL019 revealed eight patients with persistence of antibody-secreting PCs at least 25 months post-CTL019 infusion despite absence of CD19+/CD20+ B-cells. These results provide strong evidence for the existence of memory B-cell−independent, long-lived PCs in humans that contribute to long-lasting humoral immunity.[30]

GRAFT-VERSUS-HOST DISEASE

A large proportion of patients treated with CAR T-cells have previously received an allogeneic hematopoietic cell transplant.[1–3] Lack of active graft-versus-host disease (GVHD) is a frequent criterion for CAR T-cell clinical trial enrollment given the potential for exacerbation of GVHD following modified T-cell infusion.[1,2] Incorporation of the CAR is additive to a T-cell's baseline function, in which the endogenous T-cell receptor is present and cells may have alloreactivity potential. Autologous T-cell collection from patients for CAR immunotherapy production is in fact collection of allogeneic T-cells though GVHD is infrequently observed in patients treated.[24,26]

Gardner et al. found only 1 of the 27 subjects treated on their phase 1 portion of the trial, with a history of HCT, exhibited GVHD.[1] The subject was found to have grade 3 acute skin GVHD following CD19 CAR T-cell infusion, over 2 years from their HCT. The subject had been off immunosuppressive therapy for over a year before receiving immunotherapy. A skin biopsy specimen was evaluated for the modified T-cells, and only 9% of the T-cells that infiltrated the skin were felt to be CAR positive; this was in contrast to the 78% that were positive in the peripheral blood suggesting, potentially, the leading cause of the rash was due to non–CAR-transduced T-cells; however, the role the CD19 CAR T-cells may have played in the development of GVHD remains unclear. The rash resolved with prednisone therapy.[1]

The NCI and Baylor groups developed donor-derived CD19 CAR T-cell products for post-HCT patients.[19,31] The NCI group has reported the outcomes of 20 subjects treated, 6 of which obtained a complete remission and none developed GVHD.[19] Similarly, the Baylor group treated eight post-HCT subjects with donor-derived CD19 CAR T-cells. Two subjects exhibited a response, and none developed GVHD.[31] This is in contrast to donor lymphocyte infusions (DLIs), which are at increased risk of causing GVHD. The difference may be due to the CAR incorporation, and/or the cell doses are lower than those used for DLI. Thus far, obtaining T-cells from a patient that previously underwent HCT appears to be safe from a GVHD perspective; however, further research is needed to determine the safety of donor-derived CAR T-cells for posttransplant infusion. Research is currently ongoing evaluating third party, or "off-the-shelf," CAR T-cells with endogenous T-cell receptor knockout to eliminate the risk of alloreactivity.[32]

CONCLUSION AND AREAS OF FUTURE INVESTIGATION

Many of the complications associated with CAR T-cell therapy intertwine with CRS and are associated with CRS severity. As we improve upon early identification and intervention for CRS, many of these additional complications may improve. However, the mechanism underlying these associations requires further investigation. This will guide management strategies as well as prevention strategies to improve upon the safety

of the therapy as it becomes more widely available. As new targets are developed and studied, we may see different severity of adverse effects requiring, potentially, CAR-specific guidelines. Additionally, new cell manipulation techniques are being developed to allow for complex T-cell modifications for safer and potentially longer-lasting immunotherapeutic strategies. With the introduction of new complexities in T-cell immunotherapy which include not only intracellular modifications but also clinically relevant ones including different targets and modes of administration (intracranially, for example), the field will continue to challenge researchers and clinicians.

REFERENCES

1. Gardner RA, Finney O, Annesley C, et al. Intent-to-treat leukemia remission by CD19 CAR T cells of defined formulation and dose in children and young adults. *Blood.* 2017;129(25):3322–3331.
2. Maude SL, Laetsch TW, Buechner J, et al. Tisagenlecleucel in children and young adults with B-cell lymphoblastic leukemia. *N Engl J Med.* 2018;378(5):439–448.
3. Lee DW, Kochenderfer JN, Stetler-Stevenson M, et al. T cells expressing CD19 chimeric antigen receptors for acute lymphoblastic leukaemia in children and young adults: a phase 1 dose-escalation trial. *Lancet.* 2015;385(9967):517–528.
4. Gust J, Hay KA, Hanafi LA, et al. Endothelial activation and blood-brain barrier disruption in neurotoxicity after adoptive immunotherapy with CD19 CAR-T cells. *Cancer Discov.* 2017;7(12):1404–1419.
5. Santomasso BD, Park JH, Salloum D, et al. Clinical and biological correlates of neurotoxicity associated with CAR T-cell therapy in patients with B-cell acute lymphoblastic leukemia. *Cancer Discov.* 2018;8(8):958–971.
6. Henter JI, Horne A, Arico M, et al. HLH-2004: diagnostic and therapeutic guidelines for hemophagocytic lymphohistiocytosis. *Pediatr Blood Cancer.* 2007;48(2):124–131.
7. Ramos-Casals M, Brito-Zeron P, Lopez-Guillermo A, Khamashta MA, Bosch X. Adult haemophagocytic syndrome. *Lancet.* 2014;383(9927):1503–1516.
8. Cetica V, Sieni E, Pende D, et al. Genetic predisposition to hemophagocytic lymphohistiocytosis: report on 500 patients from the Italian registry. *J Allergy Clin Immunol.* 2016;137(1):188–196. e184.
9. Stepp SE, Dufourcq-Lagelouse R, Le Deist F, et al. Perforin gene defects in familial hemophagocytic lymphohistiocytosis. *Science.* 1999;286(5446):1957–1959.
10. Malinowska I, Machaczka M, Popko K, Siwicka A, Salamonowicz M, Nasilowska-Adamska B. Hemophagocytic syndrome in children and adults. *Arch Immunol Ther Exp.* 2014;62(5):385–394.
11. Teachey DT, Rheingold SR, Maude SL, et al. Cytokine release syndrome after blinatumomab treatment related

to abnormal macrophage activation and ameliorated with cytokine-directed therapy. *Blood.* 2013;121(26): 5154−5157.

12. Teachey DT, Bishop MR, Maloney DG, Grupp SA. Toxicity management after chimeric antigen receptor T cell therapy: one size does not fit 'ALL'. *Nat Rev Clin Oncol.* 2018;15(4): 218.

13. Mahadeo KM, Khazal SJ, Abdel-Azim H, et al. Management guidelines for paediatric patients receiving chimeric antigen receptor T cell therapy. *Nat Rev Clin Oncol.* 2019; 16(1):45−63.

14. Neelapu SS. An interim analysis of the ZUMA-1 study of KTE-C19 in refractory, aggressive non-Hodgkin lymphoma. *Clin Adv Hematol Oncol.* 2017;15(2):117−120.

15. Teachey DT, Lacey SF, Shaw PA, et al. Identification of predictive biomarkers for cytokine release syndrome after chimeric antigen receptor T-cell therapy for acute lymphoblastic leukemia. *Cancer Discov.* 2016;6(6):664−679.

16. Park JH, Romero FA, Taur Y, et al. Cytokine release syndrome grade as a predictive marker for infections in patients with relapsed or refractory B-cell acute lymphoblastic leukemia treated with chimeric antigen receptor T cells. *Clin Infect Dis.* 2018;67(4):533−540.

17. La Rosee P, Horne A, Hines M, et al. Recommendations for the management of hemophagocytic lymphohistiocytosis in adults. *Blood.* 2019;133(23):2465−2477.

18. Grupp SA, Kalos M, Barrett D, et al. Chimeric antigen receptor-modified T cells for acute lymphoid leukemia. *N Engl J Med.* 2013;368(16):1509−1518.

19. Brudno JN, Somerville RP, Shi V, et al. Allogeneic T cells that express an anti-CD19 chimeric antigen receptor induce remissions of B-cell malignancies that progress after allogeneic hematopoietic stem-cell transplantation without causing graft-versus-host disease. *J Clin Oncol.* 2016;34(10):1112−1121.

20. Kochenderfer JN, Dudley ME, Carpenter RO, et al. Donor-derived CD19-targeted T cells cause regression of malignancy persisting after allogeneic hematopoietic stem cell transplantation. *Blood.* 2013;122(25):4129−4139.

21. Hay KA, Hanafi LA, Li D, et al. Kinetics and biomarkers of severe cytokine release syndrome after CD19 chimeric antigen receptor-modified T-cell therapy. *Blood.* 2017; 130(21):2295−2306.

22. Gardner R, Wu D, Cherian S, et al. Acquisition of a CD19-negative myeloid phenotype allows immune escape of MLL-rearranged B-ALL from CD19 CAR-T-cell therapy. *Blood.* 2016;127(20):2406−2410.

23. Acharya UH, Dhawale T, Yun S, et al. Management of cytokine release syndrome and neurotoxicity in chimeric antigen receptor (CAR) T cell therapy. *Expert Rev Hematol.* 2019;12(3):195−205.

24. Maude SL, Frey N, Shaw PA, et al. Chimeric antigen receptor T cells for sustained remissions in leukemia. *N Engl J Med.* 2014;371(16):1507−1517.

25. Hill JA, Li D, Hay KA, et al. Infectious complications of CD19-targeted chimeric antigen receptor-modified T-cell immunotherapy. *Blood.* 2018;131(1):121−130.

26. Turtle CJ, Hanafi LA, Berger C, et al. CD19 CAR-T cells of defined CD4+:CD8+ composition in adult B cell ALL patients. *J Clin Invest.* 2016;126(6):2123−2138.

27. Kalos M, Levine BL, Porter DL, et al. T cells with chimeric antigen receptors have potent antitumor effects and can establish memory in patients with advanced leukemia. *Sci Transl Med.* 2011;3(95), 95ra73.

28. Kochenderfer JN, Dudley ME, Feldman SA, et al. B-cell depletion and remissions of malignancy along with cytokine-associated toxicity in a clinical trial of anti-CD19 chimeric-antigen-receptor-transduced T cells. *Blood.* 2012;119(12):2709−2720.

29. Kochenderfer JN, Somerville RPT, Lu T, et al. Lymphoma remissions caused by anti-CD19 chimeric antigen receptor T cells are associated with high serum interleukin-15 levels. *J Clin Oncol.* 2017;35(16):1803−1813.

30. Bhoj VG, Arhontoulis D, Wertheim G, et al. Persistence of long-lived plasma cells and humoral immunity in individuals responding to CD19-directed CAR T-cell therapy. *Blood.* 2016;128(3):360−370.

31. Cruz CRY, Micklethwaite KP, Savoldo B, et al. Infusion of donor-derived CD19-redirected-virus-specific T cells for B-cell malignancies relapsed after allogeneic stem cell transplant: a phase I study. *Blood.* 2013. blood-2013-2006-506741.

32. Qasim W, Zhan H, Samarasinghe S, et al. Molecular remission of infant B-ALL after infusion of universal TALEN gene-edited CAR T cells. *Sci Transl Med.* 2017;9(374).

CHAPTER 9

Response Assessment and Post—CAR T-Cell Therapy Management

AGNE TARASEVICIUTE, MD, PHD • MICHAEL A. PULSIPHER, MD • ALAN S. WAYNE, MD

BACKGROUND

CD19 chimeric antigen receptor-T (CAR T) cell therapy has dramatically improved the outcomes for pediatric and adult patients with short-term complete remission (CR) rates of approximately 90% in relapsed/refractory B-lineage acute lymphoblastic leukemia (ALL) and objective response rates (ORRs) of 50% in non-Hodgkin lymphoma (NHL).[1-10] Long-term, sustained remissions lasting ≥1 year after CD19 CAR T-cell therapy were demonstrated in 50% of patients with ALL and NHL.[3,9,10] CD19 CAR T-cell therapy is associated with unique side effects that require specialized short- and long-term monitoring programs. A multidisciplinary approach with expertise in the treatment of patients with CAR T-cell therapy is needed with the aim of providing systematic, comprehensive follow-up for anticipated toxicities, disease monitoring, and CAR T-cell persistence.

Initial disease response assessments following CD19 CAR T cell therapy in patients with ALL are performed within the first month, standardly between days 21 and 28 postinfusion. The testing for ALL includes bone marrow (BM) aspirate evaluation for morphology and minimal residual disease (MRD) assessment, either by multiparameter flow cytometry (MFC), polymerase chain reaction (PCR), or immunoglobulin-based next-generation sequencing (Ig-NGS). In addition, cerebrospinal fluid (CSF) is evaluated for evidence of malignant disease, and other extramedullary sites, if present, are evaluated by positron emission tomography (PET) imaging. Initial BM disease responses are characterized as either CR or CR with incomplete hematologic recovery (CRi or CRh; platelet count <100,000/μL or absolute neutrophil count [ANC] <1,000 cells/μL) and either MRD-negative (<0.01% of mononuclear cells [MNCs] by MFC) or MRD-positive (≥0.01% of MNCs by MFC) CR.

CAR T-cells are detected either via flow cytometry using antibodies for constructs producing surface markers or quantitative PCR (qPCR) assays for CAR transgene levels. However such assays are not routinely performed for the two FDA-approved CAR products.[3,4,13] A surrogate marker of CD19 CAR T-cell persistence is B-cell aplasia (BCA), which is monitored via flow cytometry as absolute CD19 counts in the peripheral blood.[3]

In NHL, disease responses are monitored via whole-body imaging techniques, including computed tomography (CT) and fluorodeoxyglucose (FDG)-positron emission tomography (PET) imaging before and after CAR T-cell therapy. Initial disease assessments in NHL are reported according to the International Working Group Response Criteria for Malignant Lymphoma (Lugano criteria) as ORR, which include CR (which also includes a complete metabolic response even with a persistent mass) and partial response (PR; a decrease by >50% in the sum of the product of the perpendicular diameters of up to six representative nodes or lesions).[14] Importantly, NHL patients with PR at initial disease assessment, usually 1—2 months post—CAR T-cell therapy, can continue to respond and convert to CR in >50% of cases.[10] Stable disease (SD) or progressive disease (PD) are other disease response categories commonly employed in the setting of NHL.[8]

After typically inpatient care of acute toxicities, including cytokine release syndrome (CRS), neurotoxicity (reviewed in Chapters This needs to be clarified based on the most up to date chapter index), and neutropenic fever/infection, subsequent management is focused on correcting and supporting any remaining complications associated with CAR T-cell therapy in an outpatient setting. This includes management of cytopenias, which may occur in up to 30%—60% of patients, with packed red blood cell (PRBC) and platelet transfusions, growth factor support with eltrombopag for persistent severe thrombocytopenia, and granulocyte colony-stimulating factor (G-CSF, filgrastim), for severe neutropenia.[15] G-CSF administration can be considered, either preemptively, at the initial onset of neutropenia, or later, after resolution of CRS, without firm data available regarding the optimal timing of administration. In addition, patients require monthly immunoglobulin (intravenous or subcutaneous) infusion for hypogammaglobulinemia as a result of BCA to maintain adequate IgG levels (>400 mg/dL). The long-term complications after CAR T-cell therapies have only recently begun to be systematically evaluated, given the relatively recent incorporation of CAR T-cells into the treatment of B-cell malignancies. These complications include prolonged cytopenias, infections, and specific organ dysfunction, such as cardiac and neurologic dysfunction as well as renal insufficiency that can persist after resolution of CRS and neurotoxicity. Such specific complications dictate the need for personalized long-term follow-up, which will become increasingly relevant as the utilization of CAR T-cell therapy increases and as more patients enter the 15-year follow-up period mandated by the FDA for recipients of gene-modified cellular therapy.

CD19 CAR T-CELL EFFICACY IN RELAPSED/REFRACTORY PEDIATRIC AND ADULT ALL (TABLES 9.1 AND 9.2)

CD19 CAR T-cell therapy induces CR in 70%–93% of adult and pediatric patients with relapsed and refractory ALL. Almost all of the morphologic CRs reported within 1 month post–CAR T-cell infusion are MRD-negative by MFC. Published studies of CARs containing the CD28 costimulation domain report CR rates of 70% in pediatric patients and 80%–83% in adults, with MRD-negative CRs in 60% of children and 67%–80% of adults.[11,2,16] Clinical trials of 4-1BB-CARs report CR rates of 81%–93% in pediatric patients and 82%–97% in adults, with MRD-negative CRs in 73%–93% of children and 78.5%–90% of adults.[1,3,4,13,17] The durability of response is CD19 CAR construct dependent, with more durable responses reported with 4-1BB-CARs compared with CD28-CARs (Tables 9.1 and 9.2).[12] In adult studies, reported event-free survival (EFS) rates range between 50% (at 8 months) and 70.5% (at 300 days) with 4-1BB-CARs versus 39%–50% (at 6 months) with CD28-CARs.[11,13,16,18,19] In pediatric studies, 1-year EFS rates of 50% have been observed with overall survival (OS) rates of 66%–76% following 4-1BB-CAR T-cell therapy, with reported leukemia-free survival (LFS) of 78.8% (at 4.8 months)

and OS of 51.6% (at 9.7 months) following CD28-CARs.[3,4,2] This important difference in the durability of response between CD28-CARs and 4-1BB-CARs has resulted in more frequent use of hematopoietic stem cell transplantation (HCT) after achieving an MRD-negative CR with CD28-CARs. In pediatric studies, 83% of patients underwent HCT following CD28-CARs compared with 10%–26% of patients after treatment with 4-1BB-CARs.[1,3,4,2] In addition, an apparent survival benefit of consolidative HCT has been observed in children who achieve an MRD-negative remission after CD19 4-1BB CAR T-cell therapy in individuals who have not previously undergone HCT.[20]

While CD19 CAR T-cell therapy results in high rates of MRD-negative remissions in relapsed/refractory ALL within the first month of therapy, the durability of these responses is less encouraging, with 1-year EFS of 50% in pediatric patients and <50% in adults (Fig. 9.1A–C). Studies exploring factors associated with continued persistence of CAR T-cells have defined multiple factors associated with durable responses: antigen burden, type of lymphodepletion chemotherapy, CAR construct type, early maximum CAR T-cell expansion, Ig-NGS MRD-negative status post–CAR T-cell therapy, and BCA lasting >6 months (Table 9.3). In a pediatric study of CD19 4-1BB-CD3ζ CAR T-cells of defined composition, i.e. 1:1 CD4:CD8 ratio, CD19 antigen burden of >15% in the BM was associated with increased persistence of BCA (Fig. 9.1E). The same study also demonstrated improved BCA duration in patients who received a combination of fludarabine and cyclophosphamide lymphodepletion, which was also confirmed in an adult study (Fig. 9.1D).[3,13] In a study of tisagenlecleucel, measurements of CAR transgene levels by qPCR revealed that earlier maximum expansion, at a median of 10 days, occurred in responding patients, compared with a delayed expansion, at a median of 20 days, in nonresponders.[4] Ig-NGS methods have been implemented to monitor MRD in pediatric and young adult patients with ALL who have received tisagenlecleucel therapy and demonstrated superior MRD detection compared with MFC, with increased lead time to morphologic relapse of 67 versus 39 days.[21] This approach using NGS-MRD testing allows earlier identification of patients at high risk for relapse and provides a window of opportunity for such patients to proceed rapidly to HCT before morphologic relapse. In addition, patients who were NGS-MRD-negative at day 28 following CD19 CAR T-cell infusion demonstrated improved duration of response with an 80% chance of remaining relapse-free at 3 years.[21] It is of critical importance to be able to distinguish CAR T-cell—

TABLE 9.1
CD19 CAR T-Cell Therapy Outcomes in Relapsed/Refractory Pediatric ALL.

Ref	NCT Institution	N	Age (years; Median)	CAR Construct (Vector)	Cell Type Transduced	Cell Dose (Cells/kg)	RESPONSE		HCT Post-CD19 CAR (Outcomes)
							CR (MRD − CR)	EFS (OS)	
Maude, NEJM, 2014[1]	NCT01626495[a] CHOP NCT01029366[b] HUP	25[a] 5[b]	5–22[a] (11) 26–60[b] (47)	4-1BB-CD3ζ (Lentivirus)	PBMC	0.76 × 10^6/kg −20.6 × 10^6kg	90%[c] (73%[c])	6 mo EFS: 67%[c] (78%[c])	3/27 pts in CR[f] (3 pts alive) (7−12 mo)
Lee, Lancet, 2015[2]	NCT01593696 NCI	20	5–27 (14)	CD28-CD3ζ (Retrovirus)	PBMC	1 × 10^6/kg − 3 × 10^6/kg[d]	70% (60%)	4.8 mo LFS: 78.8% (9.7 mo OS: 51.6%)	10/12 MRD−pts[g] (10 pts alive)
Gardner, Blood, 2017[3]	NCT02028455 SCH	45	1–25 (12)	4-1BB-CD3ζ (Lentivirus)	T-cells, 1:1 CD4: CD8 ratio	0.5 × 10^6/kg −10 × 10^6/kg	89%[e]/93%[c] (93%[c])	1 y EFS: 50.8%[c] (65.9%[c])	11/42 pts in CR (10 pts alive)
Maude, NEJM, 2018[4]	NCT02435849 Multicenter	92/75[c]	3–23 (11)	4-1BB-CD3ζ (Lentivirus)	T-cells	0.2 ×10^6/kg −5.4 × 10^6/kg	66%[e]/81%[c] (81%[c])	1 y EFS: 50%[c] (76%[c])	6/61 MRD− pts, 2/14 MRD+ pts (8 pts alive[h])

CAR, chimeric antigen receptor; *CHOP*, Children's Hospital of Philadelphia; *CR*, complete response; *EFS*, event-free survival; *HCT*, hematopoietic stem cell transplant; *HUP*, Hospital of the University of Pennsylvania; *LFS*, leukemia-free survival; *mo*, month; *MRD*, minimal residual disease; *N*, number; *NCI*, National Cancer Institute; *NCT*, National Clinical Trial number; *OS*, overall survival; *PBMCs*, peripheral blood mononuclear cells; *pts*, patients; *Ref*, reference; *SCH*, Seattle Children's Hospital; *y*, year.
[a] Pediatric cohort.
[b] Adult cohort.
[c] Infused patients.
[d] Two patients received lower doses: 0.03 × 10^6/kg and 0.48 × 10^6/kg, one patient received higher dose: 3.6 × 10^6/kg.
[e] All enrolled.
[f] Morphologic CR, 1/27 patient in CR received DLI due to MRD.
[g] 2 patients ineligible for HCT.
[h] 4 pts with no relapse and 4 patients with unknown disease status.

TABLE 9.2
CD19 CAR T-Cell Therapy Outcomes in Relapsed/Refractory Adult ALL.

Ref	NCT Institution	N	Age (years; Median)	Diagnoses (N)	CAR Construct (Vector)	Cell Type Transduced	CAR Transduction	Cell Dose	RESPONSE CR/EFS (MRD- CR)	DFS (OS)	HCT Post-CD19 CAR, Outcomes
Turtle, JCI, 2016[13]	NCT01865617 FHCRC	32/30[a]	20–73 (40)	ALL (32)	4-1BB-CD3ζ (Lentivirus)	T-cells, 1:1 CD4:CD8 ratio (CD8 Tcm (n = 16))	CD4: 79.7% (50.0%–95.9%) CD8: 84.2% (13.0%–95.6%)	1×10^5/kg –1.16 $\times 10^7$/kg CD4 1×10^5/kg –1 $\times 10^7$/kg CD8	91%[b]/97%[a] (84%[b]/90%[a])	DFS: 70.5% Cy/Flu, n = 17 300 day median F/U (OS: 43%)	13/27 MRD–pts, 8 pts alive, 3 pts died in CR, 2 pts relapsed with CD19+ disease
Brudno, JCO, 2016[16]	NCT01087294 NIH/NCI	26/20[a]	20–68 (25)	ALL (5); CLL (5); DLBCL 4; MCL (5); TFL (1)	CD28- CD3ζ (Retrovirus)	PBMC	30.8%–86.3% (Median 67.3%)	0.4×10^6/kg –8.2 $\times 10^6$/kg	30%[a]/80% (ALL) (80%[b] (ALL))	6 mo EFS: 39%[a] (1 y OS ~80%)	1/4 MRD– pts
Frey, JCO, 2016[19]	NCT02030847 NCT01029366 HUP	27	21–72 (44)	ALL (27)	4-1BB-CD3ζ (Lentivirus)	T-cells	N/A	5×10^7/kg –5 $\times 10^8$/kg	ORR: 33% (5×10^7/kg); 83% (5×10^8/kg fractionated dosing)	33% (5×10^7/kg); 50% (5×10^8/kg)	N/A
Pan, Leukemia, 2017[18]	ClinicalTrials#: ChiCTR-IIh-16008711 Hebei Yanda Lu Daopei Hospital, China	51 (42 RR, 9 MRD+)	2–68; 11 (RR), 24 (MRD+)	ALL (51)	4-1BB-CD3ζ (Lentivirus)	PBMC	RR 16.65% (1.2%–61%) MRD+ 29% (16.6% –53.6%)	0.05×10^5/kg –14 $\times 10^5$/kg	90%[c] (RR), 100% (MRD+) (85%[b] (RR), 100% (MRD+))	133 day EFS (after HCT): 85% 8 mo EFS without HCT: 50% (N/A)	27/43 MRD–pts, 12 pts alive, median 133 days post-HCT
Cao, Am J Hematol, 2018[17]	NCT02782351 Affiliated Hospital of Xuzhou Medical University, China	18[a] (10 pediatric, 8 adult)	3–15, 19 –57 (14)	ALL (18)	Humanized 4-1BB-CD3ζ (Lentivirus)	CD3+ T-cells	22.9%–55.4%	1×10^6/kg	82%[a], 92.9%[d] (78.5%[d], 33%[e])	6 mo LFS: 65.8% (6 mo OS: 71.4%)	4/12 MRD–pts, (two allogeneic, two autologous) 3 pts alive, 207 –350 days follow-up
Park, NEJM, 2018[11]	NCT01044069 MSKCC	83/53[a]	23–74 (44)	ALL (53)	CD28-CD3ζ (Retrovirus)	T-cells	30%	1×10^6/kg –3 $\times 10^6$/kg	53%[b]/83%[a] (39%[b]/67%[a])	Median EFS 6.1 mo (Median OS 12.9 mo)	16/32 MRD–pts, 1 MRD+ pt, 5 pts alive in CR, 6 pt relapses, 6 pt deaths (TRM)

ALL, acute lymphoblastic leukemia; *CAR*, chimeric antigen receptor; *CLL*, chronic lymphocytic leukemia; *Cy/Flu*, cyclophosphamide/fludarabine; *DLBCL*, diffuse large B-cell lymphoma; *EFS*, event-free survival; *FHCRC*, Fred Hutchinson Cancer Research Center; *F/U*, follow up; *HCT*, hematopoietic stem cell transplant; *HUP*, Hospital of the University of Pennsylvania; *LFS*, leukemia-free survival; *MCL*, mantle cell lymphoma; *MRD*, minimal residual disease; *MSKCC*, Memorial Sloan Kettering Cancer Center; *N*, number; *N/A*, not available; *NCI*, National Cancer Institute; *NCT*, National Clinical Trial number; *NIH*, National Institutes of Health; *ORR*, objective response rate; *OS*, overall survival; *Ref*, Reference; *RR*, relapsed/refractory; *TFL*, transformed follicular lymphoma; *TRM*, treatment-related mortality.
[a] Infused patients.
[b] All enrolled.
[c] CR or CRi (CR with incomplete hematologic recovery).
[d] First CAR infusion.
[e] Second CAR infusion.

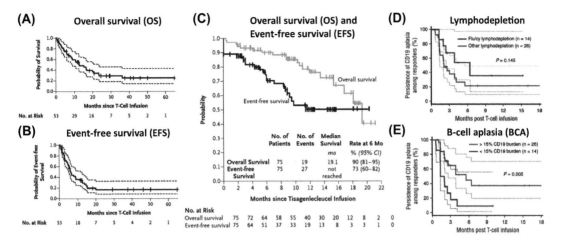

a, b: [11] Park JH, Rivière I, Gonen M, et al. Long-Term Follow-up of CD19 CAR Therapy in Acute Lymphoblastic Leukemia. *New England Journal of Medicine.* 2018;378(5):449-459. doi:10.1056/NEJMoa1709919
c: [4] Maude SL, Laetsch TW, Buechner J, et al. Tisagenlecleucel in Children and Young Adults with B-Cell Lymphoblastic Leukemia. *New England Journal of Medicine.* 2018;378(5):439-448. doi:10.1056/NEJMoa1709866
d: [3] Gardner RA, Finney O, Annesley C, et al. Intent-to-treat leukemia remission by CD19 CAR T cells of defined formulation and dose in children and young adults. *Blood.* 2017;129(25):3322-3331. doi:10.1182/blood-2017-02-769208

FIG. 9.1 Overall Survival (OS) and Event Free Survival (EFS) in pivotal CAR T-cell clinical trials.

TABLE 9.3
Factors Associated With CR and Long-Term CAR Persistence and Responses.

	Reference
Higher disease burden (BM > 5–15% CD19+)	Gardner, *Blood*, 2017,[3] Park, *NEJM*, 2018[11]
Lymphodepletion type (fludarabine/ cyclophosphamide)	Gardner, *Blood*, 2017,[3] Turtle, *JCI*, 2016[13]
Early maximum CAR T-cell expansion	Maude, *NEJM*, 2018[4]
MRD-negative status, especially by Ig-NGS (day 28)	Pulsipher, *ASH*, 2018[21]
B-cell aplasia >6 months	Gardner, *Blood*, 2017,[3] Mueller, *CCR*, 2018[22]

BM, bone marrow; *CAR*, chimeric antigen receptor; *CR*, bone marrow; *MRD*, minimal residual disease; *NGS*, next-generation sequencing.

induced CRs that will persist without any additional therapy from those that are short lived and use this distinction to avoid the toxicities of HCT in patients who may not otherwise need additional therapy.[3,4,11,21] As BCA is a pharmacodynamic surrogate marker of functional CAR T-cell persistence, early B-cell recovery within 6 months of tisagenlecleucel infusion was associated with early loss of CAR T-cells and potentially relapse (Table 9.3).[22]

LONG-TERM CD19 CAR T-CELL RESPONSES IN RELAPSED/REFRACTORY PEDIATRIC AND ADULT ALL (TABLES 9.1 AND 9.2)

Long-term responses in patients with relapsed and refractory ALL have only recently been systematically evaluated, and very few large studies report responses >1 year duration given the relatively recent introduction of this therapy in the pediatric and adult setting.[3,4,11] In pediatric studies, 1-year EFS of approximately 50% has been reported with CD19 4-1BB-CD3ζ CARs, while OS at 9.7 months was 51.6% with CD19 CD28-CD3ζ CARs.[3,4,2] HCT following treatment with CD19 4-1BB-CD3ζ CAR T-cells was performed in 10%–26% of pediatric patients in CR and resulted in 90%–100% survival.[3,4] Of 12 patients in CR following treatment with CD28-CD3ζ CAR T-cells, 10 patients (80%) received consolidative HCT, and 100%, all 10, were alive at the time of reporting.[2]

Long-term responses in older adults with relapsed and refractory ALL show similarly durable responses. In 30 patients treated with CD19 4-1BB-CD3ζ CARs, disease-free survival (DFS) was 70.5% with 300 days of median follow-up.[6] In a single institution study of adults with relapsed, refractory, or MRD + ALL treated with CD19 4-1BB-CD3ζ CARs, 8-month EFS was 50% for patients who did not receive HCT, while 133-day EFS was 85% for patients who received HCT.[18] In the largest follow-up study to date, of 53 adults treated with CD19-CD28-CD3ζ CARs, median EFS was

6.1 months, and median OS was 12.9 months.[11] In this single center study, patients with low disease burden (<5% BM blasts) had significantly improved EFS and OS compared with patients with high disease burden (≥5% BM blasts or extramedullary disease), with EFS of 10.5 versus 5.3 months and OS of 20.1 versus 12.4 months.[11] These findings are in contrast to those of 4-1BB-CD3ζ CARs, where a high disease burden (>5% or >15% BM blasts) was associated with improved CAR T-cell persistence and outcomes. The authors of the CD28-CD3ζ CAR report speculated that patients with low disease burden were more likely to achieve a high CAR T-cell to leukemia cell ratio that is required for effective disease eradication. Although multiple prior studies had correlated longer CAR T-cell persistence with improved survival, this was not the case for the CD19-CD28-CD3ζ CAR T-cell study, in which the median CAR T-cell persistence of 14 days was not associated with longer survival.[11] Studies have demonstrated T-cell–mediated rejection responses directed at murine single-chain variable fragment (scFv) CAR epitopes as contributing to limited CAR T-cell persistence, and humanized and fully human CD19 4-1BB-CD3ζ CARs have been developed.[13,23] Thus far, published data from phase 1 clinical trials is promising using humanized CD19 4-1BB-CD3ζ CARs, with 6-month LFS of 65.8% and OS of 71.4%, results that are similar to those with murine CD19 CARs, though data on CAR persistence with the humanized construct is limited.[17]

LIMITED CAR T-CELL PERSISTENCE: THERAPEUTIC OPTIONS

For patients with limited CAR T-cell persistence, a second infusion of CAR T-cells has been performed, with or without repeat lymphodepleting chemotherapy using varying intensity (sometimes increased); however, there are limited reports of engraftment and antileukemic activity.[3,13] The addition of checkpoint inhibitors, such as pembrolizumab, has been associated with CAR T-cell reexpansion, persistence, and objective responses in a subset of patients in early studies.[24] In our center, we routinely monitor BCA in patients who have received CD19 CAR T-cell therapy. For patients who demonstrate loss of BCA (absolute peripheral blood CD19+ lymphocyte count >50 cells/μL), especially within the first 6 months following infusion, we recommend a second CD19 CAR T-cell infusion followed by a checkpoint inhibitor, such as pembrolizumab.[24] If the patients continue to demonstrate poor CAR T-cell persistence and loss of BCA but remain in

MRD-negative remission (by MFC), we recommend a consolidative HCT, especially for patients who have not previously undergone HCT.

EFFICACY OF CD19 CAR T-CELL THERAPY IN ADULT NHL (TABLE 9.4)

High response rates after CD19 CAR T-cell therapy have also been demonstrated in NHL, especially in diffuse large B-cell lymphoma (DLBCL), follicular lymphoma (FL), and mantle cell lymphoma (MCL).[25] Best reported ORRs, which include CRs and PRs, range between 52% and 100%.[5,10] In an international, multicenter study of tisagenlecleucel in patients with DLBCL and transformed FL (TFL), 37 of 93 (40%) of patients achieved a CR at a median of 2 months (range 1–17 months), including 16 patients who had either SD (n = 4) or PR (n = 12) at 1 month after infusion.[10] A conversion from PR to CR occurred in 13 of 24 (54%) of patients in the study.[10] Importantly, remission at 3 months was predictive of long-term remission at 12 months, in which 28 of 35 (81%) of patients who were in remission by 3 months remained in remission at 12 months.[10]

The pivotal multicenter, phase 2, ZUMA-1 trial examined the efficacy of axicabtagene ciloleucel (CD19 CD28-CD3ζ CAR T-cells) in 101 patients with relapsed or refractory DLBCL, primary mediastinal B-cell lymphoma (PMBCL), and TFL.[8] Best ORR included CR (disappearance of measurable disease on CT scan or residual, PET negative masses) and PR (≥50% decrease in tumor burden with ongoing PET avidity) in 82% of patients, 54% of patients with CR, and 28% with PR, with a median response time of 1 month.[8] Two-year follow-up results demonstrated an OS of 51% and PFS of 39% at a median follow-up of 27.1 months.[26] In addition, the follow-up results confirmed that the responses were durable, in which 93% of patients who demonstrated a response at 12 months continued with response at 2 years.[26]

The international, phase 2 study, JULIET, using tisagenlecleucel (CD19 4-1BB-CD3ζ CAR T-cells) in patients with relapsed or refractory DLBCL demonstrated ORRs and CR rates of 52% and 40%, respectively.[10] Six-month ORRs and CR rates were 33% and 29%, respectively.[10] Remissions were durable; 1-year relapse-free survival (RFS) was 65% and OS was 49%.[10] Similar responses were also demonstrated in a multicenter phase 1 trial with lisocabtagene maraleucel (JCAR017; CD19 4-1BB-CD3ζ CAR T-cells) in patients with relapsed or refractory DLBCL: best ORRs and CR rates were 80% and 52%, respectively, and 3-month ORR was 74% in the

TABLE 9.4
CD19 CAR T-Cell Therapy in Adult NHL.

Ref	NCT/Trial/Institution	N	Diagnoses	Age (years; Median)	CD19 CAR Construct (Vector)	Cell Type Transduced	Cell Dose	RESPONSE ORR (CR)	RESPONSE PFS/RFS (OS)
Wang, *Blood*, 2016[5] DLBCL (11); MCL (5)	NCT01318317 NHL1 NCT01815749 NHL2	8 (NHL1) 8 (NHL2)	DLBCL (7) MCL (1) (NHL1) DLBCL (4) MCL (4) (NHL2)	50–75 (NHL1) (Mean 62) 23–71 (NHL2) (Mean 58)	CD3ζ—NHL1 (Lentivirus) CD28-CD3ζ—NHL2 (Lentivirus)	CD8-enriched Tcm (NHL1), "bulk" Tcm (NHL2)	NHL1: 25 × 10^6, 50 × 10^6, or 100 × 10^6 total NHL2: 50 × 10^6 or 200 × 10^6 total	NHL1: 88% (63%) NHL2: 100% (100%)	1 y PFS 50% (NHL1) 2 y PFS 50% (NHL1) 1 y PFS 75% (NHL2)
Turtle, *Science Translational Medicine*, 2016[6]	NCT01865617	32	De novo LBCL (11); TLBCL (11); FL (6); MCL (4)	36–70 (58)	4-1BB-CD3ζ (Lentivirus)	CD8 Tcm subset or bulk CD8 T-cells, 1:1 CD4:CD8 ratio	2 × 10^5/kg, 2 × 10^6/kg, or 2 × 10^7/kg	72%[a] (50%)[a] 50%[b] (8%)[b]	6 mo PFS[a] ~60% (6 mo OS[a] ~90%) 6 mo PFS[b] ~20% (6 mo OS[b] ~60%) Median PFS[b] 1.5 months
Kochenderfer, *JCO*, 2017[7]	NCT00924326	22	DLBCL (19); FL (2); MCL (1)	26–67 (54)	CD28-CD3ζ (Retrovirus)	PBMC	1 × 10^6/kg (fresh), 2 × 10^6/kg, or 6 × 10^6/kg	ORR 73% (CR 55%)	1 y PFS 63.3% *(1 y OS ~70%)*
Neelapu, *NEJM*, 2017[8]	NCT02348216 ZUMA-1 US & Israel, 22 sites	111 enrolled 101[c]	DLBCL (77), PMBCL (8), TFL (16)	23–76 (58)	CD28-CD3ζ (Retrovirus)	T-cells	2 × 10^6/kg	ORR 82% (CR 54%) 6 mo ORR 41% (6 mo ORR 36%)	1 y PFS 44% (1 y OS 59%)
Abramson, *JCO*, 2018[9]	NCT02631044 TRANSCEND NHL 001 US, 14 sites	91 65[d]	DLBCL, TFL, PMBCL	26–82 (61)	4-1BB-CD3ζ (Lentivirus)	T-cells, 1:1 CD4:CD8 ratio	DL1: 5 × 10^7 DL2: 1 × 10^8	Best ORR 74%[c] Best ORR 80%[d] *(Best CR 52%)[d]* 3 mo ORR 65%[c]–74%[d] *(3 mo CR 54%[c] –52%[d])* 6 mo ORR 50%[b] (DL2) *(6 mo CR 50%)[b] (DL2)*	1 y RFS: 42%

Continued

TABLE 9.4
CD19 CAR T-Cell Therapy in Adult NHL.—cont'd

Ref	NCT/Trial/Institution	N	Diagnoses	Age (years; Median)	CD19 CAR Construct (Vector)	Cell Type Transduced	Cell Dose	RESPONSE	
								ORR (CR)	PFS/RFS (OS)
Schuster, NEJM, 2019[10]	NCT02445248 JULIET 10 countries, 27 sites	93[e]	DLBCL, TFL	22–76 (56)	4-1BB-CD3ζ (Lentivirus)	T-cells	0.1×10^8–6×10^8 (Median: 3.1×10^8)	Best ORR 52% (Best CR 40%) 3 mo ORR 38% (3 mo CR 32%) 6 mo ORR 33% (6 mo CR 29%)	1 y RFS: 65% (1 y OS: 49%)

DL, dose level; DLBCL, diffuse large B-cell lymphoma; EFS, event-free survival; FL, follicular lymphoma; LBCL, large B-cell lymphoma; MCL, mantle cell lymphoma; N, number; NHL, non-Hodgkin lymphoma; NOS, not otherwise specified; ORR, objective response rate; OS, overall survival; PFS, progression-free survival; PMBCL, primary mediastinal B-cell lymphoma; RFS, relapse-free survival; Tcm, T central memory; TFL, transformed follicular lymphoma; TLBL, transformed large B-cell lymphoma.

[a] Cyclophosphamide/fludarabine lymphodepletion.
[b] Cyclophosphamide-based lymphodepletion without fludarabine.
[c] Total number of patients treated.
[d] Core cohort, DLBCL NOS, and high-grade lymphoma only.
[e] Main cohort (product manufactured in the United States, infusion ≥ 3 months of follow-up before the data cutoff date).

core patient cohort that included DLBCL not otherwise specified (NOS) and high-grade lymphoma only.[9] Durability of responses was similar to other CD19 CAR T-cell trials in NHL; 1-year RFS was 42%.

LONG-TERM CD19 CAR T-CELL RESPONSES IN ADULT NHL (TABLE 9.4)

In NHL, long-term, durable CAR responses were demonstrated in three recent key trials: ZUMA-1, TRANSCEND NHL, and JULIET, with 1-year PFS of 44% and 1-year RFS of 42% and 65%, respectively.[9,10,27] One-year OS was 59% in ZUMA-1 and 49% in JULIET.[8,10] Importantly, some patients without CR at 1 month postinfusion converted to CR (11 of 35 with PR; 12 of 25 with SD) as late as 15 months after treatment, and those CRs were sustained with few relapses.[8] Notably, there were no relapses observed in ZUMA-1 patients who were in CR at 1 year.[26]

POST—CAR T-CELL THERAPY MANAGEMENT

CD19 CAR T cell therapy is associated with unique toxicities and complications that require a variety of complicated management strategies in at least 50% of patients during the acute setting, and all patients require long-term follow-up monitoring after CAR T-cell therapy.[27,28] Those who receive CAR T-cell infusion in the inpatient setting are monitored in the hospital for CRS and immune effector cell—associated neurotoxicity syndrome (ICANS) until resolution of clinical and biochemical markers of toxicities. Following discharge, patients are monitored closely in the outpatient setting. For patients who receive CAR T-cells as an outpatient procedure, follow-up visits are usually conducted two to three times per week for the first 3—4 weeks to monitor for CRS, ICANS, the need for transfusions, and symptoms of infection. Almost all patients will develop fever, at which point hospitalization for monitoring and care is needed until CRS is resolved. Generally, at day 28 post—CAR T-cell therapy, disease reevaluation is performed. Patients subsequently have at least monthly visits for IVIG supplementation to manage hypogammaglobulinemia, which is a direct consequence of CD19 CAR T-cell—mediated BCA. Consensus guidelines for the management of acute CD19 CAR T-cell therapy—associated toxicities and complications have been established for pediatric and adult patients.[27—29] However, systematic, comprehensive long-term evaluation and management guidelines have not yet been developed and adopted by the CAR T-cell community.

The recommendations below are a systems-based approach guided by a comprehensive review of published reports of CD19 CAR T-cell—mediated toxicities.

RECOMMENDED EVALUATIONS AND INTERVENTIONS TIMELINE (TABLE 9.5)
Cardiovascular

Cardiac failure is listed on the package inserts as occurring in 7% of patients treated with tisagenlecleucel and in 6% of patients treated with axicabtagene ciloleucel, but it is generally transitory and there is a higher incidence of other short-term cardiovascular toxicities. Sinus tachycardia occurs often and is nonspecific but can be an early clinical sign of CRS, especially in pediatric patients. Thus, pediatric CAR T-cell management guidelines have included cardiac monitoring through resolution of CRS.[28] In a study of 93 pediatric patients receiving CD19 CAR T-cell therapy, hypotension requiring inotropic support occurred in 24 (26%) patients, with a median onset of 4.6 days postinfusion, coincident with the timing of CRS.[30] The vast majority, 88% of the patients who developed hypotension, required tocilizumab with or without steroids.[30] 6 (6%) patients required milrinone, and 10 (11%) patients had decreased systolic function on echocardiogram, which persisted until hospital discharge in 6 (6%) patients.[30] New-onset cardiac dysfunction that is persistent is rare following CD19 CAR T-cell therapy; only one patient had persistent diastolic dysfunction at the time of hospital discharge.[30] BM blast count >25%, baseline lower ejection fraction (EF), or diastolic dysfunction, but not preexisting cardiomyopathy, total body irradiation (TBI), or anthracycline dose, were identified as the key risk factors associated with the development of hypotension requiring inotropic support.[30] Understanding and further refining risk factors for cardiovascular complications is critical to identify patients who may warrant closer observation after CAR T-cell infusion. Although there are limited studies to determine the long-term cardiac effects of CAR T-cell therapy, data from these 93 pediatric patients demonstrated resolution of cardiac dysfunction in all but one patient at the 6-month follow-up timepoint.[30]

Recommendations for post—CAR cardiology follow-up

Based on the limited available data on cardiac complications of CD19 CAR T-cell therapy, consider follow-up echocardiogram and serum biomarker evaluation (e.g., brain natriuretic protein) in conjunction with

TABLE 9.5
Recommended Long-Term Follow Up Evaluations and Interventions.

aa	Labs/Studies/Medications	ASSESSMENTS AND MANAGEMENT (DAYS (D)/MONTHS (M))* D+28 through m+11	m+12	m+13 through m+180
Cardiovascular				
ECHO	Serial monitoring after d+28 for patients with decreased cardiac function at least through m+6		X	X q 12m
Cardiology follow-up	For patients with decreased cardiac function at least through m+6			
Cardiac remodeling agents, e.g., Enalapril	Per cardiology recommendations for patients with decreased cardiac function			
Hematologic				
CBC, including ALC	At least monthly d+28 through m+11		X	X q 12m
Transfusions	PRBC/Plt to maintain Hgb >8 g/dL, Plt >10,000/µL or higher levels as clinically indicated			
Filgrastim (G-CSF)	For ANC <500/µL			
Eltrombopag	For persistent thrombocytopenia requiring Plt transfusions			
Immunology				
IgG levels	Monthly starting at d+28 (if level is high preinfusion, earlier if level is low) while receiving immunoglobulin infusion to maintain IgG >400 mg/dL, target higher levels in the setting of recurrent sinopulmonary infections despite adequate IgG trough levels			
B-cell aplasia (absolute CD19 counts)	Monthly starting at d+28			
Infectious disease				
PJP prophylaxis	Pentamidine (monthly if ANC <500/µL), TMP/SMX (BID × 2 days/week if ANC >500/µL)			
Fungal prophylaxis	Fluconazole or voriconazole or posaconazole if ANC <500/µL and/or for patients with a history of suspected fungal infection			
Viral prophylaxis	Acyclovir or valacyclovir for HSV- and VZV-seropositive individuals			
Neurology				
Seizure prophylaxis	Levetiracetam through d+30 or longer if neurologic risk factors			
Neurology follow-up	Patients with a history of neurologic toxicities or dysfunction			
Neuropsychiatric assessment	q3 months d+28 through m+11		X	X[a]
Oncology				
BMA	d+28 with NGS-MRD			
LP	d+28			
FDG-PET (NHL)	m+1	m+2 and serial studies to monitor for conversion from PR to CR		

ALC, absolute lymphocyte count; *ANC*, absolute neutrophil count; *BID*, twice daily; *BMA*, bone marrow aspirate; *CBC*, complete blood count; *d*, days; *ECHO*, echocardiogram; *FDG-PET*, fluorodeoxyglucose-positron emission tomography; *G-CSF*, granulocyte colony-stimulating factor; *HSV*, herpes simplex virus; *IgG*, immunoglobulin G; *IVIG*, intravenous immunoglobulin; *LP*, lumbar puncture; *m*, months; *NGS-MRD*, next-generation sequencing minimal residual disease; *PJP*, pneumocystis jiroveci pneumonia; *Plt*, platelet; *PRBCs*, packed red blood cells; *TMP/SMX*, trimethoprim/sulfamethoxazole; *VZV*, varicella zoster virus.

*Frequency of assessments should be increased and/or management modified as clinically indicated.

[a] q3 months years 1–3, q6 months years 4–5, q12 months years 6–15.

cardiology consultation for patients with clinically evident cardiac dysfunction after CAR T-cell therapy.[30] Similar to strategies for patients who develop chemotherapy-associated heart failure, consider medications that promote reverse remodeling (e.g., enalapril) to improve cardiac function after CAR T-cell therapy for patients with CAR T-cell–associated cardiac dysfunction. This should be done in partnership with cardiology specialists. Close follow-up for such patients should continue through resolution of cardiac dysfunction, generally for 6–12 months post–CAR T-cell therapy or longer if there is evidence of persistent cardiac dysfunction.[30]

Hematology

Severe cytopenias, including anemia, thrombocytopenia, and neutropenia, may occur in 30%–60% of patients receiving CD19 CAR T-cell therapy.[15] A number of patients continue to require PRBC and platelet transfusions beyond the first month following CAR T-cell therapy. Incomplete hematologic recovery with prolonged neutropenia requiring G-CSF (filgrastim) has been described in 15% of patients by day 28 in one clinical trial of 133 adult patients with ALL, CLL, and NHL receiving CD19 CAR T-cell therapy (NCT01865617).[29] In a follow-up study of the 60 adult patients with CLL and NHL (NCT01865617), three patients (16%) developed significant cytopenias requiring transfusions, G-CSF, and erythropoietin that persisted beyond 90 days after CAR T-cell infusion that resolved at 1.7 years in one patient but persisted as severe neutropenia requiring G-CSF for 1.5 and 2 years in the other two patients.[31] In another clinical trial of CD19 CAR T-cell therapy in 35 pediatric and adult patients with ALL and NHL, late hematologic toxicities occurring beyond 42 days after infusion included neutropenia (62%), thrombocytopenia (44%), and anemia (17%).[15] The authors identified prior HCT and higher grade of CRS as risk factors strongly associated with late hematologic toxicities.[15] Grade 3 or higher cytopenias persisting beyond 30 days after infusion occurred in 28% of patients treated with axicabtagene ciloleucel, including thrombocytopenia (18%), neutropenia (15%), and anemia (3%).[32] 25%–40% of patients receiving tisagenlecleucel developed ≥ grade 3 neutropenia and 27%–40% developed thrombocytopenia that persisted beyond 28 days following infusion in JULIET and ELIANA studies.[33] Myeloid growth factors, especially granulocyte-macrophage colony-stimulating factor (GM-CSF), are not recommended during the first 21 days following tisagenlecleucel infusion or until resolution of CRS.[33] Grade 3 or higher neutropenia persisted in 17% of patients,

while ≥ grade 3 thrombocytopenia persisted in 12% of patients at 56 days following infusion in the ELIANA study.[33] Multi-institutional efforts are ongoing to capture the incidence and duration of cytopenias in patients with ALL, CLL, and NHL following CD19 CAR T-cell therapy; however, published reports are rare and currently limited to single center experiences.

Recommendations for post–CAR hematology follow-up

For patients with transfusion-dependent anemia and thrombocytopenia, we recommend PRBC transfusions to maintain Hgb >8 g/dL and platelet transfusions to maintain Plt >10,000/μL, or higher if there are signs of bleeding. In patients with persistent neutropenia, ANC <500/μL, intermittent G-CSF administration, and bacterial prophylaxis should be considered (refer to Infectious Disease (ID) section below). In patients with persistent thrombocytopenia, the mechanism for which may include interferon gamma (IFN-γ)-mediated perturbation of thrombopoietin (TPO) signaling, consider the use of the TPO mimetic, eltrombopag, to stabilize platelet counts and reduce the need for transfusions.[34]

Infectious Disease

Most of the early infectious complications that are observed in patients treated with CAR T-cell therapy are a consequence of multiple chemotherapy regimens for relapsed or refractory disease administered before CAR T-cell therapy, resulting in significant immune dysfunction and hypogammaglobulinemia.[29] In addition, lymphodepletion chemotherapy administered prior to CAR T-cell infusion can lead to further immune- and myelosuppression with increased risk of infectious complications. Treatment with corticosteroids and tocilizumab with or without other immune-targeting agents for patients experiencing severe CRS and neurotoxicity also increases the risk of infection. Thus, any patient who develops fever during presumed CRS must be treated empirically for possible infections with broad-spectrum antimicrobial agents.[29]

Hill and colleagues systematically evaluated infections in the first 90 days in 133 adult patients with ALL, CLL, and NHL who received CD19 CAR T-cell (4-1BB-CD3ζ CAR at 1:1 CD4:CD8 ratio) therapy (NCT01865617).[29] Antimicrobial prophylaxis was modeled after autologous HCT recipients and included acyclovir or valacyclovir for herpes simplex virus (HSV)–seropositive or varicella zoster virus (VZV)–seropositive patients from the start of lymphodepletion chemotherapy through ≥3 months post–CAR T-cell therapy; levofloxacin and fluconazole until ANC >500 cells/μL; and trimethoprim/sulfamethoxazole for 2 days each week starting after neutrophil engraftment until $\geq$3 months after CAR T-cell infusion, in addition to IVIG supplementation to maintain serum IgG levels >400 mg/dL.[29] 30 patients (23%) developed 43 infections in the first 28 days.[29] The most common type of infection was bacterial (17%), followed by viral (8%) and invasive fungal (3%) infection.[29] The initial infection occurred at a median of 6 days (range, 1–27 days) after the onset of CRS.[29] 5% of patients developed invasive fungal infections, and 4% of patients had life-threatening infections. Risk factors contributing to increased rate of infections were a diagnosis of ALL, $\geq$4 prior therapies, and a higher CAR T-cell dose (2 × 10^7/kg).[29] Multivariate analysis revealed that only CRS severity was associated with infection. BCA occurred in 98% of patients; by day 90, only 21% of patients had evidence of B-cell recovery, and 46% had persistent hypogammaglobulinemia.[29] There were fewer infections beyond 28 days: 17 patients (14%) had 23 infections, and viral infections were most common (9%), the majority of which were upper respiratory tract infections.[29] However, two patients without a prior history of HCT developed CMV viremia and pneumonia, respectively, while one patient developed BK cystitis.[29] Seven patients (6%) developed eight bacterial infections, half of which were bacteremia.[29] Invasive fungal infections occurred in two patients (2%) who had received prior allogeneic HCT.[29] Almost 50% of the patients with late infections had persistent malignancy, and 22% had neutropenia.[29] These findings suggest that the incidence of infection following CD19 CAR T-cell therapy is lower than in patients receiving unrelated donor myeloablative HCT but that the types of infection are similar.[29] Notably in this study, few infections that occurred after CAR T-cell therapy were life-threatening or severe; however, some infections, such as bacterial sinusitis, perirectal abscess, and invasive fungal sinusitis, were present before lymphodepletion and progressed after CAR T-cell infusion.[29] A longer-term follow-up study of 60 patients with CLL and NHL treated with CD19 CAR T-cell (4-1BB-CD3ζ CAR at 1:1 CD4:CD8 ratio) therapy (NCT01865617) who were beyond 90 days after infusion, with a median follow-up of 1 year, demonstrated 138 late infections occurring in 31 patients.[31] The majority of late infections were mild with 80% successfully managed in the outpatient setting.[31] Respiratory infections accounted for 77% of infections, followed by bacterial infections, and rarely, fungal infections.[31]

Recommendations for post–CAR ID follow-up

We recommend a thorough ID evaluation for patients receiving CAR T-cell therapy to evaluate prior infectious history and any current infections. We also recommend administration of antimicrobial prophylaxis during periods of neutropenia and peak immunosuppression to prevent common infectious complications. Specific recommendations include PJP prophylaxis with pentamidine, especially during neutropenia, followed by trimethoprim/sulfamethoxazole (TMP/SMX) upon count recovery through at least 3 months post–CAR T-cell therapy or until the CD4 count exceeds 200/μL, whichever is longer. Fungal prophylaxis should include either fluconazole or a broader-spectrum azole such as voriconazole or posaconazole for patients with a history of or suspected fungal infections. In addition, viral prophylaxis with acyclovir or valacyclovir is recommended for HSV- and/or VZV-seropositive individuals.

Immunology

Hypogammaglobulinemia is common and expected following CAR T-cell therapy with variable duration based on CAR T-cell persistence and associated BCA, lasting for months to years. In adult patients with CLL and NHL treated with CD19 CAR T-cell (4-1BB-CD3ζ CAR at 1:1 CD4:CD8 ratio) therapy (NCT01865617), hypogammaglobulinemia beyond 90 days after infusion was common and occurred in 60% of patients.[31] Hypogammaglobulinemia is a risk factor for recurrent infections, as demonstrated in patients with humoral immune deficiency, resulting in upper and lower respiratory tract infections (sinusitis, bronchitis, or pneumonia) or gastrointestinal tract infections (parasitic or bacterial gastroenteritis), as well as joint or skin infections.[35,36]

Recommendations for post–CAR immunology follow-up

We recommend monthly testing of IgG levels and immunoglobulin (IV or subcutaneous) supplementation to maintain trough IgG levels >400 mg/dL and higher trough levels for patients who develop recurrent sinopulmonary infections while receiving immunoglobulin replacement.[36]

Neurology

Neurologic toxicity/ICANS occurs in 40%–50% of patients receiving CD19 CAR T-cell therapy.[37] In 133 adult patients treated with CD19 CAR T-cell therapy, 53 (40%) patients developed neurologic toxicity, clinically characterized by delirium with preserved alertness, headache, decreased level of consciousness, language disturbance, and infrequently, focal neurologic deficits, ataxia, and seizures.[38] Acute brain MRI abnormalities were evident in only 30% of patients with neurologic toxicity who underwent such imaging.[38] In the majority of patients, neurologic toxicities resolved by day 28.[38]

Recommendations for post–CAR neurology follow-up

We recommend baseline neurology evaluation for all patients with a history of neurologic toxicity with prior therapy or with CNS dysfunction and associated brain MRI findings. In addition, we recommend a baseline neurocognitive and neuropsychologic assessment, especially for children and young adults who may experience neurologic toxicities that can affect future knowledge acquisition and school performance. Following CAR T-cell therapy, we recommend routine use of the ICANS screening tools, the Cornell Assessment of Pediatric Delirium (CAPD; for children <12 years old or for children >12 years old with baseline developmental delay) and the Immune Effector Cell–Associated Encephalopathy (ICE) score for children ≥12 years old and adults, to monitor for any neurologic changes. Antiseizure prophylaxis with levetiracetam should be instituted at the start of lymphodepletion chemotherapy and continued for 30 days for all patients. For patients with prior CNS disease or seizure history, we recommend neurology follow-up to help determine the duration of levetiracetam therapy.

Other, Less Common Organ Toxicities Following CAR T-Cell Therapy: Pulmonary, Renal, Hepatic, Graft-Versus-Host Disease

Pulmonary toxicity is mainly observed during CRS, manifesting clinically as hypoxia. Additional pulmonary complications include infectious complications (refer to ID section above), for which patients should undergo focused testing including blood cultures, serum markers (e.g., beta-D-glucan, galactomannan for fungal infections), and sputum and endotracheal tube secretion or bronchoalveolar lavage testing to identify a possible infectious source. In addition, post-HCT patients should continue to undergo pulmonary function testing (PFT) for routine post-HCT long-term follow-up.

Renal toxicity is also mainly observed during CRS, complicated by tumor lysis syndrome in patients with high disease burden. No systematic studies have evaluated the duration of acute kidney injury (AKI) in post-CAR T-cell patients, but chronic renal insufficiency is possible. In patients with elevated serum creatinine, proteinuria, and/or hypertension, we recommend close monitoring and follow-up of renal function, maintaining adequate hydration, treatment of hypertension and nephrology consultation as needed.

Hepatotoxicity can be observed during CRS, commonly in the setting of hemophagocytic lymphohistiocytosis (HLH) with coagulopathy. This may persist after CAR T-cell therapy and can be exacerbated by concurrent hepatotoxic medications. There are no studies that identify the incidence and prevalence of hepatic dysfunction in patients post–CAR T-cell therapy. We recommend routine liver function test monitoring and avoiding the administration of hepatotoxic medications whenever possible.

For post-HCT patients receiving allogeneic-derived CAR T-cell therapy, patients should be monitored for the development of acute and chronic graft-versus-host disease (GVHD). In various clinical trials using allogeneic CD19 CAR T-cells, which included 132 patients with B-cell malignancies, acute GVHD developed in 4% of patients and chronic GVHD in 3% of patients.[39] With such a low incidence, and the subjective nature of clinical GVHD diagnosis, it is unclear whether this is true GVHD. Monitoring for the development of GVHD will become even more critical as nonautologous universal, off-the-shelf, CAR T-cell therapies become more widely utilized. One such approach, UCART19, a non–HLA-matched CD19 CAR T-cell product with gene-edited T-cell receptor alpha and CD52 is currently in clinical trials (NCT02808442). In 20 pediatric and adult patients with relapsed/refractory ALL treated with UCART19, two patients developed grade 1 acute skin GVHD following CAR T-cell infusion, which was responsive to steroids.[40]

Long-Term Follow-Up After CAR T-Cell Therapy (for More Details, Refer to Chapter 14)

The FDA mandates 15 years of follow-up for patients who have received gene-modified cellular therapy.[23] Given the relatively recent introduction of CAR T-cell therapy for the treatment of B-cell malignancies, coordinated and comprehensive registry efforts will need to be prioritized and evaluation guidelines established and revised to collect data about the specific side effects of CAR T-cell therapy and their duration as well as to optimize and expand the use of CAR T-cell therapy.

CONCLUSION

With the expected increased use of CAR T-cell therapy for relapsed/refractory hematologic and other malignancies, detailed guidelines for disease response assessment and posttherapy management will be critical to optimize outcomes. The majority of data guiding the current recommendations are derived from reports and experience with CD19 CAR T-cell therapy. As CAR constructs targeting antigens other than CD19 enter the clinic in the future, the large experience with CD19 CARs provide a starting point from which to consider post-CAR management recommendations. However, it is expected that other CARs will have antigen-specific toxicities that will require special consideration and may differ from the CD19-directed CAR T-cells. As CAR T-cell therapy becomes optimized to minimize toxicity, more sensitive molecularly based methods will be used to determine persistence of therapeutic response and for early detection of disease recurrence. Finally, standardized, organ-specific guidelines will be crucial for long-term management of patients after CAR T-cell therapy.

REFERENCES

1. Maude SL, Frey N, Shaw PA, et al. Chimeric antigen receptor T cells for sustained remissions in leukemia. *N Engl J Med.* 2014;371(16):1507−1517. https://doi.org/10.1056/NEJMoa1407222.
2. Lee DW, Kochenderfer JN, Stetler-Stevenson M, et al. T cells expressing CD19 chimeric antigen receptors for acute lymphoblastic leukaemia in children and young adults: a phase 1 dose-escalation trial. *The Lancet.* 2015;385(9967):517−528. https://doi.org/10.1016/S0140-6736(14)61403-3.
3. Gardner RA, Finney O, Annesley C, et al. Intent-to-treat leukemia remission by CD19 CAR T cells of defined formulation and dose in children and young adults. *Blood.* 2017;129(25):3322−3331. https://doi.org/10.1182/blood-2017-02-769208.
4. Maude SL, Laetsch TW, Buechner J, et al. Tisagenlecleucel in children and young adults with B-cell lymphoblastic leukemia. *N Engl J Med.* 2018;378(5):439−448. https://doi.org/10.1056/NEJMoa1709866.
5. Wang X, Popplewell LL, Wagner JR, et al. Phase 1 studies of central memory-derived CD19 CAR T-cell therapy following autologous HSCT in patients with B-cell NHL. *Blood.* 2016;127(24):2980−2990. https://doi.org/10.1182/blood-2015-12-686725.
6. Turtle CJ, Hanafi L-A, Berger C, et al. Immunotherapy of non-Hodgkin's lymphoma with a defined ratio of CD8+ and CD4+ CD19-specific chimeric antigen receptor−modified T cells. *Sci Transl Med.* 2016;8(355):355ra116. https://doi.org/10.1126/scitranslmed.aaf8621.
7. Kochenderfer JN, Somerville RP, Lu T, et al. Lymphoma remissions caused by anti-CD19 chimeric antigen receptor T cells are associated with high serum interleukin-15 levels. *J Clin Oncol.* 2017;35(16):1803−1819.
8. Neelapu SS, Locke FL, Bartlett NL, et al. Axicabtagene ciloleucel CAR T-cell therapy in refractory large B-cell lymphoma. *N Engl J Med.* 2017;377(26):2531−2544. https://doi.org/10.1056/NEJMoa1707447.
9. Abramson JS, Gordon LI, Palomba ML, et al. Updated safety and long term clinical outcomes in TRANSCEND NHL 001, pivotal trial of lisocabtagene maraleucel (JCAR017) in R/R aggressive NHL. *J Clin Oncol.* 2018;36(15_suppl 1):7505. https://doi.org/10.1200/JCO.2018.36.15_suppl.7505.
10. Schuster SJ, Bishop MR, Tam CS, et al. Tisagenlecleucel in adult relapsed or refractory diffuse large B-cell lymphoma. *N Engl J Med.* 2019;380(1):45−56. https://doi.org/10.1056/NEJMoa1804980.
11. Park JH, Rivière I, Gonen M, et al. Long-term follow-up of CD19 CAR therapy in acute lymphoblastic leukemia. *N Engl J Med.* 2018;378(5):449−459. https://doi.org/10.1056/NEJMoa1709919.
12. Long AH, Haso WM, Shern JF, et al. 4-1BB costimulation ameliorates T cell exhaustion induced by tonic signaling of chimeric antigen receptors. *Nat Med.* 2015;21(6):581−590.
13. Turtle CJ, Hanafi L-A, Berger C, et al. CD19 CAR−T cells of defined CD4+:CD8+ composition in adult B cell ALL patients. *J Clin Invest.* 2016;126(6):2123−2138. https://doi.org/10.1172/JCI85309.
14. Cheson BD, Fisher RI, Barrington SF, et al. Recommendations for initial evaluation, staging, and response assessment of Hodgkin and non-Hodgkin lymphoma: the Lugano classification. *J Clin Oncol.* 2014;32(27):3059−3067. https://doi.org/10.1200/JCO.2013.54.8800.
15. Fried S, Avigdor A, Bielorai B, et al. Early and late hematologic toxicity following CD19 CAR-T cells. *Bone Marrow Transplant.* February 2019. https://doi.org/10.1038/s41409-019-0487-3.
16. Brudno JN, Somerville RPT, Shi V, et al. Allogeneic T cells that express an anti-CD19 chimeric antigen receptor induce remissions of B-cell malignancies that progress after allogeneic hematopoietic stem-cell transplantation without causing graft-versus-host disease. *J Clin Oncol.* 2016;34(10):1112−1121. https://doi.org/10.1200/JCO.2015.64.5929.
17. Cao J, Wang G, Cheng H, et al. Potent anti-leukemia activities of humanized CD19-targeted Chimeric antigen receptor T (CAR-T) cells in patients with relapsed/refractory acute lymphoblastic leukemia. *Am J Hematol.* 2018;93(7):851−858. https://doi.org/10.1002/ajh.25108.
18. Pan J, Yang JF, Deng BP, et al. High efficacy and safety of low-dose CD19-directed CAR-T cell therapy in 51 refractory or relapsed B acute lymphoblastic leukemia patients. *Leukemia.* 2017;31(12):2587−2593. https://doi.org/10.1038/leu.2017.145.
19. Frey NV, Shaw PA, Hexner EO, et al. Optimizing chimeric antigen receptor (CAR) T cell therapy for adult patients with relapsed or refractory (r/r) acute lymphoblastic leukemia (ALL). *J Clin Oncol.* 2016;34(15_suppl 1):7002. https://doi.org/10.1200/JCO.2016.34.15_suppl.7002.
20. Summers C, Annesley C, Bleakley M, et al. Long term follow-up after SCRI-CAR19v1 reveals late recurrences as well as a survival advantage to consolidation with HCT after CAR T cell induced remission. *Blood.* 2018;132(suppl_1):967. https://doi.org/10.1182/blood-2018-99-115599.

21. Pulsipher M, Han X, Quigley M, et al. Molecular detection of minimal residual disease precedes morphological relapse and could be used to identify relapse in pediatric and young adult B-cell acute lymphoblastic leukemia patients treated with tisagenlecleucel. *Blood.* 2018; 132(suppl_1):1551. https://doi.org/10.1182/blood-2018-99-115460.

22. Mueller KT, Waldron E, Grupp SA, et al. Clinical Pharmacology of tisagenlecleucel in B-cell acute lymphoblastic leukemia. *Clin Cancer Res.* 2018;24(24):6175–6184. https://doi.org/10.1158/1078-0432.CCR-18-0758.

23. Jensen MC, Popplewell L, Cooper LJ, et al. Antitransgene rejection responses contribute to attenuated persistence of adoptively transferred CD20/CD19-specific chimeric antigen receptor redirected T cells in humans. *Biol Blood Marrow Transplant.* 2010;16(9):1245–1256. https://doi.org/10.1016/j.bbmt.2010.03.014.

24. Maude SL, Hucks GE, Seif AE, et al. The effect of pembrolizumab in combination with CD19-targeted chimeric antigen receptor (CAR) T cells in relapsed acute lymphoblastic leukemia (ALL). *J Clin Oncol.* 2017; 35(15_suppl l):103. https://doi.org/10.1200/JCO.2017.35.15_suppl.103.

25. Brudno JN, Kochenderfer JN. Chimeric antigen receptor T-cell therapies for lymphoma. *Nat Rev Clin Oncol.* 2017; 15(1):31–46. https://doi.org/10.1038/nrclinonc.2017.128.

26. Neelapu S, Ghobadi A, Jacobson C, et al. 2-Year follow-up and high-risk subset analysis of Zuma-1, the pivotal study of axicabtagene ciloleucel (Axi-Cel) in patients with refractory large B cell lymphoma. *Blood.* 2018;132(suppl_1): 2967. https://doi.org/10.1182/blood-2018-99-111368.

27. Neelapu SS, Tummala S, Kebriaei P, et al. Chimeric antigen receptor T-cell therapy—assessment and management of toxicities. *Nat Rev Clin Oncol.* 2017;15(1):47–62. https://doi.org/10.1038/nrclinonc.2017.148.

28. Mahadeo KM, Khazal SJ, Abdel-Azim H, et al. Management guidelines for paediatric patients receiving chimeric antigen receptor T cell therapy. *Nat Rev Clin Oncol.* August 2018. https://doi.org/10.1038/s41571-018-0075-2.

29. Hill JA, Li D, Hay KA, et al. Infectious complications of CD19-targeted chimeric antigen receptor-modified T cell immunotherapy. *Blood.* October 2017. https://doi.org/10.1182/blood-2017-07-793760.

30. Burstein DS, Maude S, Grupp S, Griffis H, Rossano J, Lin K. Cardiac profile of chimeric antigen receptor T cell therapy in children: a single-institution experience. *Biol Blood Marrow Transplant.* 2018;24(8):1590–1595. https://doi.org/10.1016/j.bbmt.2018.05.014.

31. Cordeiro A, Bezerra E, Hill J, et al. Late effects of CD19-targeted CAR-T cell therapy. *Blood.* 2018;132(suppl_1): 223. https://doi.org/10.1182/blood-2018-99-112023.

32. *Yescarta (Axicabtagene Ciloleucel) [Package Insert].* Santa Monica, CA: Kite Pharma, Inc.; 2018.

33. *Kymriah (Tisagenlecleucel) [Package Insert].* East Hanover, NJ: Novartis Pharmaceuticals Corporation; 2018.

34. Alvarado LJ, Huntsman HD, Cheng H, et al. Eltrombopag maintains human hematopoietic stem and progenitor cells under inflammatory conditions mediated by IFN-γ. *Blood.* 2019;133(19):2043–2055. https://doi.org/10.1182/blood-2018-11-884486.

35. Tomuleasa C, Fuji S, Berce C, et al. Chimeric antigen receptor T-cells for the treatment of B-cell acute lymphoblastic leukemia. *Front Immunol.* 2018;9. https://doi.org/10.3389/fimmu.2018.00239.

36. Doan A, Pulsipher MA. Hypogammaglobulinemia due to CAR T-cell therapy. *Pediatr Blood Cancer.* 2018;65(4): e26914. https://doi.org/10.1002/pbc.26914.

37. Gust J, Taraseviciute A, Turtle CJ. Neurotoxicity associated with CD19-targeted CAR-T cell therapies. *CNS Drugs.* 2018;32(12):1091–1101. https://doi.org/10.1007/s40263-018-0582-9.

38. Gust J, Hay KA, Hanafi L-A, et al. Endothelial activation and blood-brain barrier disruption in neurotoxicity after adoptive immunotherapy with CD19 CAR-T cells. *Cancer Discov.* 2017;7(12):1404–1419. https://doi.org/10.1158/2159-8290.CD-17-0698.

39. Smith M, Zakrzewski J, James S, Sadelain M. Posttransplant chimeric antigen receptor therapy. *Blood.* 2018; 131(10):1045–1052. https://doi.org/10.1182/blood-2017-08-752121.

40. Benjamin R, Graham C, Yallop D, et al. Preliminary data on safety, cellular kinetics and anti-leukemic activity of UCART19, an allogeneic anti-CD19 CAR T-cell product, in a pool of adult and pediatric patients with high-risk CD19+ relapsed/refractory B-cell acute lymphoblastic leukemia. *Blood.* 2018;132(suppl 1):896. https://doi.org/10.1182/blood-2018-99-111356.

CHAPTER 10

Relapse Management and Role for Consolidative Hematopoietic Stem Cell Transplantation Following CAR T-Cell Therapy*

HANEEN SHALABI, DO • NIRALI N. SHAH, MD, MHSC

INTRODUCTION

Treatment strategies for children and young adults with relapsed and/or refractory acute lymphoblastic leukemia (ALL) have evolved significantly, from a historical reliance on intensive combination antineoplastic therapy to targeted genetically modified cell-based therapies. Hundreds of trials utilizing CAR T-cells are currently ongoing globally.[1] In fact, the success of CAR T-cells in clinical trials has led to the FDA approval of tisagenlecleucel and axicabtagene ciloleucel for use in relapsed refractory cases of children with ALL and/or adults with lymphoma.[2,3] While the results for inducing remission in this high-risk patient population are impressive, long-term durable remissions are achievable in only a fraction of patients. This section will focus on relapses post-CAR T therapy, efficacy of second infusions, alternative CAR targets, and the role of consolidative allogeneic bone marrow transplant post-CAR T therapy.

Relapses Post-Chimeric Antigen Receptor T Therapy

As data mature in the CAR T-cell field, and longer follow-up is available, a high relapse rate has emerged as a significant problem postremission induction.[2-7] At 12-month post-CAR therapy, many studies are reporting relapse rates in up to 50% of patients with B-cell ALL, independent of the antigen targeted, and a median progression-free survival of approximately 6 months in those with diffuse large B-cell lymphoma treated with CD19-28z CAR.[2,3,6,8,9] In general, relapses post-CAR occur in two broad categories, early antigen-positive relapse in the setting of loss of CAR T-cell persistence, which typically occurs <6 months postinfusion, and antigen-negative relapse, which reportedly has a later onset >6 months postinfusion.[10]

Types of relapse

Antigen-positive relapse. Antigen-positive relapse typically occurs early after CAR T-cell infusion, with loss of persistence or T-cell failure cited as the main drivers.[10-12] Several studies suggest that CAR T-cell persistence, measured by B-cell aplasia, of at least 3−6 months is needed to provide ongoing antileukemia surveillance.[6,10,11] The optimal duration of CAR T-cell persistence is yet to be fully determined, and persistence can be affected by numerous factors, including T-cell exhaustion or costimulatory domains associated with the construct of the CAR T-cells.[10,12-16] T-cell senescence and exhaustion in the setting of CAR T-cell therapy can occur due to exposure to the tumor microenvironment where inhibitory cytokines, such as PD-1, affect response of CAR T-cells by causing downregulation of the immune system response and inhibition of T-cell function, which in turn impairs effectiveness of CAR T-cells in targeting disease.[16,17] Additionally, signaling through the endogenous T-cell receptor can negatively impact the persistence and efficacy of CD8+ CAR T-cells by promoting exhaustion and apoptosis of CD8+ CAR T-cells.[18] Finally, antigen-independent tonic signaling by CAR T-cells can increase differentiation and promote an exhaustion phenotype, thereby decreasing cytotoxic potency of CAR cells.[13,19]

In preclinical models, incorporation of 4-1BB costimulation seemed to abate the problem of tonic signaling

---

*Contributed by Haneen Shalabi & Nirali N. Shah is under Public domain as the contributors are US Government employees.

Chimeric Antigen Receptor T-Cell Therapies for Cancer. https://doi.org/10.1016/B978-0-323-66181-2.00010-X

and CAR exhaustion phenotype, as compared with CD28z costimulation.[13] In clinical trials, it has become evident that CD28 costimulation facilitates more rapid and higher peak T-cell expansion, which also predisposes T-cells to early exhaustion, which leads to poor long-term T-cell persistence as a result of activation-induced cell death.[10,13,15] In contrast, 4-1BB costimulation is associated with a slower expansion rate, lower peak level, a diminished risk of T-cell exhaustion, and more prolonged persistence following adoptive transfer.[10,13] Also, CAR constructs utilizing the costimulatory domain CD28z have demonstrated comparable efficacy in antileukemia activity as compared with constructs that have 4-1BB; however, these have demonstrated less persistence than those CAR constructs that incorporate the 4-1BB domain,[14,15] with a median duration of persistence of 30 versus 168 days.[2,14,15] Many other costimulatory domains are currently being investigated in clinical trials; however, no consensus has been reached regarding which domain is most optimal with regard to CAR persistence and antileukemia activity.

Many investigators are now looking into ways to improve upon CAR T-cell activity and persistence, both by improving upon CAR T manufacturing and independent strategies to bolster persistence. Approaches currently under clinical investigation include development of armored CAR T-cells that secrete proinflammatory cytokines (e.g., IL-12), which would modulate the tumor microenvironment, creating a more accepting niche for CAR T-cells to flourish, a particularly attractive strategy in solid tumor where achieving that initial expansion has been difficult.[20] Incorporation of other costimulatory molecules (CD40L, CD80, or 4-1BBL) to modulate tumor immunophenotype is also being explored, in an effort to improve tumor immunogenicity and thus further optimize the efficacy of CAR T-cells.[20,21] Alternatively, combinatorial approaches utilizing checkpoint inhibitors with CAR T-cells are being utilized to extend CAR T-cell effects by attempting to decrease CAR T-cell exhaustion and improve upon expansion and persistence.[22] Clinical evidence in pediatric patients with B-cell malignancies using checkpoint inhibitors in combination with CAR T-cell therapy demonstrated safety and early signs of efficacy in patients who either had B-cell recovery or had bulky extramedullary disease.[23] Additional cases in the literature have been noted in a patient with lymphoma who had an augmented CAR response with significant tumor reduction and lymphocytosis following administration of a PD-1 inhibitor.[24] Clinical trials are now being established to test these strategies systematically.

Other strategies currently under study in attempts to bolster persistence of CAR T-cells include post-CAR vaccines, which has recently been tested in a small multicenter trial.[25] Interestingly, donor Epstein-Barr virus (EBV)-specific T-cells transduced with a first-generation CD19 CAR were used in pediatric B-ALL patients posttransplant, if they had a molecular relapse or prophylactically if it was a second transplant.[25] The initial cohort demonstrated poor expansion and persistence; however, after addition of an EBV-directed vaccine, although expansion remained poor, median persistence of CAR T-cells in the vaccine group was significantly longer than those who did not receive vaccinations, 56 days (range: 0−221) versus 0 days (range: 0−28), $P = .06$, respectively.[25] Thus, this study identifies a potential for enhancing persistence with vaccinations. Additional areas of investigation include incorporating antigen-presenting cells (APCs) in T-cell–based immunotherapies to bolster efficacy and enhance persistence of these treatments.[26−28] A study currently in clinical trial utilizes T-cell APCs at various timepoints following CD19 CAR T-cell treatment to determine whether the APCs will lead to reengagement and quantitative reexpansion of CAR cells and whether this can lead to improved persistence and decrease the risk of antigen-positive relapse (Clinicaltrials.gov NCT03186118).

Reinfusion strategies can also be utilized as a mechanism to enhance or prolong remission or to treat antigen-positive relapse; however, this has been met with limited success. Additionally, it is unclear when to use a reinfusion and whether it is primarily for treatment of relapsed disease or for relapse prevention. Accordingly, no consensus criteria regarding who is eligible for reinfusions post-CAR have been established. Although some aspects may be protocol specific, the majority of providers have been considering reinfusions for patients who have lost CAR T persistence >30 days postinitial infusion with antigen-positive disease, alternatively for treatment of recurrence of normal B-precursors or hematogones.[6,29] Patients eligible for reinfusion on these protocols include those that tolerated the prior dose, without significant dose-limiting toxicities or clinically significant adverse events. Other points include consideration of patient response to initial therapy and duration from first infusion; perhaps a patient is more likely to respond to a reinfusion if they had an initial response to therapy and/or if the primary infusion was far removed from the second infusion, which could play a factor in the role of immune-mediated rejection.[30]

Additionally, many clinical trials have utilized a reinfusion strategy in the setting of early B-cell recovery, with varying outcomes. The largest report of reinfusions to date by Gardner et al. was of 10 patients who initially had a response after first infusion of CD19 CAR T-cells, nine of whom had MRD-negative remissions. Of these 10 patients, 8 received a reinfusion for loss of CAR T-cells, of which only 2 experienced CAR expansion, with only 1 having a complete response.[6] Lee et al. reported on three patients who received a second infusion between 2 and 5.5 months after the initial infusion with CD19-28z CAR T-cells, with no patients having an objective response.[15] An additional study demonstrated that five patients treated with a reinfusion of CD19 CAR T-cells did not have expansion or any antitumor activity with the second infusion.[31]

Due to the underwhelming response investigators anecdotally noted with reinfusions, modification of dosing of CAR T-cells or intensifying lymphodepletion has been a strategy that some groups are utilizing to overcome potential immune-mediated rejection. Work done by Turtle et al. demonstrated that a potential reason for nonresponse in patients who underwent a reinfusion was T-cell rejection directed at epitopes encoded by the murine CAR transgene.[31] The group was able to demonstrate anti-CAR-specific CD8+ T-cell response in all five patients who failed to have expansion or persistence. Increased lymphodepletion has been utilized as a strategy to mitigate rejection of CAR T-cells in the host. Two groups have demonstrated preliminary data that suggest that increased chemotherapy prior to a reinfusion led to enhanced antitumor activity and persistence of CAR T-cells.[30,32] Other groups have initiated clinical trials that involve a humanized CD19 CAR T construct to overcome murine-based rejection, with early signals suggesting this approach can be successful.[33]

Antigen-negative relapse. One of the biggest barriers to durable remissions following single-antigen targeted therapy is relapse with antigen-negative disease. This has been seen in other targeted therapies, such as blinatumomab, and poses a significant problem in the field of adoptive cellular therapy, with antigen escape accounting for the majority of cases of relapse.[2,34,35] Mechanisms to date that have been reported to cause loss of CD19 surface epitope include alternative splicing of the CD19 isoform and disruption of the transportation of CD19 to the cell surface.[36–38] One study that compared leukemia samples pre- and post-CD19 CAR T therapy revealed the emergence of de novo genomic alterations, primarily affecting exon 2.[36] On the other hand, a different study demonstrated that CD19 isoforms that enabled resistance to CD19-directed immunotherapy were present at initial diagnosis, thus suggesting that this evolved as a dominant clone after therapy, rather than a causative event due to therapy-related immune pressure.[37] This remains an active area of ongoing research.

Interestingly, complete loss of antigen may not be necessary for leukemia cells to evade the immune system in the post-CAR treatment setting. For instance, diminution of CD22 antigen expression, following CD22 CAR T therapy, was shown to be enough of a quantitative change for patients to relapse despite ongoing CD22 positive disease, in the setting of persistent CAR T-cells.[9]

The rates of antigen-negative escape in patients with lymphoma thus far have been poorly defined, although cases have been reported post-CAR T-cell therapy.[39,40] A majority of patients who have relapsed lymphoma post-CAR treatment do not undergo additional biopsy sampling, thus making it difficult to ascertain how many relapses are due to antigen modulation. Additionally, tissue expression of surface proteins CD19 and/or CD22 is less quantitative due to reliance on immunohistochemical staining, making it difficult to determine the true mechanism of relapse in patients who do not have paired biopsy samples. Also, tumor heterogeneity may predispose patients to have a suboptimal response to therapy and/or emergence of antigen-negative disease—a potentially larger problem in solid tumors where CAR T-cell therapy remission to the extent of those in B-cell malignancies has yet to be achieved.

Lineage switch. Persistence of CAR T-cells can generate constant immune pressure against the antigen targeted, thus creating a unique mechanism of resistance, due to inherent leukemia plasticity. Preclinical data have demonstrated that lineage switch, as a mechanism of CAR resistance, can occur as a result of intrinsic cell reprogramming, by inducing loss of B-cell transcription factors, thereby blocking B-cell developmental pathways.[41] Clinically, lineage switch has been demonstrated in few cases, most notably in patients with *KMT2A* or mixed lineage leukemia (*MLL*)—rearranged leukemia. One recent publication reported on seven patients with *KMT2A/MLL*-rearranged ALL who were treated with CD19 CAR T-cells, all of whom achieved a complete remission. One-month postinfusion, two of seven patients developed acute myeloid leukemia, with further studies demonstrating that, in at least one case, the AML was clonally related to their original B-ALL. The other case in this small series did not identify the previous gene rearrangement, suggesting that perhaps the myeloid relapse occurred from an immature clone.[42]

Alternative Targets

Based on these reports of antigen modulation or negativity contributing to patient relapse, identification and optimization of alternative targets remains paramount to this field. In a first-in-human trial of an alternative B-cell target, our group has demonstrated safety and feasibility utilizing a CD22-directed CAR T-cell approach.[7] Similar potency and antileukemia activity were seen in those that were immunotherapy naïve, as well as those who received CD19-directed therapy. Additionally, this was the first study to demonstrate that patients who developed antigen-negative escape post-CD19 CAR could be salvaged via an alternative antigen targeted.[7] Though, as previously mentioned, antigen modulation of CD22 emerged as a major cause of relapse post-CD22 CAR T therapy.

Given the problem of antigen-negative relapse with single-antigen targeted therapies, CAR protocols are now investigating the use of dual-antigen targeted CAR T-cells in an attempt to decrease relapse rates. In this regard, confirmation of activity of a single-antigen CD22-targeted strategy played an important role in moving this construct into combinatorial strategies. Multiple studies are being conducted to optimize the structure of a multitargeted CAR. This can be achieved by coexpressing two different CARs on one T-cell (cotransduction), infusing two CAR T-cell products, each targeting a different antigen (coinfusion), use of a vector that encodes two separate CARs on the same cell (bicistronic), or incorporating two scFvs into one single chain (bispecific or tandem) (Fig. 10.1).[43] One of the first bispecific or dual targeted CAR constructs was a single-chain CAR-targeting CD19 and human epidermal growth factor receptor 2 (HER2/neu) known as the TanCAR.[44] This single-chain bispecific receptor was designed to trigger T-cell activation if either CD19 or HER2 was encountered. Antigen loss was also seen with this construct, as these two antigens are not coexpressed on the same cell.[44] Several clinical trials are currently ongoing with multitargeted CAR T-cells, and follow-up will help determine whether these approaches are adequate in preventing antigen-negative escape in these high-risk subpopulations.

Ruella et al. showed that by utilizing different CD19/CD123 CAR T-cell manufacturing approaches in in vitro models, with either cotransduction, coinfusion, or biscistronic CARs, antigen-negative escape could be mitigated and prevented.[45] Other CAR constructs that have used a single-chain, bispecific scFvs include a CD19/CD20 that was shown to have robust T-cell responses if either cell expressed CD19 or CD20, working as an OR-gate strategy.[46] Early results from a phase 1 bispecific trial in patients with non-Hodgkin's lymphoma using CD19/CD20 tandem

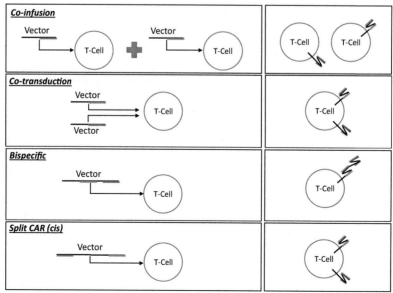

FIG. 10.1 Multiantigen-targeting strategies. (Image courtesy of Terry Fry, Haiying Qin, and Sneha Ramakrishna.)

receptor CAR T-cells demonstrate preliminary efficacy, and in those that have since relapsed, biopsies illustrate retained CD19/CD20 expression.[47] Fry et al. developed a bispecific CD19/CD22 CAR construct that showed efficacy in vitro, and phase 1 clinical trials using this construct are currently underway in pediatric and adult patients with relapsed/refractory B-cell malignancies (ClinicalTrials.gov NCT03241940/NCT03233854/NCT03448393). Preliminary phase 1 data have demonstrated efficacy of this CAR T construct with 4/4 pediatric patients with ALL and 3/7 adult patients with B-cell malignancies having a complete response.[48,49] Interim analysis of a novel CAR construct utilizing a bicistronic approach for CD19/CD22 was recently shown to be safe and feasible in a phase 1/2 study in pediatric patients with B-ALL with early signals of efficacy with 4/4 patients achieving MRD-negative CR, with the longest follow-up at 4 months.[50] Additional preclinical work toward developing a trivalent CAR T product against CD19, CD20, and CD22 demonstrated the ability to effectively target primary ALL cell lines with varying antigen profiles and prevent CD19-negative relapses.[51]

Role of Consolidative Hematopoietic Stem Cell Transplant Post-CAR T Therapy

Prior to the era of CAR T-cell therapy, the well-established standard of care in patients with high-risk or relapsed/refractory ALL was to attain a remission and proceed with a consolidative allogeneic hematopoietic stem cell transplant (HSCT) for long-term cure. With a fraction of patients attaining long-term cure with CAR T-cell therapy alone; however, the role of HSCT in the era of CAR T-cell therapy is less clear. Many providers contemplate using CAR T-cell−induced remissions as a bridge to HSCT, with substantial data supporting the curative intent of HSCT. Certainly, with the emergence of antigen-negative escape, and relapse in up to 50% of patients within 1-year post-CAR T-cell therapy, a rationale for consideration of a consolidative allo-HSCT is well supported. Reports from two groups who used a CD19-28z CAR demonstrated a high degree of B-ALL patients who underwent a consolidative transplant following CAR-induced remission with overall improved outcomes.[14,15,52] Davila et al. reported on 16 patients with B-ALL, a majority who did not have a previous transplant, treated with the 19-28z CAR T-cells, with 7/16 (44%) of patients undergoing transplant, and with no relapses noted at a median time of follow-up of 64 days (range: 43−121 days). Lee et al. also showed that relapse was significantly more common in subjects who did not have an HSCT after CAR therapy compared with those who did (6/7%; 85.7% vs. 2/21%; 9.5%, P = .0001).[52] Additionally, Gardener et al. described 11 patients who underwent HSCT after receiving CD19-41BB CAR T-cells, and only 2/11 patients relapsed, both of whom had next-generation sequence-positive detectable disease at the time of transplant.[6] More recent data from this latter group more clearly supported the role of a first HSCT in patients who had achieved a CAR-induced remission, while the role for a second transplant was less certain.[53] On the other hand, Park et al. reported on 17 of 44 patients who proceeded to transplant after attaining a complete remission post-CAR T infusion, with 12/17 patients experiencing relapse or death posttransplant.[8] This study ultimately concluded that there was no difference in overall or event-free survival in those that proceeded to transplant versus those that did not. Notably, the differences between the outcomes from the two groups may also reflect more favorable outcomes of HSCT in a pediatric population versus HSCT in an older age group that was reflective of the data presented by Park.

Nevertheless, providers are trying to determine which patients are at risk of post-CAR relapse, thus warranting referral to HSCT. In a multivariable modeling analysis, Hay et al. illustrated that prelymphodepletion, higher platelet count, and lower LDH, in addition to utilization of a fludarabine/Cytoxan regimen, identified patients who had improved disease-free survival (DFS). Additionally, adjusting for these factors, those that received an HSCT post-CD19 CAR had improved DFS.[54] Other potential useful factors for referral to transplant include whether this is a first or second HSCT and how long patient has B-cell aplasia, i.e., CAR T persistence, postinfusion. However, none of these parameters will successfully predict when antigen-negative relapse may emerge. Thus, the role of HSCT needs to be more well defined and is likely a stronger consideration in patients who do not have a prior HSCT history and those that received shorter-acting CAR T-cells.[55] As CAR T-cell therapies evolve to treat other hematologic conditions, HSCT may also serve as a reservoir stem cell source in situations where there may be concern for myeloid aplasia, i.e., with AML antigen-directed CAR T-cell trials. An upcoming CD33 CAR T-cell trial, for instance, has been written specifically with the goal for CAR T-cells to serve as a bridge to HSCT. In this case, HSCT is planned to be used for both consolidative therapies to prevent antigen-negative escape, which could be an even greater problem with myeloid targeting, and is also being used as a safety parameter should there be prolonged myeloid aplasia to provide a stem cell source (Clinicaltrials.gov NCT03971799) Ultimately, while HSCT has an established role in hematologic malignancies, the optimal utilization of CAR T-cells will need to be more clearly defined in these conditions, for those diseases or for patients in whom HSCT does not have a role; optimizing the ability to achieve durable CAR T-cell–induced remission remains a long-term goal.

CONCLUSIONS

With the high-remission induction rate of CAR T-cell therapy in B-cell malignancies, understanding the limitations to this therapy is critical in determining why remission may not be durable for all. Ultimately, many challenges remain in the field of CAR T-cells, and current research efforts are focused on optimization of constructs, improving durability of remission, and establishing treatment of relapse. Lessons learned from the experiences with B-cell targeting will inform the field regarding CAR T-cell therapies in other diseases, with a major consideration of preventing antigen-negative relapses and optimizing multiantigen-targeting approaches.

DISCLAIMER

The content of this publication does not necessarily reflect the views of policies of the Department of Health and Human Services, nor does mention of trade names, commercial products, or organizations imply endorsement by the US government.

REFERENCES

1. Hartmann J, Schussler-Lenz M, Bondanza A, Buchholz CJ. Clinical development of CAR T cells-challenges and opportunities in translating innovative treatment concepts. *EMBO Mol Med.* 2017;9(9):1183–1197.
2. Maude SL, Laetsch TW, Buechner J, et al. Tisagenlecleucel in children and young adults with B-cell lymphoblastic leukemia. *N Engl J Med.* 2018;378(5):439–448.
3. Neelapu SS, Ghobadi A, Jacobson CA, et al. 2-Year follow-up and high-risk subset analysis of Zuma-1, the pivotal study of axicabtagene ciloleucel (Axi-Cel) in patients with refractory large B cell lymphoma. *Blood.* 2018;132.
4. Locke FL, Neelapu SS, Bartlett NL, et al. Phase 1 results of ZUMA-1: a multicenter study of KTE-C19 anti-CD19 CAR T cell therapy in refractory aggressive lymphoma. *Mol Ther.* 2017;25(1):285–295.
5. Park JH, Riviere I, Wang XY, et al. Durable long-term survival of adult patients with relapsed B-ALL after CD19 CAR (19-28z) T-cell therapy. *J Clin Oncol.* 2017:35.
6. Gardner RA, Finney O, Annesley C, et al. Intent-to-treat leukemia remission by CD19 CAR T cells of defined formulation and dose in children and young adults. *Blood.* 2017;129(25):3322–3331.
7. Fry TJ, Shah NN, Orentas RJ, et al. CD22-targeted CAR T cells induce remission in B-ALL that is naive or resistant to CD19-targeted CAR immunotherapy. *Nat Med.* 2018; 24(1):20–28.
8. Park JH, Riviere I, Gonen M, et al. Long-term follow-up of CD19 CAR therapy in acute lymphoblastic leukemia. *N Engl J Med.* 2018;378(5):449–459.
9. Fry TJ, Shah NN, Orentas RJ, et al. CD22-targeted CAR T cells induce remission in B-ALL that is naive or resistant to CD19-targeted CAR immunotherapy. *Nat Med.* 2017; 24(1):20–28.
10. Maude SL, Frey N, Shaw PA, et al. Chimeric antigen receptor T cells for sustained remissions in leukemia. *N Engl J Med.* 2014;371(16):1507–1517.
11. Gardner RA, Finney O, Smithers H, et al. Prolonged functional persistence of CD19CAR t cell products of defined CD4:CD8 composition and transgene expression determines durability of MRD-negative ALL remission. *J Clin Oncol.* 2016;34(15).
12. Mackall CL. Enhancing the efficacy of CAR T cells. *Blood.* 2017:130.
13. Long AH, Haso WM, Shern JF, et al. 4-1BB costimulation ameliorates T cell exhaustion induced by tonic signaling of chimeric antigen receptors. *Nat Med.* 2015;21(6):581–590.
14. Davila ML, Riviere I, Wang X, et al. Efficacy and toxicity management of 19-28z CAR T cell therapy in B cell acute lymphoblastic leukemia. *Sci Transl Med.* 2014;6(224): 224ra25.
15. Lee DW, Kochenderfer JN, Stetler-Stevenson M, et al. T cells expressing CD19 chimeric antigen receptors for acute lymphoblastic leukaemia in children and young adults: a phase 1 dose-escalation trial. *Lancet.* 2015; 385(9967):517–528.
16. Kasakovski D, Xu L, Li Y. T cell senescence and CAR-T cell exhaustion in hematological malignancies. *J Hematol Oncol.* 2018;11(1):91.
17. Cherkassky L, Morello A, Villena-Vargas J, et al. Human CAR T cells with cell-intrinsic PD-1 checkpoint blockade resist tumor-mediated inhibition. *J Clin Invest.* 2016; 126(8):3130–3144.
18. Yang Y, Kohler ME, Chien CD, et al. TCR engagement negatively affects CD8 but not CD4 CAR T cell expansion and leukemic clearance. *Sci Transl Med.* 2017;9(417).
19. Gomes-Silva D, Mukherjee M, Srinivasan M, et al. Tonic 4-1BB costimulation in chimeric antigen receptors impedes T cell survival and is vector-dependent. *Cell Rep.* 2017; 21(1):17–26.
20. Yeku OO, Purdon TJ, Koneru M, Spriggs D, Brentjens RJ. Armored CAR T cells enhance antitumor efficacy and overcome the tumor microenvironment. *Sci Rep.* 2017;7(1):10541.
21. Jackson HJ, Brentjens RJ. Overcoming antigen escape with CAR T-cell therapy. *Cancer Discov.* 2015;5(12):1238–1240.
22. Yoon DH, Osborn MJ, Tolar J, Kim CJ. Incorporation of immune checkpoint blockade into chimeric antigen

receptor T cells (CAR-Ts): combination or built-in CAR-T. *Int J Mol Sci.* 2018;19(2).

23. Li AM, Hucks GE, Dinofia AM, et al. Checkpoint inhibitors augment CD19-directed chimeric antigen receptor (CAR) T cell therapy in relapsed B-cell acute lymphoblastic leukemia. *Blood.* 2018:132.

24. Hill BT, Roberts ZJ, Rossi JM, Smith MR. Marked Re-expansion of chimeric antigen receptor (CAR) T cells and tumor regression following Nivolumab treatment in a patient treated with axicabtagene ciloleucel (axi-cel; KTE-C19) for refractory diffuse large B cell lymphoma (DLBCL). *Blood.* 2017:130.

25. Rossig C, Pule M, Altvater B, et al. Vaccination to improve the persistence of CD19CAR gene-modified T cells in relapsed pediatric acute lymphoblastic leukemia. *Leukemia.* 2017;31(5):1087—1095.

26. Hasan AN, Selvakumar A, O'Reilly RJ. Artificial antigen presenting cells: an off the shelf approach for generation of desirable T-cell populations for broad application of adoptive immunotherapy. *Adv Genet Eng.* 2015;4(3).

27. Turtle CJ, Riddell SR. Artificial antigen-presenting cells for use in adoptive immunotherapy. *Cancer J.* 2010;16(4): 374—381.

28. Butler MO, Hirano N. Human cell-based artificial antigen-presenting cells for cancer immunotherapy. *Immunol Rev.* 2014;257(1):191—209.

29. Maude SL, Teachey DT, Porter DL, Grupp SA. CD19-targeted chimeric antigen receptor T-cell therapy for acute lymphoblastic leukemia. *Blood.* 2015;125(26):4017—4023.

30. Shalabi H, Shah NN, Fry TJ, et al. Intensification of lymphodepletion optimizes CAR Re-treatment efficacy. *Blood.* 2017;130.

31. Turtle CJ, Hanafi LA, Berger C, et al. CD19 CAR-T cells of defined CD4+:CD8+ composition in adult B cell ALL patients. *J Clin Invest.* 2016;126(6):2123—2138.

32. Turtle CJ, Hanafi LA, Berger C, et al. Rate of durable complete response in ALL, NHL, and CLL after immunotherapy with optimized lymphodepletion and defined composition CD19 CAR-T cells. *J Clin Oncol.* 2016;34(15).

33. Maude SL, Barrett DM, Rheingold SR, et al. Efficacy of humanized CD19-targeted chimeric antigen receptor (CAR)-modified T cells in children and young adults with relapsed/refractory acute lymphoblastic leukemia. *Blood.* 2016;128(22).

34. Topp MS, Kufer P, Gokbuget N, et al. Targeted therapy with the T-cell-engaging antibody blinatumomab of chemotherapy-refractory minimal residual disease in B-lineage acute lymphoblastic leukemia patients results in high response rate and prolonged leukemia-free survival. *J Clin Oncol.* 2011;29(18):2493—2498.

35. Majzner RG, Mackall CL. Tumor antigen escape from CAR T-cell therapy. *Cancer Discov.* 2018;8(10):1219—1226.

36. Sotillo E, Barrett DM, Black KL, et al. Convergence of acquired mutations and alternative splicing of CD19 enables resistance to CART-19 immunotherapy. *Cancer Discov.* 2015;5(12):1282—1295.

37. Fischer J, Paret C, El Malki K, et al. CD19 isoforms enabling resistance to CART-19 immunotherapy are expressed in B-all patients at initial diagnosis. *J Immunother.* 2017;40(5):187—195.

38. Braig F, Brandt A, Goebeler M, et al. Resistance to anti-CD19/CD3 BiTE in acute lymphoblastic leukemia may be mediated by disrupted CD19 membrane trafficking. *Blood.* 2017;129(1):100—104.

39. Neelapu SS, Locke FL, Bartlett NL, et al. Axicabtagene ciloleucel CAR T-cell therapy in refractory large B-cell lymphoma. *N Engl J Med.* 2017;377(26):2531—2544.

40. Shalabi H, Kraft IL, Wang HW, et al. Sequential loss of tumor surface antigens following chimeric antigen receptor T-cell therapies in diffuse large B-cell lymphoma. *Haematologica.* 2018;103(5):e215—e218.

41. Jacoby E, Nguyen SM, Fountaine TJ, et al. CD19 CAR immune pressure induces B-precursor acute lymphoblastic leukaemia lineage switch exposing inherent leukaemic plasticity. *Nat Commun.* 2016;7:12320.

42. Gardner R, Wu D, Cherian S, et al. Acquisition of a CD19-negative myeloid phenotype allows immune escape of MLL-rearranged B-ALL from CD19 CAR-T-cell therapy. *Blood.* 2016;127(20):2406—2410.

43. Shah NN, Maatman T, Hari P, Johnson B. Multi targeted CAR-T cell therapies for B-cell malignancies. *Front Oncol.* 2019:9.

44. Grada Z, Hegde M, Byrd T, et al. TanCAR: a novel bispecific chimeric antigen receptor for cancer immunotherapy. *Mol Ther Nucleic Acids.* 2013:2.

45. Ruella M, Barrett DM, Kenderian SS, et al. Dual CD19 and CD123 targeting prevents antigen-loss relapses after CD19-directed immunotherapies. *J Clin Invest.* 2016; 126(10):3814—3826.

46. Zah E, Lin MY, Silva-Benedict A, Jensen MC, Chen YY. T cells expressing CD19/CD20 bispecific chimeric antigen receptors prevent antigen escape by malignant B cells. *Cancer Immunol Res.* 2016;4(6):498—508.

47. Shah NN, Zhu FL, Taylor C, et al. A phase 1 study with point-of-care manufacturing of dual targeted, tandem anti-CD19, anti-CD20 chimeric antigen receptor modified T (CART-T) cells for relapsed, refractory, non-Hodgkin lymphoma. *Blood.* 2018:132.

48. Schultz LM, Davis KL, Baggott C, et al. 1 study of CD19/CD22 bispecific chimeric antigen receptor (CAR) therapy in children and young adults with B cell acute lymphoblastic leukemia (ALL). *Blood.* 2018:132.

49. Hossain N, Sahaf B, Abramian M, et al. Phase I experience with a Bi-specific CAR targeting CD19 and CD22 in adults with B-cell malignancies. *Blood.* 2018:132.

50. Amrolia PJ, Wynn R, Hough R, et al. Simultaneous targeting of CD19 and CD22: phase I study of AUTO3, a bicistronic chimeric antigen receptor (CAR) T-cell therapy, in pediatric patients with relapsed/refractory B-cell acute lymphoblastic leukemia (r/r B-all): Amelia study. *Blood.* 2018:132.

51. Fousek K, Watanabe J, George A, et al. Targeting CD19-negative relapsed B-acute lymphoblastic leukemia using trivalent CAR T cells. *Mol Ther.* 2018;26(5):298.

52. Lee DW, Stetler-Stevenson M, Yuan CM, et al. Long-term outcomes following CD19 CAR T cell therapy for B-all are superior in patients receiving a fludarabine/

cyclophosphamide preparative regimen and post-CAR hematopoietic stem cell transplantation. *Blood*. 2016; 128(22).

53. Summers C, Annesley C, Bleakley M, Dahlberg A, Jensen MC, Gardner R. Long term follow-up after SCRI-CAR19v1 reveals late recurrences as well As a survival advantage to consolidation with HCT after CAR T cell induced remission. *Blood*. 2018;132(Suppl 1):967.

54. Hay KA, Gauthier J, Hirayama AV, et al. Multivariable modeling of disease and treatment characteristics of adults with B-all in MRD-negative CR after CD19 CAR-T cells identifies factors impacting disease-free survival. *Blood*. 2018:132.

55. Shalabi H, Stetler-Stevenson M, Yuan C, et al. Chimeric antigen receptor T-cell (CAR-T) can render patients with ALL into PCR-negative remission and can be an effective bridge to transplant (HCT). *Biol Blood Marrow Transplant*. 2018; 24(3):S25−S26.

CHAPTER 11

Promising Chimeric Antigen Receptors for Non-B-Cell Hematological Malignancies, Pediatric Solid Tumors, and Carcinomas

JACOB S. APPELBAUM, MD, PHD • NAVIN PINTO, MD • RIMAS J. ORENTAS, PHD

INTRODUCTION

The success of chimeric antigen receptor (CAR) T-cell therapy for relapsed/refractory acute lymphoblastic leukemia and non-Hodgkin lymphoma has led to interest in developing CAR T-cell treatments for other malignancies. The modular nature of the CAR brought hope that simply replacing the FMC63 antigen-binding domain of CD19 CAR T-cells with other antigen-binding domains would rapidly yield new therapies, bringing cellular immunotherapy to myeloid leukemias, CD19-negative lymphoid leukemias, myeloma, and other hematologic malignancies as well as solid tumors. The reality has been more sobering but is not without promise. Key principles for the success or failure of CAR therapies are beginning to emerge, allowing researchers to prioritize and evaluate new CAR designs more efficiently.

In this chapter, we briefly outline key challenges in preclinical development of CAR T-cell therapies, i.e., laboratory findings that may correlate with successful clinical trials, and identify some areas where further development of preclinical models is needed. Next, we proceed to review promising CAR T-cell therapies in development, organized by disease type.

In addition to an increased diversity of antigen targets, needed improvements in CAR T-cell technology can be identified through examining causes of CAR T-cell failure. CAR T-cell failure can be divided into four broad categories: (1) unacceptable toxicity, (2) emergence of antigen-negative tumor, (3) lack of CAR T-cell persistence, and (4) insufficiently effective T-cell antitumor response (in which both CAR T-cells and tumor cells exist simultaneously within a patient). The ability of preclinical laboratory testing to identify CAR products likely to fail (or conversely to identify CAR T-cell products likely to succeed) is limited. Each of these failure mechanisms points to needed improvements in preclinical assessments and engineering.

With increased understanding of the mechanisms leading to CAR T-cell failure comes the need for increasingly sophisticated model systems to interrogate these mechanisms. Models for toxicity as well as technologies for understanding the mechanisms for antigen-negative tumor escape may be specific for each antigen.[1] Whereas initial preclinical data supporting safety were limited to immunostaining tissue arrays to describe levels of antigen expression, now transgenic mouse models engineered to express human CD19 from the murine CD19 locus can report on cytokine release[1] and neurotoxicity.[1,2] In vitro T-cell reactivity likely accurately predicts the sensitivity of CAR T-cells to the targeted antigen, but sustained antigen response requires not only efficient signaling through the CAR receptor but also the generation of long-lived memory and the absence of anergy/exhaustion. CAR T-cell loss can, in some cases, be mediated through the generation of immune responses to the transgenic CAR protein,[3] and efforts to minimize this phenomenon through the use of humanized proteins are ongoing.

Models to predict persistent CAR T-cell function are more challenging to generate. In vivo differentiation into memory phenotype may serve as a surrogate for CAR T-cell continued activity; however, the validity of this endpoint is not proven. Mice transplanted with human hematopoietic cells do not express T-cell mitogens derived from nonhematopoietic cells (such as endothelial cells). Furthermore, manufacturing techniques, including the amount of viral vector used, transduction efficiency, the addition of cytokines or the use of drug selection during in vitro manufacture, use of defined ratios of $CD4^+$ and $CD8^+$ T-cells, the length of in vitro culture and degree of expansion allowed, the use of naïve, memory, or mixed populations of T-cells as starting material, use of other cell types (such as natural killer [NK] cells) as effector cells (i.e., CAR-NK cells) as well as the structure of the viral construct including promoter, antigen binding, transmembrane, and signaling domains of the CAR receptor all influence the reactivity, persistence, and perhaps most importantly, the phenotype of the cellular product.

Benchmarks for successful manufacturing, often restricted to viability, sterility, and transduction efficiency, differ from trial to trial and institution to institution, making cross-trial and cross-institutional comparisons difficult and confounding attempts to analyze the contribution of phenotypes within the infused cell product on eventual patient outcomes. Streamlining and standardizing manufacturing process and increasing the diversity of targetable antigens promise to bring the next generation of CAR T-cell therapies to a broader patient base.

As critical features of cellular products are difficult to define prior to human trials, data from initial first-in-human experience are critical to identify promising CAR constructs. For this reason, except in cases with preclinical results that are exceptional or inform the field generally, we have restricted our review of promising chimeric antigen receptors for non—B-cell hematological malignancies, pediatric solid tumors, and carcinomas to those constructs with available human data.

HEMATOLOGIC MALIGNANCY
Acute Myeloid Leukemia

Acute myeloid leukemia (AML) is a hematopoietic stem cell neoplasm with a poor prognosis. In adults, while induction chemotherapy can induce remissions in >80% of patients, relapse remains common, and the overall 5-year survival is only 26%.[4] Risk stratification, based on cytogenetic and molecular characterization, as well as response to initial therapy (i.e., the presence or absence of measurable residual disease) can predict patients likely to relapse in the absence of a hematopoietic stem cell transplant. There is no standard therapy for relapsed or refractory disease, and hence, the bar for success is low.

A challenge specific to AML is that, to date, all tumor-associated antigens (TAAs) are expressed on hematopoietic stem or stem/progenitor cells.[5] Multiomics analytic attempts at identifying AML-associated tumor antigens failed to identify a single antigen restricted to AML-initiating cells and absent from hematopoietic stem cells. As a result, there has been a secondary focus on multiplexed CAR T-cells, i.e., designs that require two antigens or the presence of one antigen and the absence of another to trigger CAR T reactivity.

CD33

The stem cell surface antigen CD33 was identified as the target of the antibody L4F3, which showed binding to and elimination of leukemic blasts (but preservation of stem/progenitor cells) in vitro upon the addition of complement.[6] High impact studies using genetic lineage tracing and serial transplantation identified CD33 as a marker of stem cells capable of transferring leukemia to immunodeficient mice (so-called leukemia-initiating cells [LICs]) in some, but not all, patients.[7,8] Higher-affinity anti-CD33 clones were used to engineer the approved antibody-drug conjugate (ADC) gemtuzumab ozogamacin.[9,10] Initially in relapsed patients,[11] then in combination with induction regimens, gemtuzumab showed efficacy in some trials,[12,13] but not in others.[14,15] Retrospective cross-trial comparisons showed that trial design and drug dosing varied along with toxicity; retrospective evaluation identified a subset of patients with low levels of CD33 expression that did not benefit from addition of gemtuzumab.[16,17] Thus, CD33 was among the first recognized targets of antileukemic antibodies in AML.

Early studies in adoptive T-cell therapy applied a single-chain variable fragment (scFv) derived from a rat-anti-human CD33 antibody to a first-generation CAR design (i.e., CD33 scFv-CD28 transmembrane domain-*CD3ζ* signaling domain) to generate retroviral vector (RV)—transduced cytokine-induced killer cells.[18] These cells showed modest in vitro efficacy but were not tested in patients. Subsequent studies using second-generation CAR designs (i.e., including a CD28 or 4-1BB costimulatory domain in addition to CD3ζ) showed improved cytokine release, higher rates of in vitro tumor killing, and, when injected into immunodeficient mice, elimination of tumor xenografts.[19,20] These studies formed the basis of preclinical testing and FDA approval for clinical trials. Subsequent mouse studies have developed combination CRISPR/CAR strategies wherein hematopoietic cells are rendered resistant to CD33 CAR T-cells through inactivation of CD33 by CRISPR. This strategy would reduce or eliminate the concern for myelosuppression by CD33 CAR T-cells, but gene-edited hematopoietic stem cell transplants remain a technology[21,22] still in development.

Despite the preclinical efficacy of CD33 CAR T-cells, patient experience has been limited. A single report of one 41-year-old male patient with AML describes the clinical experience following escalated doses of a cellular product manufactured from 90 mL of peripheral blood that was comprised nearly entirely of CD8 T-cells. Following treatment, the patient developed elevated levels of IL-6, TNFα, IL-8, IL-10, and IFNγ and worsened pancytopenia that fluctuated inversely with the patient's fever. Two weeks after infusion, the patients' marrow blasts had decreased from 50% to <6%, after which the blast fraction increased, resulting in relapse.[23] Transient hyperbilirubinemia was observed but resolved without specific intervention. Levels of CAR T DNA measured in both peripheral blood and marrow remained high, implying CAR T-cell persistence. To gain insight to the mechanism of relapse, the authors found CAR T-cells recovered from the patient retained the ability to kill CD33[+] target cell lines ex vivo. Nevertheless, the immunophenotype of the AML blasts at the time of relapse remained CD33[+], suggesting a mechanism of immune escape that was either specific to the blasts or the in vivo environment.

An alternative approach using an NK cell line transduced with a CD33 CAR construct showed in vitro efficacy and tolerability in three patients, but none achieved a complete remission without measurable residual disease. Despite transplantation in the two responding patients, both relapsed: one after 15 months and the second after 4 months.[24] Other phase I trials are in progress, including a trial at the University of Texas MD Anderson Cancer Center, but have yet to report outcomes.

CD123

The IL-3 receptor (CD123) is an early stem cell marker that efficiently defines LICs.[25,26] In humans, the fraction of AML cases expressing CD123 in early progenitor populations ranges from 70% to >95%.[27,28] In vitro treatment of leukemic marrow samples with an antibody to CD123 eliminated the LIC population through targeted complement activation.[26] This led to suggestions that, in most cases, all or nearly all of the LIC population was CD123[+].

Attempts to target CD123 in myeloid neoplasms include an engineered dual-affinity molecule CD123 × CD3 (flotetuzumab) that retargets T-cells as well as a ligand-toxin conjugate linking IL3 to diphtheria toxin (SL-401, tagraxofusp). Flotetuzumab

showed modest efficacy in initial phase 1 studies, with 5 of 27 (18.5%) of patients treated at the recommended phase 2 dose showing complete response or complete response with incomplete count recovery. In a related neoplasm, blastic plasmacytoid dendritic cell neoplasm (BPDCN), high CD123 expression is a diagnostic hallmark and outcomes are very poor, with median overall survival ranging from 2 to 10 months depending on immunophenotype.[29] A planned interim analysis of a single-arm phase 2 trial evaluated 47 patients with BPDCN treated with tagraxofusp found complete remission rates above 80%, high rates of subsequent stem cell transplantation rates, and 18 and 24 month survival rates of 59% and 52%, respectively.[30] These data were sufficient for the FDA to approve the drug for BPDCN, and trials in other myeloid leukemias are ongoing.

The clinical experience with CD123 CAR T-cells is limited, but promising. Initial studies conducted at City of Hope Cancer Center (Duarte, CA), identified a second-generation CAR utilizing a CD28 costimulatory domain that, when transduced into T-cells via lentiviral vector (LV), showed activity against CD123-expressing targets,[31] including primary patient AML samples in vitro. Mouse xenograft models showed transient reductions in tumor bulk following CAR T-cell administration and delayed mortality. In addition, treatment of cord blood samples with CD123 CAR T-cells did not reduce the number of colony-forming units, suggesting the safety of this approach.

The first reported trial of CD123 CAR T-cells[32] treated seven patients, six with refractory AML following allogeneic stem cell transplant and one with BPDCN. Escalating doses (50 × 10[6] cells, 2 pts; or 200 × 10[6] cells, 4 pts) of CAR T-cells were administered following fludarabine plus cyclophosphamide lymphodepletion. Importantly the authors reported that there were no treatment-related cytopenias. One of the two patients treated at the lower dose achieved a CR (blast percentage 0.9%) after two infusions of CAR T-cells; two patients treated at the higher dose achieved a CR without MRD and were subsequently treated with a second allogeneic stem cell transplant. The remaining four patients did not respond to treatment.

Safety concerns, based on preclinical data that more potent CD123-targeted CARs prevented or impaired human hematopoiesis in mouse xenograft models,[33] led researchers at the University of Pennsylvania to develop a system in which T-cells were electroporated with RNA encoding the CAR, resulting in transient activity. In a phase 1 clinical trial, involving seven patients with AML (four with prior allo-HSCT), only two of six patients received all planned doses due to manufacturing challenges, and all five patients who were treated with CAR T-cells had disease progression before day 28, with no observed expansion of CAR T-cells within the blood or reduction in the number of circulating CD123-positive cells.[34] These results led the authors to indicate their intention to abandon the strategy of RNA-based CAR T-cell manufacture in favor of elimination of lentivirus-transduced CAR T-cells using alemtuzumab followed by rescue allogeneic transplant.[35,36]

Others have focused on further preclinical design strategies that tune levels of expression and CAR affinity to distinguish tumor from normal cells[37] or to incorporate inducible suicide switches.[38] A single report of a safety switch containing CD123 CAR T enhanced with CD27 costimulation (CD123 scFv—CD28 transmembrane—4-1BB—CD27—CD3ζ—iCasp9) was tested in a single 47-year-old male patient. The patient had FLT3[+] AML that had relapsed following allogeneic transplant. The patient was conditioned with cyclophosphamide prior to administration of 1.8×10^6 CAR T-cells/kg. On day 8 postinfusion, the patient developed severe cytokine release syndrome (CRS), accompanied by high levels of IL-6 and TNFα that was controlled by tocilizumab. Bone marrow examination 20 days following infusion showed a decrease in blast fraction from 59% to 45%.[39] The authors report that this result warrants further investigation.

Clinical trials investigating CD123 CAR T-cells are currently registered at MD Anderson Cancer Center, University of Pennsylvania, Cornell Weill Cancer Center and City of Hope in addition to 12 institutions in China. The use of dual-targeted CD123 × CD19 CAR T-cells has been reported in three patients with refractory acute lymphocytic leukemia and appears tolerable and efficacious (all three patients achieved a complete remission, two of which were MRD negative); however the relative contribution of CD19 and CD123 CAR targeting is unclear.[40]

CLL1/CLEC12A

C-type lectin-like molecule 1 (CLL1/CLEC12A) is a surface glycoprotein that is expressed on approximately 90% of leukemic cells with early/progenitor phenotype.[41] Both an unbiased phage-display/cloning approach[42] and a comprehensive multiomics approach[5] identified this protein as highly expressed on both leukemic blasts and LICs and absent or minimally expressed on hematopoietic stem cells. Immunophenotyping showed expression of CLL1 on committed CD33[+]CD34[+] myeloid cells in bone marrow and peripheral blood, specifically granulocytes and monocytes as well as mature and precursor dendritic cells, but not

lymphocytes or NK cells. No other tissues analyzed expressed CLL1 mRNA.[42] In addition, reengrafting normal HSC failed to express CLL1, whereas engrafting AML blasts showed expression of CLL1 with the ratio of CLL1[+] to CLL1[−] cells among CD34[+] CD38[−] cells predictive of the time to relapse.[43]

Three groups have provided preclinical data describing CAR constructs targeting CLL1, which have activity against in vitro targets and prolonged survival of xenografted NOD/SCID/IL2-gamma knockout (NSG) mice.[44–46] In one case, the authors used a standard second-generation CAR construct (scFv-CD8 transmembrane domain-41BB-CD3ζ)[46]; in another, the authors used a murine costimulatory domains and a backbone that incorporated both CD28 and 41BB costimulatory domains[44]; and in the third case, the authors used a standard second-generation CAR construct with an added iCasp9 (inducible caspase-9) safety switch.[45] All showed effective killing and tumor elimination. Using NSG mice that additionally express GM-CSF, IL3, and stem cell factor (NSG-S), Kenderian et al. showed CLL1-targeted CAR T-cells can eliminate a leukemic stem cell population that is resistant to chemotherapy.[47]

In vivo studies with CLL1-targeted CAR T-cells are limited to a single case series of compound CD33-CLL1 CAR T-cells in which an LV encoding two complete CAR constructs joined by a cleavable linker (P2A) was used. A single pediatric patient with Fanconi anemia that had progressed to AML and was refractory to five cycles of chemotherapy was treated with lymphodepletion followed by two doses of compound CD33-CLL1 CAR T-cells (1×10^6 per kg, days 1 and 2). On day 12, the patient's blast count was 98% and developed signs of mild CRS, and then 7 days later, the repeat marrow showed a complete remission without measurable residual disease[48] and the patient was subsequently treated with a nonmyeloablative allogeneic stem cell transplant. Outcomes for additional patients reported to have been treated are not yet publicly available.

Lewis-Y/CD44

Early studies designed second-generation CAR constructs to the Lewis-Y antigen, a carbohydrate with increased expression on leukemic blasts. The numerous challenges of targeting carbohydrate antigens include the following: glycosylated structures are present on nearly all mammalian cells, detection of the target difucosylated oligosaccharide depends on the specificity of the antibody, and RNA expression and routine mass spectrometry cannot detect the specific stereochemistry recognized by anti-Lewis-Y antibodies. Nevertheless, differential glycosylation is common on tumors,[49] and generation of positive cell lines (and a negative control) can be accomplished by introduction of the FUT2 gene responsible for fucosyltransferase[50] activity. However, this enzyme may mediate glycosylation of multiple glycolipids, carbohydrates, and proteins. CD44 is one of several proteins modified by fucosylation, copurifies with Lewis-Y,[51] and has been associated with stemness and invasive properties of various tumors, including ovarian and breast carcinoma,[52–54] in part mediated by increased expression of adhesion molecules and increased secretion of metalloproteinases. CD44 binds to various glycans (including hyaluronic acid) and specific spliced isoforms, i.e., those that include exon 6, are further enriched on AML and myeloma[55] and maybe required for bone marrow homing and in vivo tumorigenesis.[56]

A second-generation CAR composed of an anti-Lewis-Y scFv fused to a CD28 transmembrane and costimulatory domain followed by *CD3ζ* showed activity against both ovarian cancer[57] and AML cell lines[58] in vitro and in mouse xenografts. Importantly, these studies demonstrated minimal off-target effects, as measured by lack of reactivity against autologous neutrophils that express approximately 20% the amount of Lewis-Y antigen that breast cancer cell expresses.[57] A phase 1 trial enrolled five patients with relapsed AML.[58] One patient died during an attempt at reinduction and did not receive CAR T-cells. Patient conditioning was with fludarabine (30 mg/m^2 days 1–5) and high-dose cytarabine (2 g/m^2 days 1–5), and the cell product was infused following marrow recovery in patients with residual disease. The four infused patients received between 1.5 and 9.2 × 10^6 transduced CAR T-cells per kg. Two of the four patients had postinfusion reaction that included neutropenia in one patient and fevers and chills in a second. Two patients had stable disease (one with stable MRD that lasted 23 months, the other with relapse at day 49), and one patient has a transient reduction in blasts followed by relapse after 28 days. A fourth patient had a cytogenetic complete remission but relapsed 5 months after infusion. The fourth infused patient had no benefit. A fraction of the CAR T-cells labeled with indium showed tracking to sites of disease in the three patients with discernible benefit; furthermore, the two patients with the greatest benefit also had the most robust CAR T-cell expansion, though interestingly the patient with the complete response did not show high levels of serum cytokines. Samples obtained at relapse showed expression of Lewis-Y antigen at levels comparable with levels observed at diagnosis. None of the patients reported in the manuscript were described to have completed an allogeneic stem cell transplant following therapy, which may have provided some benefit.

Current trials of Lewis-Y-targeted CAR T-cells are limited to a single site in China and a trial by the original authors treating solid tumors. Improvements in CAR T-cell manufacture may lead to improved responses and outcomes. Severe CRS was not seen, and this may be interpreted either as evidence of safety, or of a somewhat inert product. Preclinical studies investigating CAR constructs targeting CD44v6 were reported,[55,59] but these have not been explored in patients. The field seems to have paused, but interest in this CAR construct may be resurrected if improved designs could be identified using more sophisticated preclinical models.

NKG2D

In response to genotoxic or metabolic stress including malignant transformation, cells may increase expression of one or several of eight ligands bound by NKG2D, an activating protein receptor whose expression is mostly limited to cytotoxic lymphocytes, including NK cells, NKT-cells, γδ T-cells, and CD8$^+$ T-cells.[60] NKG2D ligands all share structural homology to the α1 and α2 domains of MHC class 1 but exhibit extensive allelic diversity (i.e., one ligand, MICA, has 109 alleles).

While activation of endogenous NKG2D proceeds with induction of a switch in RNA isoform, which results in a protein capable of binding adaptor molecules that in turn activate PI3 kinase, the CAR design tested by the Nikifarow and colleagues[61] is distinct: to maintain sensitivity to the wide variety of NKG2D ligands, the entire NKG2D protein (rather than an scFv) was used as the targeting moiety and the *CD3ζ* domain without a costimulatory domain was fused to the cytoplasmic tail. The recombinant NKG2D/*CD3ζ* fusion protein bound the endogenous adaptor protein Dap10, which provides an additional costimulatory signal to RV-transduced T-cells. Preclinical studies showed robust cytokine production from transduced T-cells, lysis of NKG2D ligand-expressing tumor cells lines, and limited inhibition by soluble NKG2D ligands.[62,63] Perhaps most interestingly, immunodeficient mice that had eliminated xenografted tumors following adoptive transfer of NKG2D-CAR-T-cells were resistant to tumor rechallenge.[63] A recent phase 1 trial[61] featured 14 patients, 12 of whom provided T-cells for CAR manufacture, of which 7 had AML. Patients with prior allogeneic transplant were excluded. Because inflammation may increase NKG2D ligand expression on normal tissues, no lymphodepleting chemotherapy was used prior to cell infusion as an additional safety parameter. No infusion reactions, CRS, neurotoxicity, colitis, or pneumonitis was observed, and all adverse events of grade ≥3 were attributed to underlying disease. No objective clinical response was seen in any patient, and all went on to receive additional therapy. Three patients experienced short-lived (3−6 months) stable disease under conditions in which progression was expected.

Because of the wide variety of tumors found to express NKG2D ligands, the safety of the initial clinical studies, and the efficacy seen in preclinical mouse studies, further investigations are ongoing.

NK/T-Cell Leukemias

Because most recognized T-cell leukemia antigens are expressed on normal T-cells, targeting T-cell leukemias using chimeric antigen receptor is challenged by the occurrence of fratricide—wherein cells transduced with the CAR recognize expression of the cognate TAA on normal T-cells causing the cells to kill each other. In addition, special safety considerations exist, as viral transduction of leukemic T-cells during CAR manufacture may have unknown consequences, and could lead to tonic growth signals in addition to antigen negativity.[64] In addition, antigen expression on normal T-cells within the host may lead to activation of host T-cells and elimination of the adoptively transferred cells in a manner similar to bispecific T-cell engager antibodies.[65] Antigen identification is also a challenge: Fry et al. recently reviewed potential antigens for adoptive immunotherapy of T-cell ALL and identified CD5 as a potential antigen,[66] whereas a strategy based on comparisons of transcript abundance found additional targets including TALLA-1, $CD3\delta$, as well as CD1, CD52, CD37, and CD98.[67] Effects of immunodepletion using CAMPATH, which targets CD52, are well described,[68,69] but targeting other antigens may be challenged by expression on normal tissues.

Nevertheless, T-cell leukemia is a high-risk malignancy requiring extended treatment,[70] and those failing induction therapy are left with very few options; e.g. only two of seven patients achieving CR2 in one study,[71] and more than half of patients dying within 3 months in a second study attempting salvage transplant in patients with active disease but fewer than 25% blasts.[72]

NK/T-cell lymphomas also express CD56 (NCAM). As this antigen is expressed on neuroblastoma, and

may be amenable to immune targeting, it is discussed under neuroblastoma in this chapter.

CD30/CD37

Some TAAs are shared between T-cell and B-cell neoplasms, including CD30 and CD37.[73] The CD30-targeted immunoconjugate brentuximab vedotin has shown efficacy in CD30-expressing T-cell lymphomas including angioimmunoblastic T-cell lymphoma and anaplastic large-cell lymphoma[74]; however, subtypes of peripheral T-cell lymphoma show variable expression of CD30 and decreased responses to brentuximab. These data suggest that CAR targeting of this antigen may be more potent. Constructs targeting the CD37 antigen have been shown to be effective in vitro[73] but have not been tested in patients with T-cell malignancies.

CD30-directed CARs has been tested in two phase 1 trials and shown tolerability and success.[75,76] The first trial,[76] conducted in China, used an LV to deliver a CAR construct containing a 4-1BB costimulatory domain. Eighteen patients with non-Hodgkin lymphoma (one of which was anaplastic large-cell lymphoma) were infused following one of four chemotherapy conditioning regimens, the most frequent of which was fludarabine/cyclophosphamide; however, the patient with ALCL did not receive pretherapy conditioning. A 57% reduction in skin lesions was noted, and the patient was judged to have a partial response that lasted 3 months. Two patients had adverse events of grade ≥3, both of which were judged to be due to disease and/or prior chemotherapy. Thus, this treatment showed safety and promise.

The second trial[75] included nine patients, two with anaplastic large-cell lymphoma. This CD30 construct used a CD28 costimulatory domain, CAR T-cells were manufactured via RV and were infused without chemotherapy conditioning. No adverse events related to CAR T-cell infusion were documented, and no cases of CRS were observed. Of nine patients, three achieved a complete remission following CAR T-cell therapy, two of which extended beyond 2 years. Three patients had transient stable disease or partial responses but progressed within 6 months, and three did not benefit from treatment. There was an inverse correlation between soluble CD30 at the time of infusion and peak CAR T-cell expansion, suggesting that soluble antigen may dampen CAR T-cell reactivity in vivo, even though soluble antigen did not block CAR T-cell reactivity in preclinical testing. The authors also examined PD1 expression on CAR T-cells but found no correlation between expression levels and response. In sum, expanding the indication of the CAR product already tested in NHL may be one strategy to deliver the promise of this technology to patients with T-cell leukemia.

CD7

While coexpression of a CAR protein and the cognate tumor antigen has been shown to lead to retention of the tumor antigen within the endoplasmic reticulum,[64,77] an alternate approach is to intentionally delete the tumor antigen as well as the T-cell receptor from allogeneic T-cells constructing a "universal" product that would not result in graft-versus-host disease.[78–80] While CD7 is expressed on ~30% of AML cells and nearly all T-cell leukemias, there is controversy as to whether the population of LICs is CD7 positive[81] or CD7 negative[82]; its coexpression on normal T-cells prevents production of CD7-directed CAR T-cells via the above mechanism. A recent study described preclinical data showing the feasibility of combining CRISPR-mediated gene editing and viral transduction to produce CD7^{KO} CD7 CAR T-cells.[83,84] These cells were efficiently transduced (>70%), successfully gene edited, and reactive against tumor cell lines in vitro and in vivo. In murine models of T-cell[83] and myeloid leukemias,[84] the CAR T-cells showed protection. This approach may be more widely adopted, and a clinical trial is planned.

CD5

Early studies using CAR T-cells directed at CD5 and carrying a CD28 costimulatory domain showed resistance to fratricide through increased BCL-2 expression and downregulation of surface CD5 expression. These cells showed reactivity against CD5-expressing tumor cell lines and primary tumors; xenografted mice treated with CD5 CAR T-cells showed initial tumor clearance followed by recurrence.[77] These studies are being followed up with further attempts at engineering CD5^{KO} T-cells[85] similar to the description of CD7 above and with a clinical trial, which has not yet reported outcomes.

CD4

Pinz et al. generated CAR T-cells directed at the CD4 antigen by selecting CD8$^+$ T-cells for transduction.[86] Cells isolated from normal peripheral blood or from umbilical cord blood showed reactivity against CD4$^+$ tumor cell lines and delayed tumor progression in mouse xenograft models. One challenge to this approach is that patients would be expected to develop immune suppression similar to that seen in the CD4-depleting viral infection HIV. Thus, the authors developed a transduced NK cell approach using the same CAR backbone

but using a GMP-qualified NK cell line (NK-92) as the effector cell. These cells react similarly to CAR-transduced T-cells but persist in vivo for approximately 2 weeks.[87] The authors report that transduction of NK-92 cells resulted in in vitro killing of CD4$^+$ tumor cell lines and delayed tumor progression in mouse xenograft models but showed no toxicity to hematopoietic stem cells when assessed by methylcellulose colony formation.[88] These results are being followed up in a clinical trial.

PEDIATRIC SOLID TUMORS

Neuroblastoma

Neuroblastoma is the most common extracranial solid tumor in children, the most common tumor in infancy and accounts for 15% of pediatric cancer-related deaths.[89] Patients with high-risk neuroblastoma, characteristically toddlers with metastatic disease and/or patients with biologically unfavorable disease, account for the vast majority of neuroblastoma-related deaths. Despite aggressive multimodal therapy, only approximately 50% of patients with high-risk neuroblastoma will survive long term.[90] Because of the poor overall statistics for high-risk neuroblastoma, adoptive cell therapies for this indication have been well investigated.

GD2

One of the most exciting recent advances in high-risk neuroblastoma came with the incorporation of immunotherapy targeting the neuroblastoma antigen disialoganglioside (GD2). This target is uniformly expressed on tumor cells,[91] and a randomized phase 3 study incorporating the chimeric monoclonal antibody dinutuximab after consolidative myeloablative chemotherapy demonstrated a 20% improvement in event-free survival compared with patients receiving standard-of-care therapy.[92] Toxicities associated with this therapy were significant, however, and up to 40% of patients experience grade 3 or greater neuropathic pain, likely from antibody binding and complement activation on peripheral nerves, which also express surface GD2.[93]

Based on both the promise and limitations of antibody-based immunotherapies, CAR T-cells targeting GD2 have been a long-standing interest in neuroblastoma. Investigators at Baylor College of Medicine were the first to present preclinical models of a first-generation CAR (containing only the CD3ξ endodomain without any other costimulatory domains) with in vitro antineuroblastoma activity.[94] The first clinical trial incorporating this GD2 CAR attempted to enhance costimulatory activity via engagement of the native TCR by transducing the CAR into Epstein-Barr virus (EBV)–specific CD8[+] cytotoxic T lymphocytes (CTLs). Persistence of the adoptively transferred product was enhanced in EBV-specific CTLs compared with CAR-transduced polyclonal T-cells, and persistence was enhanced by the presence of CD4[+] or CD45RO[+]CD62L[+] central memory T-cells in the adoptively transferred product. Of 19 patients treated, 2 patients experienced long-term remissions, but all patients eventually developed progressive disease, and time to progression correlated with CAR T-cell persistence.[95,96]

The use of viral-specific T-cells is appealing because it leverages native TCR functionality and theoretically provides physiologic stimulation. However, preclinical data suggest that target engagement simultaneously through a CAR and a TCR can lead to decreased persistence and T-cell exhaustion.[97] Most CAR constructs now use embedded costimulation. In preclinical studies, a third-generation CAR containing both the CD28 and OX40 costimulatory domains demonstrated that incorporation of tandem costimulation domains increased T-cell expansion and improved cytokine release.[98,99] This third-generation CAR construct was evaluated in a single-institution phase 1 study at Baylor where patients with relapsed or refractory disease were treated in one of three cohorts: GD2 CAR T-cells alone, GD2 CAR T-cells following lymphodepleting chemotherapy with fludarabine and cyclophosphamide (Flu/Cy), and GD2 CAR T-cells following Flu/Cy and the anti-PD-1 checkpoint inhibitor pembrolizumab. While subjects who received lymphodepleting chemotherapy and checkpoint blockade had increased persistence when compared with those who did not receive these therapies, antineuroblastoma efficacy was limited in all cohorts with no objective responses seen.[100] While persistence appeared to improve with the addition of costimulatory domains, clinical activity did not appear to improve compared with first-generation CARs or viral-specific CARs. Others have postulated that the scFv used for this CAR construct, 14g2a, can aggregate on the surface of CAR T-cells and lead to tonic signaling and T-cell exhaustion and that specific costimulatory molecules may accelerate this process.[101,102]

In an effort to overcome obstacles encountered with the 14G2a scFv, including tonic signaling and a risk for antibody-mediated CAR rejection from patients with previous exposure to the 14g2a-based chimeric antibody dinutuximab, investigators have looked at alternate scFvs to target GD2. Based on promising preclinical activity of an alternative CAR construct incorporating the humanized murine scFv KM8138 fused to the CD28 costimulatory domain and the CD3ξ endodomain,[103,104] investigators in the United Kingdom are enrolling patients with relapsed and refractory neuroblastoma to receive this second-generation CAR. Preliminary results of this trial presented in abstract format demonstrated minor clinical responses, limited CAR persistence, and CRS in one patient.[105]

Despite the challenges faced by GD2 CAR, it is an active area of continued focus. Several approaches to improve persistence and antineuroblastoma activity are ongoing. Investigators in Shenzen, China, are evaluating a fourth-generation CAR (including CD27, CD28, and 4-1BB costimulatory domains fused to the CD3ξ endodomain) in patients with relapsed/refractory neuroblastoma and have presented early findings, which include two near-complete regressions of bulky disease and a 15% partial response rate in the first 34 patients treated.[106] In addition, optimization of the GD2 scFv to improve binding affinity and decrease aggregation to improve antitumor activity has been evaluated. Investigators at the Children's Hospital of Philadelphia created two novel GD2 binders based off of the 14G2a construct. Changes to both the scFv linker and affinity structures were evaluated, and the high-affinity scFv GD2-E101K led to increased cytokine production and antineuroblastoma activity in vitro compared with 14G2a. However, in vivo xenograft experiments of GD2-E101K induced a fatal encephalopathy in all CAR-treated mice.[107] This study highlights one potential risk of creating highly specific CAR binders in solid tumors, where TAAs usually have some normal tissue expression and off-tumor on-target toxicities remain a challenge.

L1-CAM (CD171)

Based on the known toxicity profile of GD2-targeted therapies and the concern that a CAR that is effectively able to effectively target GD2 may have significant neurotoxic effects, our group has evaluated an alternative CAR target in neuroblastoma, L1-CAM or CD171. L1-CAM expression has been associated with recurrent NB[108] and found to correlate with tumor progression and metastasis in several types of cancer, including colon carcinoma,[109] malignant glioma,[110] cutaneous malignant melanoma,[111] ovarian carcinoma,[112–114] prostate cancer,[115] renal cell carcinoma,[116] and uterine carcinoma.[117] Furthermore, L1-CAM has been found to participate in the regulation of tumor cell differentiation, proliferation, migration, and invasion.[109,117–120]

City of Hope in collaboration with Fred Hutchinson Cancer Research Center (FHCRC) and Seattle Children's Hospital (SCH) performed the first-in-human pilot study and assessed the feasibility of isolating and the safety of infusing, autologous CD8[+] cytolytic T lymphocytes coexpressing a first-generation CD171-specific CE7 CAR and the selection-suicide expression enzyme HyTK in children with recurrent/refractory NB.[121] The CAR used in that trial was developed by using a single-chain antibody extracellular domain (scFv) derived from the L1-CAM-specific murine CE7 hybridoma.[122] This chimeric immunoreceptor, CE7, is specific for an epitope in the extracellular domain of L1-CAM present on NB cells and, to a limited extent, on adrenal medulla and sympathetic ganglia.[123] Meli et al. found that inhibition of glycosylation in NB cells leads to a loss of cell surface binding sites for mAb chCE7,[124] suggesting that CE7mAb binds to an epitope on L1-CAM that is selective for tumor L1-CAM and dependent on glycosylation. Although this first clinical study was designed to maximize patient safety, tumor response was observed. No patient experienced grade 4 or 5 adverse events associated with the administration of the genetically altered T-cells, nor were overt toxicities to tissues known to express L1-CAM, such as the central nervous system, adrenal medulla, and sympathetic ganglia, observed. Four of the six patients treated in that study had detectable levels of transferred T-cells 1 week after the first infusion. Interestingly, the patient who experienced a partial tumor response following adoptive transfer showed persistence of the transferred T-cells up to 6 weeks after the second infusion. The patient was also the only patient to have minimal residual/stable disease upon administration of the first infusion. Among the six patients who underwent adoptive T-cell therapy, one experienced prolonged survival, succumbing to disease four-and-a-half years after the first infusion.[121]

Based on these encouraging preliminary results, patients are being actively enrolled on a follow-up study targeting CE7 at SCH. The study is evaluating three different CAR constructs in three different therapeutic arms: a second-generation 4-1BB CE7 CAR (arm A), a third-generation 4-1BB-CD28tm CE7 CAR (arm B), and a second-generation 4-1BB CE7 CAR incorporating the full-length IgG4 spacer domain (arm C). The goal of this study is to evaluate the safety and efficacy of each CAR construct and, within the confines of a phase 1 trial, understand differences in persistence and efficacy of each of the CAR constructs. At the time of publication, enrollment is ongoing (NCT02311621).

Other targets
Anaplastic lymphoma kinase. Anaplastic lymphoma kinase (*ALK*) is a receptor tyrosine kinase responsible for regulation of cellular proliferation and differentiation

with relatively restricted expression during fetal neuronal development.[125,126] Activating mutations in *ALK* were identified in pedigrees of families with multiple generations as a neuroblastoma oncogene.[127] In addition, somatic aberrations in *ALK* (activating mutations, amplification) have been identified as oncogenic drivers and potential therapeutic targets for kinase inhibition.[128,129] In addition, 15%–20% of neuroblastomas without activating mutations overexpress wild-type ALK,[130] making it an attractive target for immunotherapy.

An ALK CAR incorporating scFvs from previously described ALK antibodies[131] demonstrated antineuroblastoma activity in vitro but had limited activity in xenograft models. Investigations into the lack of in vivo activity suggested that the low antigen density of cell surface ALK was likely below a threshold required for CAR activation.[132] This experience highlights the importance of antigen density for CAR activation; the mere presence of a cancer-specific cell surface antigen may be insufficient for CAR activation.

B7-H3 (CD276)
B7-H3 (CD276) is a minor immune checkpoint highly expressed on a wide variety of pediatric solid and central nervous system malignancies with limited expression in normal tissues.[133–136] Overexpression of B7-H3 is associated with poor prognosis in a variety of cancers,[137] likely due to its role in immune evasion.[138] These characteristics make B7-H3 an attractive immunotherapeutic target.

Early-phase clinical trials with B7-H3-targeting monoclonal antibodies have demonstrated encouraging results in patients with advanced cancers.[139] 8H9, a murine-derived monoclonal antibody recognizing B7-H3, has been in clinical trials for neuroblastoma for more than 10 years. Omburtamab, an 8H9 conjugated to radioactive iodide is being investigated for relapsed CNS neuroblastoma (NCT00089245).[140,141]

Investigators at the University of North Carolina generated CAR T-cells targeting B7-H3 and found that they controlled the growth of pancreatic ductal adenocarcinoma, ovarian cancer, and neuroblastoma in vitro and in orthotopic and metastatic xenograft mouse models, including a patient-derived xenograft. They found that 4-1BB costimulation promoted lower PD-1 expression in CARs and resulted in superior antitumor efficacy when compared with CD28 costimulated CARs. Based on the cross-reactivity of the B7-H3 CAR with murine B7-H3, B7-H3 CARs were able to significantly control tumor growth in a syngeneic tumor model without evident toxicity.[142]

GPC2

GPC2 is a glypican protein involved in growth and differentiation of axons in developing nervous tissues.[143–145] In an evaluation comparing differential expression of cell surface proteins between tumor and normal tissues, GPC2 has been reported twice as one of the most differentially expressed proteins, making it a potentially attractive target for CAR T-cell–based immunotherapy.[67,146] Investigations led by Bosse et al. demonstrated significantly decreased survival in neuroblastoma patients with tumors expressing high levels of GPC2 and that an anti-GPC2 ADC had strong antitumor activity in a neuroblastoma patient-derived xenograft (PDX) mouse model.[146] The National Institutes of Health generated second-generation CARs containing heavy chain–only scFvs against GPC2 with 4-1BB costimulation. Anti-GPC2 CARs demonstrated both in vitro activity against neuroblastoma cell lines and in vivo activity against a disseminated neuroblastoma xenograft tumor model.[147] These encouraging preliminary results warrant further investigations in patients with neuroblastoma.

NCAM/CD56

NCAM (CD56) is a glycoprotein important in neural development that is overexpressed in neuroblastoma.[148] However, CD56 is also expressed on some normal tissues, including NK cells. A phase 1/2 study of the CD56 ADC IMGN901 in adults with relapsed/refractory CD56+ found a reasonable toxicity profile of targeting CD56 with modest response rates, most notably in Merkel cell carcinoma.[149] Based on the manageable toxicity profile of the CD56 ADC and the high and homogeneous expression of CD56 on neuroblastoma, investigators at MD Anderson developed a second-generation CAR (CD28 costimulation) directed against CD56. The CAR was able to control tumor growth in a neuroblastoma xenograft but had a limited survival benefit.[150] CD56 CAR T-cells are being studied in clinical trials for relapsed multiple myeloma (NCT03473496) and for relapsed AML (NCT03473457), and further investigation in neuroblastoma may be warranted based on these first-in-human experiences.

Sarcomas

Sarcomas are a diverse group of malignancies originating in bone and connective tissues that account for approximately 15% of pediatric cancers. Common pediatric sarcomas include osteosarcoma, Ewing sarcoma, and rhabdomyosarcoma. While most children with localized disease will be cured with conventional chemotherapy, surgery, and/or radiation, patients with recurrent or metastatic disease continue to have an exceedingly poor prognosis.[151]

Because of the diversity of tissues of origin, identifying pansarcoma TAAs has been challenging. Traditional histology-restricted CAR trials have been limited in sarcoma, and there is an emerging shift toward basket trials: histology independent trials that focus on the presence of a threshold TAA expression as an eligibility requirement.

GD2

GD2 is also of interest in sarcoma based on its expression in most osteosarcomas as well as some Ewing sarcomas and rhabdomyosarcomas.[152–154] Based on the encouraging preclinical and early clinical data with GD2 CARs in neuroblastoma, others have sought to reproduce these results in sarcoma. While a third-generation GD2 CAR (CD28 and OX40 costimulation) had in vitro activity against osteosarcoma cell lines, it had no in vivo activity in mouse xenograft experiments. Interestingly, sarcoma xenografts, but not neuroblastoma xenografts, induced robust murine monocytic and granulocytic myeloid-derived suppressor cell (MDSCs) infiltrates. Administration of all-*trans* retinoic acid (ATRA) reduced the MDSC infiltrate and partially restored GD2 CAR activity in vivo.[154] These experiments highlight the importance of the immunosuppressive tumor microenvironment present in most pediatric solid tumors that will likely also need to be targeted in order for adoptive therapies to have effect. Investigators at Baylor College of Medicine, who pioneered GD2 CAR therapy, are currently evaluating GD2 CARs (expressed in VZV-specific CTLs) in patients with GD2-positive sarcomas and neuroblastoma (NCT01953900).

HER2

HER2 (ERBB2), a receptor tyrosine kinase in the ErbB family of membrane-bound growth factor receptors, is expressed in over 70% of osteosarcomas but at much lower levels than HER2-amplified tumors like breast cancer.[155] HER2-specific CAR T-cells demonstrated potent antitumor effects in osteosarcoma xenograft models.[155] Despite a case of fatal pneumonitis in an adult colon cancer patient attributable to HER2 CARs at the Surgery Branch of the NCI,[156] HER2 CARs appeared safe in a phase 1/2 study of HER2-positive sarcomas.[157] In early published reports of the first 19 patients treated on this ongoing phase 1/2 study (NCT00902044), persistence appeared to be dose dependent, with detectable persistence for at least 6 weeks in seven of the nine evaluable patients who received greater than 1×10^6 HER2.CARs/m^2. While no objective responses were seen, four patients experienced stable disease and one patient had a tumor resection, which demonstrated >90% tumor necrosis. In addition, HER2 CARs were detectable in 2/2 tumors removed and evaluated for CAR persistence despite no evidence of peripheral blood persistence, suggesting that CARs were capable of trafficking to and expansion at sites of disease.[157] This study highlights an additional challenge in solid tumor CAR development: in contrast to leukemia studies, where CAR T-cell persistence in peripheral blood can be easily monitored and can serve as an important biomarker of response,[158] peripheral blood persistence studies in solid tumors may not be as reliable if CARs traffic to sites of disease.

FOLR1/2

Folate receptors (FRs) are membrane-bound surface proteins that bind folates and folate conjugates with high affinity. FRs are frequently overexpressed in a number of human malignancies including cancers of the ovary, lung, endometrium, kidney, breast, bladder, and brain. In a screen of FR isoform expression by mRNA in both normal and malignant tissues, an osteosarcoma sample was among the cancers with the highest FRα (FOLR1) expression. Expression of either isoform was extremely limited in healthy tissues, making it an attractive immunotherapeutic target.[159] Using immunohistochemical methodology (IHC), 78.5% of a series of 107 osteosarcoma tumors had FRα mRNA expression.[160]

Our group has developed a CAR T adaptor molecule (CAM)–based therapy that uses the small bispecific molecule, EC17 (folic acid coupled with FITC isomer I via an ethylenediamine linker).[161] In this setting, EC17 effectively "paints" FR$^+$ tumors with the FITC antigen to attract anti-FL(FITC-E2) CAR T-cells, which drive their proliferation and activate a robust immune response. In preclinical evaluations with tumor-bearing mice, EC17 penetrated solid tumors quickly and was retained due to its high affinity for the FR, whereas unbound EC17 was rapidly cleared from the blood and did not bind to receptor-negative tissues. When combined with a second-generation anti-FITC CAR (4-1BB costimulation), EC17 triggered CAR activation and cytolytic activity. Maximal cytolytic potential correlated with both functional FR levels (in a semilog fashion) and the amount of effector cells present. Tumor-bearing mice treated with EC17 and anti-FITC CARs did develop CRS, but severe CRS could be easily mitigated or prevented by applying intermittent dosing and/or dose titration of EC17. In addition, mice experiencing severe CRS were able to be rapidly rescued with the administration intravenous sodium fluorescein, which displaced bound EC17 from the CAR.[162] These experiments highlight additional safety features that may be important to mitigate toxicities and provide a platform for more universal CAR creation by creating constructs that bind to exogenously administered targets capable of binding to TAAs.

Epidermal growth factor receptor

The epidermal growth factor receptor (EGFR or HER1) is a cell surface tyrosine kinase receptor that is expressed in a diverse group of epithelial and nonepithelial tissues and broadly associated with cell proliferation and differentiation. Expression of wild-type EGFR and activating mutations are described in many solid tumors, such as lung, pancreatic, glioblastoma, head, and neck cancers, as well as a number of predominantly pediatric tumors, including bone and soft tissue sarcomas and neuroblastoma.[163–165] In the setting of malignancy, EGFR expression has been associated with aggressive disease, chemotherapy resistance, and increased metastatic potential.[165,166] Therefore, it has been the focus of numerous targeted cancer therapy initiatives over the past decade, primarily manifest in two groups of agents: tyrosine kinase inhibitors (TKIs) and anti-EGFR antibodies.[167] Employment of these agents has yielded some promising results, but they are not necessarily effective against all cancer-associated EGFR mutations or tumors with overexpression of wild-type EGFR and are frequently associated with notable off-target toxicities due to the expression of EGFR in normal tissue.[168]

The unique EGFR monoclonal antibody (mAb) 806 selectively binds to an epitope on the extracellular portion of human EGFR expressed on the surface of tumor cell.[169] Though this antibody was raised against the deletion mutant EGFRvIII commonly present in glioblastomas and some other adult solid tumors, it also binds to wild-type EGFR that is untethered on the cell surface, which accounts for approximately 10% of EGFR expressed by cancer cells due to aberrant post-translational processing that is not present in nonmalignant EGFR-expressing cells.[169–172] A phase 1 trial utilizing a radiolabeled chimeric version of this antibody in varied tumor types confirmed reliable tumor tissue uptake with no evidence of toxicity related to uptake in normal tissues known to express EGFR.[172] A more recent phase 1 trial in adults with solid tumors characterized by EGFRvIII mutation or wild-type EGFR overexpression studied the effects of a humanized mAb 806, ABT-806. Treatment was well tolerated with an acceptable adverse event profile. Two subjects achieved prolonged stable disease.[173] Given tumor specificity of this antibody, its ability to recognize an epitope on cells with a variety of EGFR aberrations, and favorable toxicity profile in multiple adult trials, humanized mAb 806 is an attractive candidate for use in the development of an EGFR-specific CAR for employment in adoptive T-cell therapy for EGFR-expressing relapsed or refractory pediatric solid tumors, and our group is evaluating the safety and efficacy of this CAR construct in patients with EGFR⁺ solid tumors (NCT03618381).

Other targets

Other studies that have demonstrated positive results in sarcoma cell lines or mouse models with CAR T-cells include B7-H3,[142] IGF1R, and ROR1.[174] Clinical trials testing these approaches are eagerly awaited.

CARCINOMAS

The application of CAR-modified T-cells to adult solid tumors, the cancers that comprise the majority of oncologic disease burden in the world, has yet to meet with any modicum of success that approaches that seen in B-cell malignancy. Worldwide, the cancers that account for the greatest amount of morbidity and mortality are found in the lung, breast, colorectal tissue, stomach, liver, prostate, and skin (nonmelanoma) (World Health Organization, Cancer Key Facts, September 12, 2018, www.who.int/news-room/fact-sheets/detail/cancer).

Public health interventions, such as vaccination against human papilloma virus (HPV) and hepatitis B virus (HBV), could prevent greater than 1 million cancer cases each year.[175] Approximately 15% of all cancers are associated with infections of *Helicobacter pylori*, HPV, HBV, hepatitis C virus, and Epstein-Barr virus. This vast burden of disease associated with infectious etiology impacts our discussion of CAR T immunotherapy in two ways. First, the current value of developing what is currently an expensive and resource-intensive process must be balanced against other interventions focused on prevention. Second, viral-associated cancers encode a set of nongenomic (viral) target antigens and have an inflammatory milieu that may be fundamentally different from non–viral-associated cancers. Significant progress has been made using T-cell receptor–based approaches for both EBV- and HPV-associated cancers.[176–178] Moreover, commercially, the most advanced product for the adoptive immunotherapy of solid tumors is the recombinant TCR specific for the NY-ESO 1 antigen, developed by Adaptimmune

(acquired by GSK and marketed as GSK3377794/NY-ESO SPEAR T-cell therapy), being tested in a range of malignancies including ovarian cancer, non–small cell lung cancer (NSCLC) synovial sarcoma, melanoma, and multiple myeloma. This level of clinical success has yet to be realized for CAR T approaches in solid tumors. Nevertheless, enthusiasm for a number of CAR T targets is high. What remains to be seen is if the level of specificity with TCRs targeting either viral or cancer neoantigens can be approached using CAR T. We will discuss the most common approaches to the major solid tumors in adults and also look at alternative approaches that target the immune cell milieu and non–marrow-derived stroma that comprise the tumor lesion as well.

LUNG CANCER

The most significant advance in lung cancer therapy in decades has been the FDA approval of the immune checkpoint inhibitors, antibodies that target tumor-expressed proteins or their ligands on T-cells, blocking antiactivation signals to T-cells. In NSCLC, anti-PD1 (pembrolizumab) is standard therapy. Anti-PD1 has also been proposed to be given in combination with mesothelin-specific CARs[179] Also available are other anti-PD1 antibodies (nivolumab), anti-PDL-1 antibody (atezolizumab), and the anti-CTLA-4 antibody, ipilimumab. Adult cancers differ from pediatric cancer in the accumulation of numerous neoantigens during carcinogenesis that serve as tumor-specific T-cell antigens to which an active T-cell response can develop, once negative signals have been eliminated. Throughout this entire section, it should be assumed that some manner of blocking these negative signals will be required for effective antitumor immunity mediated either by TCR-based or CAR-based approaches.

Mesothelin

Originally a target proposed for mesothelioma, the mesothelin protein has been found to be expressed in 60%–65% of lung cancers in addition to 85%–90% of mesotheliomas.[180] The mesothelin protein is not broadly expressed on normal mesothelial cells, giving rise to its potential as a target for CAR T-cells.[180] Concerns with on-target yet off-tumor activity for CARs targeting mesothelin led to an innovative clinical trial in which mRNA encoding for the CAR was electroporated into activated T-cells, which were subsequently infused into patients, a departure for the use of retroviral or lentiviral gene vectors normally used in CAR T production.[181] The approach was well-tolerated and there were indications of T-cell activity. Long-term effects or persistence could not be expected for this approach, as the CAR T transcript is only temporarily expressed. Subsequent clinical testing remained mindful of the potential cytotoxicity of an anti-mesothelin CAR, and in one CAR T trial, therapeutic cells were administered with a nonmyeloablative conditioning regimen (fludarabine on days −7 to −3 at 25 mg/m^2/day and cyclophosphamide on days −7 and −6 at 60 mg/kg) combined with IL-2 (aldesluekin) (NCT01583686). While this study at the National Institutes of Health and a similar study focusing on pleural disease at Memorial Sloan-Kettering Cancer Center are progressing, more attention has focused on alternative mesothelin epitopes targeted by the CAR T-binding domain and defining the interaction of mesothelin with MUC16.

Mesothelin has an extracellular cleavage site, resulting in a membrane-bound remnant and a soluble protein known as megakaryocyte potentiating factor (MPF), a decline in which serves as a biomarker for disease response.[182] Designing CARs to target mesothelin needs to take into account whether the antibody or recombinant scFv used to create the binding domain targets the most membrane distal region I (as do SS1P- and HN1-scFv-based CARs), region II, or region III, or a more global conformational epitope.[183] Region I is also known to interact with MUC16/CA125, which may account for variable binding activity in different tumor types.[184] Mesothelin-specific CAR T-cells have also been proposed for pancreatic cancer where it is expressed in 80%–85% of cases, as well as in ovarian cancer and in cholangiocarcinoma.[180]

MET

The hepatocyte growth factor (HGF) receptor MET (MNNG-HOS transforming gene) is expressed in a majority of malignant pleural mesotheliomas and has proved a tractable target in murine models of this disease.[185] Interestingly, the targeting moiety of the CAR in this study was not an scFV, but a specific ligand of MET, encoding the NK1 isoform of HGF. MET is also expressed in NSCLC, breast, gastric, and liver cancer and has the potential for being a broadly applicable target.

BREAST CANCER

CAR T-cells are being considered for triple-negative breast cancer (TNBC), where fewer therapeutic options exist, along with relapsed or refractory disease. TNBC is estrogen and progesterone receptor negative and does not express therapeutically relevant levels of HER2 (human epidermal growth factor receptor, the target of Herceptin antibody [trastuzumab]).[186] As no targeted therapies exist for TNBC, new approaches are badly needed. For breast cancer, both mesothelin and folate receptor targeting have been proposed. As mesothelin was discussed above, we will focus on the folate receptor.

Folate Receptor

In normal tissues, folate receptor-alpha (FOLR1) expression is limited to the apical surface of polarized epithelial cells.[187] This restriction is lost upon oncologic transformation, and thus, FOLR1 is available for either antibody- or CAR-based targeting in numerous cancers of epithelial origin. Importantly, estrogen receptor binding has been found to downregulate FOLR1 expression, which is reversed by tamoxifen, while TNBC is associated with increased FOLR1 expression.[188] In the first study of patient xenografts in a murine model, it was demonstrated that anti-FOLR1 CAR T-cells are effective against TNBC, yet are highly dependent of the level of FOLR1 expression.[189] This highlights a growing theme in solid tumor immune-based therapeutics wherein the overall expression level of target that is known to be variable may need to be taken into consideration before initiating a new therapeutic approach. Alternatively, a combination approach might be taken where two or more CAR T targets are expressed. The B-cell antigen CD22 is also expressed at limiting levels in CAR T failure with CD22 CARs, and preliminary studies have shown that small molecules like bryostatin have the ability to upregulate CD22 expression levels.[190] The tumor biology behind the mechanisms of target expression level modulation that can lead to CAR T escape is nascent field and should yield exciting new findings.

TEM8/ANTXR1

TEM8 was originally described as a membrane protein associated with tumor vasculature in colorectal carcinoma[191] but has recently been described as a CAR T target in TNBC.[192] Further research has demonstrated that TEM8, which binds to the extracellular matrix (ECM) component—cleaved collagen alpha 3(VI), is overexpressed in breast cancer in comparison with normal tissue and is associated with cells having a breast cancer-stem cell phenotype.[193,194] While a TEM8-CAR has only been evaluated in mouse PDX models to date, the near identity of the mouse and human TEM8 lends added confidence to the safety of its rapid evaluation in human trials.

MUC1

Mucin-1 (MUC1) is unique among TAAs in that its differentiation from normal tissue is not based on expression level per se, but on the exposure of a unique epitope due to hypoglycosylation. MUC1 is a large protein with tandem repeated sequences carrying O-linked glycosylation that is dysregulated due to its overexpression in a variety of adenocarcinomas, thus creating a tumor-specific form of the molecule.[195] The development of a CAR T effective against tumor-expressed MUC1 highlights that in addition to an active antigen-binding domain, the inclusion of a flexible elongated "hinge" domain between the binder and the transmembrane region of the CAR generates a more active construct.[196] A more restricted MUC1-binding domain that binds to aberrant-glycoprotein conjugates (the MUC1 Tn glycoform) has recently been tested in a pancreatic xenograft model and may also be applicable in breast cancer.[197] These studies highlight that the specific cancer-expressed forms of a CAR T target and the structural components of the CAR molecule itself interact in precise ways. Biophysical rules to describe this interaction have yet to be formulated.

PROSTATE

The two CAR targets uniquely considered for prostate cancer are prostate-specific membrane antigen (PSMA) and prostate stem cell antigen (PSCA). Other general carcinoma-specific CARs worth considering for prostate cancer, especially in combinatorial approaches, include MUC1, Her2, and EpCAM.

Prostate-Specific Membrane Antigen

PSMA is a multiply spliced membrane protein and encodes both membrane-bound and cytosolic forms[198] The ratio of membrane to cytosolic forms dramatically increases in prostate cancer cells.[199] The established secretion of TGF-beta by prostate cancer was countered in animal models by the co-expression of a PMSA-specific CAR construct and a dominant-negative[200] TBF-beta receptor. This approach led to a current clinical trial featuring this combined approach (NCT03089203). In another murine model, the effectiveness of a PMSA-directed CAR was enhanced by the inclusion of an anti-human PD-1 antibody, which allowed for more effective CAR T penetration of the lesion.[201]

PSMA not only serves as a prostate cancer specific target antigen, but also as a tumor specific antigen generally upregulated on tumor-associated vasculature. In a recent study, a CAR based on the anti-PSMA scFv J951 was demonstrated to profoundly disrupt tumor associated vasculature in a mouse model of ovarian cancer, which lead to secondary destruction of tumor cells and a decrease in tumor burden.[202]

Prostate Stem Cell Antigen

PSCA encodes for a unique cell surface glycoprotein that bears homology only to stem cell antigen 2, a member of the Thy-1/Ly6 family of proteins.[203] PSCA has been reported to demonstrate increased staining in concordance with a higher Gleason score, tumor stage, universal expression in bone metastases, and linkage to progression of androgen independence.[204] A large histopathological study did not validate these associations but nevertheless confirms that PSCA is a viable candidate CAR target.[205] A PSCA-targeting CAR was evaluated in bone metastatic xenografts in immunocompromised mice and showed strong antitumor activity.[206] This model also supported the inclusion of a 4-1BB signaling domain in the CAR-signaling domain, which prevented rapid T-cells exhaustion and increased antitumor effectiveness.

COLORECTAL TISSUE

More than 90% of colorectal carcinomas are classified as adenocarcinomas. As with lung cancers, antibody-based approaches are currently being employed with some success against this disease, including those against checkpoint molecules (PD-1/PD-L1), tumor surface antigens (EGFR, HER2, CEA), and tumor vasculature (VEGF/VEGFR2). In addition to broad carcinoma approaches (see Fig. 11.1), the newly recognized surface antigen, GUCY2C, is being targeted. Colorectal carcinoma can be subdivided into at least four major groups by either gene expression profiling or pathological analysis of the immune cell context of the lesion. The microsatellite-enriched subgroup (CMS1) expresses genes associated with CTLs and is a candidate for checkpoint blockade therapy. The poor prognosis CMS4 group (mesenchymal subtype) expresses genes enriched for inflammatory markers, lymphocytes, fibroblasts, and monocytic cells, while the intermediate risk types CMS2 (canonical) and CMS3 (metabolic subtype) present with a less inflammatory gene signature.[207,208] Each subtype expresses a unique set of targets and will likely require a unique set of interventions, while the group with microsatellite enrichment already has already been shown to respond to antibody-based immune checkpoint treatment.[209]

GUCY2C

GUCY2 (guanylate cyclase 2C, GUC2C, DIAR6, MUCIL) is a transmembrane protein recently recognized as a potential target for CAR T in model systems.[210] In normal intestinal epithelium, GUCY2YC expression is restricted to the apical membrane. Expression is found in more than 95% of colorectal cancer metastases, which no longer maintain membrane-polarized expression.[211,212]

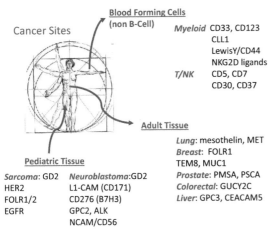

CAR-T Therapeutic Candidates

Cancer Sites

Blood Forming Cells (non B-Cell)

Myeloid CD33, CD123
CLL1
LewisY/CD44
NKG2D ligands
T/NK CD5, CD7
CD30, CD37

Adult Tissue

Lung: mesothelin, MET
Breast: FOLR1
TEM8, MUC1
Prostate: PMSA, PSCA
Colorectal: GUCY2C
Liver: GPC3, CEACAM5

Pediatric Tissue

Sarcoma: GD2
HER2
FOLR1/2
EGFR

*Neuroblastoma:*GD2
L1-CAM (CD171)
CD276 (B7H3)
GPC2, ALK
NCAM/CD56

FIG. 11.1 Promising chimeric antigen receptor (CAR) T approaches according to cancer site. The major cancer sites, and the cancers to which promising CAR therapeutics are currently or about to enter clinical trials, are illustrated. Targets with only laboratory-based approaches are not shown, nor are those with known severe toxicity. Remarkable for not being shown are tumor stroma—associated targets and cancer stem cell targets, which await safe and effective targeting strategies.

LIVER CANCER

The majority of primary liver cancers are classified as hepatocellular carcinoma (HCC) or intrahepatic cholangiocarcinoma. Fibrolamellar carcinoma and hepatoblastoma, primarily pediatric, are considered rare.[213] As in lung cancer, anti-PD1 therapeutic approaches are now an approved therapeutic approach, lending support to the immune sensitivity of these tumors.[214] Nevertheless, liver tumor-specific, and more general carcinoma marker—targeted approaches are being developed for CAR T-based therapy for liver cancer.

GPC3

Glypican-3 (GPC3) is a heparan sulfate proteoglycan that is highly expressed in HCC and is being evaluated as a target in both immunotoxin and bispecific antibody approaches.[215,216] Currently, GPC3 CARs are at the preclinical stage, but the restriction of GPC3 expression to HCC, activity of CAR T in xenograft models,[217] and synergy with PD-1 blockade[218] portend a number of clinical trials opening soon (NCT02395250, NCT02905188).

Carcinoembryonic Antigen (CEACAM5)

Carcinoembryonic antigen (CEA)—specific CAR T-cells are under active study in clinical trials. One of these trials was very broad, encompassing breast, colorectal, gastric, lung, ovarian, pancreatic, and unspecified adult solid tumors (NCT01212887). The CAR in this trial features the MFE23 scFv and is used in the context of cyclophosphamide and fludarabine preconditioning and IL-2 treatment. The CAR construct itself only expressed a CD3-zeta chain and thus is a first-generation CAR. Lung toxicity was seen in a patient at the highest dose level, leading to cessation of this trial.[219] Although the toxicity was not severe or long term, perhaps due to the short persistence of the CEA-CAR-T product, it did highlight the possibility of on-target off-tumor toxicity. In another CEA-CAR-T trial, T-cells were administered to patients with CEA-positive liver metastases by hepatic artery infusion (NCT01373047). In the published summary of this phase 1 trial, no systemic toxicity was seen. The study differed from the previous one in that a second-generation CD28-CD3zeta CAR was used, the hMN14 scFv was used, and there was no chemotherapeutic preconditioning. Although a meaningful response was seen in a minority of patients (increased survival or decreased serum CEA), there may indeed be a therapeutic window whereby CEA-specific CARs can be safely and effectively used.[220]

STOMACH CANCER

Gastric cancer is known to be linked to both diet and *H. pylori* infection.[221] *H. pylori* activates a chronic inflammatory response in associated mucosal lymphoid tissues, directly activates NF-κB, and upregulates IL-8 in gastric epithelial cells, leading to gastric carcinogenesis.[222] Not as much detailed work has been carried out with gastric cancer with respect to unique CAR target antigens. The major targets proposed for gastric cancer are CEA and MUC1, both discussed above in other tissue histopathologies. FOLR1 is also expressed on 30% of gastric cancers[223] and may also serve as a CAR target antigen.[223]

SKIN CANCER (NONMELANOMA)

Basal cell carcinoma is the most common malignancy in the world. Although it has a low mortality rate, the incidence is rising and significant morbidity can arise through local tissue destruction.[224] Although having a lower incidence rate, cutaneous squamous cell carcinoma will result in 1 million cases in the United States this year. Although most cases can be treated locally, the overall incidence is rising, and metastatic relapse and death can occur (approximately 9000 cases per year).[225] The reported improvement in outcome with patients treated with cetuximab[226] indicates the presence of targetable EGFR on the squamous cell carcinoma surface. In 2018, a monoclonal antibody to PD-1 (Cemiplimab) became the first approved drug for cutaneous squamous cell carcinoma, demonstrating again the ability of the immune system to impact disease progression.

E-cadherin

The expression of E-cadherin (CDH1, CD324, LCAM) is a major distinguishing factor between adenoma and carcinoma.[227] Mutated forms are found in stomach, pancreas, colorectal, ovarian, and breast cancer, highlighting that maintenance of tissue architecture governs the biology of the lesion and the ability to invade adjacent tissue.[227] The expression of E-cadherin on invasive squamous cell carcinoma may provide another CAR T target for this disease.[228]

THE IMMUNOSUPPRESSIVE TUMOR CELLULAR ARCHITECTURE

In addition to the transformed cancer cells in and of themselves, the tumor lesion is also composed of tumor-associated fibroblasts (TAFs), tumor-associated macrophages (TAMs), MDSCs, T-regulatory cells (Tregs), and tumor-associated vasculature all of which produce soluble factors and an ECM known to protect tumor cells from immune surveillance. These nontransformed cells, often referred to as tumor stroma, produce cytokines, chemokines, and metabolic by-products (and also deplete the tumor milieu of metabolites required for effective T-cell function), which block the effective activation and expansion of antitumor T-cells. Through the production of an aberrant lesional tissue architecture also includes the production of extracellular proteins such as collagens or glycosaminoglycans that misdirect T-cell migration.

Cancer-Associated Fibroblasts

Cancer-associated fibroblasts (CAFs) are normal tissue components that have been subverted by cancer cells to produce factors that promote cancer growth, angiogenesis, and invasion including specific collagen types, growth factors, enzymes, and other soluble factors that significantly alter the ECM.[229,230] The discovery of the expression of fibroblast-activating protein (FAP) was met with enthusiasm as it is expressed in nearly all tumors lesions, on a set of TAFs.[206] However, when FAP-specific CAR T-cells were tested in animal models,

significant toxicity against bone marrow stem cells was noted. FAP expression was also found on human marrow cells.[231] Gene expression analysis of CAFs has revealed a specific immunosuppressive signature but has yet to yield specific other tumor-specific extracellular markers beyond the collagen subtype COL11A1.[232]

CAFs from invasive adenocarcinoma of the lung were found in approximately 30% of analyzed specimens to express **podoplanin**.[233] Interestingly, podoplanin has been shown to be expressed in orthotopic glioblastomas in mice and can be effectively targeted by CAR T.[234] Thus, it may serve to be a CAR T target in multiple applications. Chondroitin sulfate proteoglycan 4 (**CSPG4**, also referred to as high-molecular-weight melanoma-associated antigen [HMW-MAA], neuron-glial antigen 2 [NG2], a chondroitin sulfate glycosaminoglycan) is another promising CAR T target present in tumor stroma, although safety has yet to be established due to its expression on normal tissue.[235]

Tumor Vasculature

A number of antibody-based reagents have been found to impact angiogenesis and preferentially act against cancer. The clinically approved antibody to vascular endothelial growth factor A (VEGF-A), bevacizumab (Avastin), was recently used in an animal model of neuroblastoma in combination with GD2-specific CAR T.[236] The combination of both agents was required to treat engrafted IMR-32 or the HTLA-230 cell lines in immunocompromised mice. Targeting the same signaling axis, CAR T-cells specific for both VEGFR-2 and VEGFR-1 have demonstrated activity in animal models.[237,238] A full analysis of clinical safety and efficacy for these targets has yet to be published.

Myeloid-Derived Suppressor Cell

MDSC is a general term for immature granulocytic and monocytic cell types that accumulate in tumor lesions and actively suppress T-cell activity. The primary goal for the CAR T therapist has been to subvert MDSC activity with agents such as retinoic acid, which differentiates MDSC, making them less immunosuppressive or blocking soluble factors they produce.[154,239] In a murine model of liver metastases, CEA-specific CAR T-cells were found to be subverted by an expansion of liver-resident MDSC.[240] These effects were countered by a combination of blocking the PD-L1 and neutralizing GM-CSF (which recruits MDSC to the metastatic lesion).

Soluble Factors

The cytokines and chemokines produced in a tumor lesion can arise from the tumor itself, CAFs, MDSCs, or lymphocytes that have been misdirected to produce factors that suppress rather than enhance tumor immunity, such as those produced by T-regulatory cells. One elegant example of subverting these negative tumor signals and turning them to the T effector cell's advantage was the creation of a chimeric cytokine receptor wherein the extracellular domain of the IL-4 receptor was linked to the intracellular signaling domain of IL-7, thus protecting anti-MUC1-CAR-T from exhaustion and amplifying their antitumor activity.[241] Any number of these combinations could be created to subvert the specific cytokines present in a particular lesion. Moreover, including chemokine receptors as part of the gene expression package present in the CAR construct may also aid in directing CAR T to the tumor site.

CANCER STEM CELL MARKERS

Advances in cancer biology have led to the recognition that two related processes of dedifferentiation are at work in cancer lesions. One is the epithelial-to-mesenchymal transition (EMT), and the other is the recognition that there are cancer cells within a lesion that are resistant to chemotherapy and have distinct stem cell–like properties. Cancer stem cell (CSC) markers that are broadly expressed in solid tumors could potentially serve as CAR T targets. **CD24** has been proposed as a marker for colorectal carcinoma cells that are have stem cell-like properties and which have a propensity to undergo EMT.[242] Similarly, CD24 has been described as a CSC marker in ovarian carcinoma, and CAR-based clinical approaches have been proposed.[243] CD44 variant 6 (**CD44v6**) is expressed on a broad range of epithelial and hematologic CSCs.[244] Its limited expression on normal stem cells in the marrow may allow for selective targeting of tumors.[245] Recent translational studies have proposed its application in hematologic malignancies and indicate potential efficacy in solid tumors as well.[246,247] The expression of **CD133** on a broad array of epithelial CSCs has already led to phase 1 clinical trial in patients with CD133-positive liver, pancreatic, and colorectal cancer.[248] No drastic toxicity was noted, and the apparent safety of this approach supports further exploration of CD133 as a CAR T target. In a single case report, a patient with cholangiocarcinoma received a combined product of CD133- and EGFR-specific CAR T. The off-tumor effects, which included subcutaneous hemorrhages, necessitated the administration of steroids to control CAR T toxicity.[249]

CONCLUSION

CAR-based therapy for non–B-cell malignancy remains an area of great expectation. The vast unmet medical need that cancer presents is an opportunity to develop new methods of engineering CAR T activity and control. We have outlined the most clinically relevant targets expressed outside of B-cell and CNS malignancy. The most rapid progress is anticipated for AML and T-cell malignancy. Although targets specificity is essential, new technologies have been developed that, on their own or in concert with hematopoietic stem cell transplantation, will allow CD33, CD123, CD5, and CD7 to be effectively targeted. Outside of hematologic malignancy, the field is still in early development. Credible targets are being pursued in pediatric solid tumors and include HER2, FOLR1/2, EGFR, CD276 (B7H3), and GPC2. In adult carcinomas, these targets and others such as mesothelin, PSMA, MUC1, and GPC3 are also being targeted. What is not known is how T-cells will need to be engineered to overcome the immunosuppressive tumor microenvironment, how this will differ between tumor types and perhaps even between patients, and whether tumor-associated stromal cells will also need to be targeted. The next 5 years will yield important answers to these questions. The time to aggressively test CAR T approaches in the most challenging solid tumor types has arrived, and new advances for our patients are our much-hoped-for and anticipated result.

REFERENCES

1. Ruella M, June CH. Predicting dangerous rides in CAR T-cells: bridging the gap between mice and humans. *Mol Ther.* 2018;26:1401–1403. https://doi.org/10.1016/j.ymthe.2018.05.005.
2. Taraseviciute A, Tkachev V, Ponce R, et al. Chimeric antigen receptor T-cell–mediated neurotoxicity in nonhuman primates. *Cancer Discov.* 2018;8:750–763. https://doi.org/10.1158/2159-8290.CD-17-1368.
3. Turtle CJ, Hay KA, Hanafi L-A, et al. Durable molecular remissions in chronic lymphocytic leukemia treated with CD19-specific chimeric antigen receptor–modified T-cells after failure of Ibrutinib. *J Clin Orthod.* 2017;35:3010–3020. https://doi.org/10.1200/JCO.2017.72.8519.
4. Estey E. Acute myeloid leukemia: 2016 update on risk-stratification and management. *Am J Hematol.* 2016;91:824–846. https://doi.org/10.1002/ajh.24439.
5. Perna F, Berman SH, Soni RK, et al. Integrating proteomics and transcriptomics for systematic combinatorial chimeric antigen receptor therapy of AML. *Cancer Cell.* 2017;32:506–519.e5. https://doi.org/10.1016/j.ccell.2017.09.004.

6. Bernstein ID, Singer JW, Andrews RG, et al. Treatment of acute myeloid leukemia cells in vitro with a monoclonal antibody recognizing a myeloid differentiation antigen allows normal progenitor cells to be expressed. *J Clin Investig.* 1987;79:1153–1159. https://doi.org/10.1172/JCI112932.

7. Shlush LI, Mitchell A, Heisler L, et al. Tracing the origins of relapse in acute myeloid leukaemia to stem cells. *Nature.* 2017;547:104–108. https://doi.org/10.1038/nature22993.

8. Shlush LI, Zandi S, Mitchell A, et al. Identification of pre-leukaemic haematopoietic stem cells in acute leukaemia. *Nature.* 2014;506:328–333. https://doi.org/10.1038/nature13038.

9. Hamann PR, Hinman LM, Hollander I, et al. A potent and selective anti-CD33 Antibody–Calicheamicin conjugate for treatment of acute myeloid leukemia. *Bioconjug Chem.* 2002;13:47–58. https://doi.org/10.1021/bc010021y.

10. Sievers EL, Appelbaum FR, Spielberger RT, et al. Selective ablation of acute myeloid leukemia using antibody-targeted chemotherapy: a phase I study of an anti-CD33 calicheamicin immunoconjugate: presented in part at the 1997 annual meeting of the American Society of clinical Oncology, Denver, CO; the 1997 European cancer Conference, Hamburg, Germany; and the 1997 Annual meeting of the American Society of Hematology, San Diego, CA. *Blood.* 1999;93:3678–3684.

11. Sievers EL, Larson RA, Stadtmauer EA, et al. Efficacy and safety of gemtuzumab ozogamicin in patients with CD33-positive acute myeloid leukemia in first relapse. *J Clin Orthod.* 2001;19:3244–3254. https://doi.org/10.1200/JCO.2001.19.13.3244.

12. Candoni A, Martinelli G, Toffoletti E, et al. Gemtuzumab-ozogamicin in combination with fludarabine, cytarabine, idarubicin (FLAI-GO) as induction therapy in CD33-positive AML patients younger than 65 years. *Leuk Res.* 2008;32:1800–1808. https://doi.org/10.1016/j.leukres.2008.05.011.

13. Castaigne S, Pautas C, Terré C, et al. Effect of gemtuzumab ozogamicin on survival of adult patients with de-novo acute myeloid leukaemia (ALFA-0701): a randomised, open-label, phase 3 study. *The Lancet.* 2012;379:1508–1516. https://doi.org/10.1016/S0140-6736(12)60485-1.

14. Petersdorf SH, Kopecky KJ, Slovak M, et al. A phase 3 study of gemtuzumab ozogamicin during induction and postconsolidation therapy in younger patients with acute myeloid leukemia. *Blood.* 2013;121:4854–4860. https://doi.org/10.1182/blood-2013-01-466706.

15. Burnett AK, Hills RK, Milligan D, et al. Identification of patients with acute myeloblastic leukemia who benefit from the addition of gemtuzumab ozogamicin: results of the MRC AML15 trial. *J Clin Orthod.* 2011;29:369–377. https://doi.org/10.1200/JCO.2010.31.4310.

16. Lamba JK, Chauhan L, Shin M, et al. CD33 splicing polymorphism determines gemtuzumab ozogamicin response in de novo acute myeloid leukemia: report from randomized phase III Children's oncology group trial AAML0531. *J Clin Orthod.* 2017;35:2674–2682. https://doi.org/10.1200/JCO.2016.71.2513.

17. Laszlo GS, Harrington KH, Gudgeon CJ, et al. Expression and functional characterization of CD33 transcript variants in human acute myeloid leukemia. *Oncotarget.* 2016;7:43281–43294. https://doi.org/10.18632/oncotarget.9674.

18. Marin V, Pizzitola I, Agostoni V, et al. Cytokine-induced killer cells for cell therapy of acute myeloid leukemia: improvement of their immune activity by expression of CD33-specific chimeric receptors. *Haematologica.* 2010;95:2144–2152. https://doi.org/10.3324/haematol.2010.026310.

19. Kenderian SS, Ruella M, Shestova O, et al. CD33 directed chimeric antigen receptor T-cell therapy as a novel preparative regimen prior to allogeneic stem cell transplantation in acute myeloid leukemia. *Biol Blood Marrow Transplant.* 2015;21:S25–S26. https://doi.org/10.1016/j.bbmt.2014.11.013.

20. Kenderian SS, Ruella M, Shestova O, et al. CD33-specific chimeric antigen receptor T-cells exhibit potent preclinical activity against human acute myeloid leukemia. *Leukemia.* 2015;29:1637–1647. https://doi.org/10.1038/leu.2015.52.

21. Eichler F, Duncan C, Musolino PL, et al. Hematopoietic stem-cell gene therapy for cerebral adrenoleukodystrophy. *N Engl J Med.* 2017;377:1630–1638. https://doi.org/10.1056/NEJMoa1700554.

22. Thompson AA, Walters MC, Kwiatkowski J, et al. Gene therapy in patients with transfusion-dependent β-thalassemia. *N Engl J Med.* 2018;378:1479–1493. https://doi.org/10.1056/NEJMoa1705342.

23. Wang Q, Wang Y, Lv H, et al. Treatment of CD33-directed chimeric antigen receptor-modified T-cells in one patient with relapsed and refractory acute myeloid leukemia. *Mol Ther.* 2015;23:184–191. https://doi.org/10.1038/mt.2014.164.

24. Tang X, Yang L, Li Z, et al. First-in-man clinical trial of CAR NK-92 cells: safety test of CD33-CAR NK-92 cells in patients with relapsed and refractory acute myeloid leukemia. *Am J Cancer Res.* 2018;8:1083–1089.

25. Jordan CT, Upchurch D, Szilvassy SJ, et al. The interleukin-3 receptor alpha chain is a unique marker for human acute myelogenous leukemia stem cells. *Leukemia.* 2000;14:1777–1784. https://doi.org/10.1038/sj.leu.2401903.

26. Jin L, Lee EM, Ramshaw HS, et al. Monoclonal antibody-mediated targeting of CD123, IL-3 receptor α chain, eliminates human acute myeloid leukemic stem cells. *Cell Stem Cell.* 2009;5:31–42. https://doi.org/10.1016/j.stem.2009.04.018.

27. Al-Mawali A, Pinto AD, Al-Zadjali S. CD34+CD38-CD123+ cells are present in virtually all acute myeloid leukaemia blasts: a promising single unique phenotype for minimal residual disease detection. *AHA.* 2017;138:175–181. https://doi.org/10.1159/000480448.

28. Haubner S, Perna F, Köhnke T, et al. Coexpression profile of leukemic stem cell markers for combinatorial targeted therapy in AML. *Leukemia*. 2019;33:64. https://doi.org/10.1038/s41375-018-0180-3.

29. Martín-Martín L, López A, Vidriales B, et al. Classification and clinical behavior of blastic plasmacytoid dendritic cell neoplasms according to their maturation-associated immunophenotypic profile. *Oncotarget*. 2015;6:19204–19216. https://doi.org/10.18632/oncotarget.4146.

30. Pemmaraju N, Lane AA, Sweet KL, et al. Tagraxofusp in blastic plasmacytoid dendritic-cell neoplasm. *N Engl J Med*. 2019;380:1628–1637. https://doi.org/10.1056/NEJMoa1815105.

31. Mardiros A, Santos CD, McDonald T, et al. T-cells expressing CD123-specific chimeric antigen receptors exhibit specific cytolytic effector functions and antitumor effects against human acute myeloid leukemia. *Blood*. 2013;122:3138–3148. https://doi.org/10.1182/blood-2012-12-474056.

32. Budde L, Song JY, Kim Y, et al. Remissions of acute myeloid leukemia and blastic plasmacytoid dendritic cell neoplasm following treatment with CD123-specific CAR T-cells: a first-in-human clinical trial. *Blood*. 2017;130:811.

33. Gill S, Tasian SK, Ruella M, et al. Preclinical targeting of human acute myeloid leukemia and myeloablation using chimeric antigen receptor-modified T-cells. *Blood*. 2014;123:2343–2354. https://doi.org/10.1182/blood-2013-09-529537.

34. Cummins KD, Frey N, Nelson AM, et al. Treating relapsed/refractory (RR) AML with Biodegradable anti-CD123 CAR modified T-cells. *Blood*. 2017;130:1359.

35. Tasian SK, Kenderian SS, Shen F, et al. Optimized depletion of chimeric antigen receptor T-cells in murine xenograft models of human acute myeloid leukemia. *Blood*. 2017;129:2395–2407. https://doi.org/10.1182/blood-2016-08-736041.

36. Tasian SK, Kenderian SS, Shen F, et al. Efficient termination of CD123-redirected chimeric antigen receptor T-cells for acute myeloid leukemia to mitigate toxicity. *Blood*. 2015;126:565.

37. Arcangeli S, Rotiroti MC, Bardelli M, et al. Balance of anti-CD123 chimeric antigen receptor binding affinity and density for the targeting of acute myeloid leukemia. *Mol Ther*. 2017;25:1933–1945. https://doi.org/10.1016/j.ymthe.2017.04.017.

38. Straathof KC, Pulè MA, Yotnda P, et al. An inducible caspase 9 safety switch for T-cell therapy. *Blood*. 2005;105:4247–4254. https://doi.org/10.1182/blood-2004-11-4564.

39. Luo Y, Chang L-J, Hu Y, Dong L, Wei G, Huang H. First-in-Man CD123-specific chimeric antigen receptor-modified T-cells for the treatment of refractory acute myeloid leukemia. *Blood*. 2015;126:3778.

40. Tu S, Deng L, Huang R, et al. A novel chimeric antigen receptor T-cells therapy strategy that dual targeting CD19 and CD123 to treat relapsed acute lymphoblastic leukemia after allogeneic hematopoietic stem cell transplantation. *Blood*. 2018;132:4015. https://doi.org/10.1182/blood-2018-99-118526.

41. van Rhenen A, Moshaver B, Kelder A, et al. Aberrant marker expression patterns on the CD34+CD38−stem cell compartment in acute myeloid leukemia allows to distinguish the malignant from the normal stem cell compartment both at diagnosis and in remission. *Leukemia*. 2007;21:1700–1707. https://doi.org/10.1038/sj.leu.2404754.

42. Bakker ABH, van den Oudenrijn S, Bakker AQ, et al. C-type lectin-like molecule-1: a novel myeloid cell surface marker associated with acute myeloid leukemia. *Cancer Res*. 2004;64:8443–8450. https://doi.org/10.1158/0008-5472.CAN-04-1659.

43. van Rhenen A, van Dongen GAMS, Kelder A, et al. The novel AML stem cell–associated antigen CLL-1 aids in discrimination between normal and leukemic stem cells. *Blood*. 2007;110:2659–2666. https://doi.org/10.1182/blood-2007-03-083048.

44. Wang J, Chen S, Xiao W, et al. CAR-T-cells targeting CLL-1 as an approach to treat acute myeloid leukemia. *J Hematol Oncol*. 2018;11:7. https://doi.org/10.1186/s13045-017-0553-5.

45. Tashiro H, Sauer T, Shum T, et al. Treatment of acute myeloid leukemia with T-cells expressing chimeric antigen receptors directed to C-type lectin-like molecule 1. *Mol Ther*. 2017;25:2202–2213. https://doi.org/10.1016/j.ymthe.2017.05.024.

46. Laborda E, Mazagova M, Shao S, et al. Development of A Chimeric antigen receptor targeting C-type lectin-like molecule-1 for human acute myeloid leukemia. *Int J Mol Sci*. 2017;18:2259. https://doi.org/10.3390/ijms18112259.

47. Kenderian SS, Ruella M, Shestova O, et al. Targeting CLEC12A with chimeric antigen receptor T-cells can overcome the chemotherapy refractoriness of leukemia stem cells. *Biol Blood Marrow Transplant*. 2017;23:S247–S248. https://doi.org/10.1016/j.bbmt.2016.12.413.

48. Liu F, Cao Y, Pinz K, et al. First-in-Human CLL1-CD33 compound CAR T-cell therapy induces complete remission in patients with refractory acute myeloid leukemia: update on phase 1 clinical trial. *Blood*. 2018;132:901. https://doi.org/10.1182/blood-2018-99-110579.

49. Sakamoto J, Furukawa K, Cordon-Cardo C, et al. Expression of Lewisa, Lewisb, X, and Y blood group Antigens in human colonic tumors and normal tissue and in human tumor-derived cell lines. *Cancer Res*. 1986;46:1553–1561.

50. Yan L, Lin B, Gao L, et al. Lewis (y) antigen overexpression increases the expression of MMP-2 and MMP-9 and invasion of human ovarian cancer cells. *Int J Mol Sci*. 2010;11:4441–4452. https://doi.org/10.3390/ijms11114441.

51. Gao L, Yan L, Lin B, et al. Enhancive effects of Lewis y antigen on CD44-mediated adhesion and spreading of human ovarian cancer cell line RMG-I. *J Exp Clin Cancer Res*. 2011;30:15. https://doi.org/10.1186/1756-9966-30-15.

52. Barkeer S, Chugh S, Batra SK, Ponnusamy MP. Glycosylation of cancer stem cells: function in stemness, tumorigenesis, and metastasis. *Neoplasia.* 2018;20:813—825. https://doi.org/10.1016/j.neo.2018.06.001.

53. Pachón-Peña G, Donnelly C, Ruiz-Cañada C, et al. A glycovariant of human CD44 is characteristically expressed on human mesenchymal stem cells: human MSCs display a distinct CD44 glycosignature. *Stem Cells.* 2017;35:1080—1092.   https://doi.org/10.1002/stem.2549.

54. Blanas A, Sahasrabudhe NM, Rodríguez E, van Kooyk Y, van Vliet SJ. Fucosylated antigens in cancer: an alliance toward tumor progression, metastasis, and resistance to chemotherapy. *Front Oncol.* 2018;8. https://doi.org/10.3389/fonc.2018.00039.

55. Casucci M, di Robilant BN, Falcone L, et al. Co-expression of a suicide gene in CAR-redirected T-cells enables the safe targeting of CD44v6 for leukemia and myeloma eradication. *Blood.* 2012;120:949.

56. Casucci M, Falcone L, Camisa B, et al. CD44v6 is required for in vivo tumorigenesis of human AML and MM cells: role of microenvironmental signals and therapeutic implications. *Blood.* 2013;122:605.

57. Westwood JA, Smyth MJ, Teng MWL, et al. Adoptive transfer of T-cells modified with a humanized chimeric receptor gene inhibits growth of Lewis-Y-expressing tumors in mice. *Proc Natl Acad Sci.* 2005;102:19051—19056.   https://doi.org/10.1073/pnas.0504312102.

58. Peinert S, Prince HM, Guru PM, et al. Gene-modified T-cells as immunotherapy for multiple myeloma and acute myeloid leukemia expressing the Lewis Y antigen. *Gene Ther.* 2010;17:678—686.   https://doi.org/10.1038/gt.2010.21.

59. Casucci M. 465. Dual transgenesis of T-cells with a CD44v6 CAR and a suicide gene for the safe eradication of myeloid leukemia and myeloma. *Mol Ther.* 2012;20:S180—S181.   https://doi.org/10.1016/S1525-0016(16)36269-4.

60. Lanier LL. NKG2D receptor and its ligands in host defense. *Cancer Immunol Res.* 2015;3:575—582. https://doi.org/10.1158/2326-6066.CIR-15-0098.

61. Baumeister SH, Murad J, Werner L, et al. Phase I trial of autologous CAR T-cells targeting NKG2D ligands in patients with AML/MDS and multiple myeloma. *Cancer Immunol Res.* 2019;7:100—112. https://doi.org/10.1158/2326-6066.CIR-18-0307.

62. Zhang T, Barber A, Sentman CL. Generation of antitumor responses by genetic modification of primary human T-cells with a chimeric NKG2D receptor. *Cancer Res.* 2006;66:5927—5933.   https://doi.org/10.1158/0008-5472.CAN-06-0130.

63. Zhang T, Lemoi BA, Sentman CL. Chimeric NK-receptor—bearing T-cells mediate antitumor immunotherapy. *Blood.* 2005;106:1544—1551. https://doi.org/10.1182/blood-2004-11-4365.

64. Ruella M, Xu J, Barrett DM, et al. Induction of resistance to chimeric antigen receptor T-cell therapy by transduction of a single leukemic B cell. *Nat Med.* 2018;24:1499. https://doi.org/10.1038/s41591-018-0201-9.

65. Scherer LD, Brenner MK, Mamonkin M. Chimeric antigen receptors for T-cell malignancies. *Front Oncol.* 2019;9:134. https://doi.org/10.3389/fonc.2019.00126.

66. Shalabi H, Angiolillo A, Fry TJ. Beyond CD19: opportunities for future development of targeted immunotherapy in pediatric relapsed-refractory acute leukemia. *Front Pediatr.* 2015;3. https://doi.org/10.3389/fped.2015.00080.

67. Orentas RJ, Nordlund J, He J, et al. Bioinformatic description of immunotherapy targets for pediatric T-cell leukemia and the impact of normal gene sets used for comparison. *Front Oncol.* 2014;4. https://doi.org/10.3389/fonc.2014.00134.

68. Waldmann H, Hale G. CAMPATH: from concept to clinic. *Philos Trans R Soc B Biol Sci.* 2005;360:1707—1711. https://doi.org/10.1098/rstb.2005.1702.

69. Kharfan-Dabaja MA, Nishihori T, Otrock ZK, Haidar N, Mohty M, Hamadani M. Monoclonal antibodies in conditioning regimens for hematopoietic cell transplantation. *Biol Blood Marrow Transplant.* 2013;19:1288—1300. https://doi.org/10.1016/j.bbmt.2013.04.016.

70. Seibel NL, Steinherz PG, Sather HN, et al. Early postinduction intensification therapy improves survival for children and adolescents with high-risk acute lymphoblastic leukemia: a report from the Children's Oncology Group. *Blood.* 2008;111:2548—2555. https://doi.org/10.1182/blood-2007-02-070342.

71. Raetz EA, Borowitz MJ, Devidas M, et al. Reinduction platform for children with first marrow relapse of acute lymphoblastic Leukemia: a Children's Oncology Group Study [corrected]. *J Clin Oncol.* 2008;26:3971—3978. https://doi.org/10.1200/JCO.2008.16.1414.

72. Gaynon PS, Harris RE, Altman AJ, et al. Bone marrow transplantation versus prolonged intensive chemotherapy for children with acute lymphoblastic leukemia and an initial bone marrow relapse within 12 months of the completion of primary therapy: children's Oncology Group study CCG-1941. *J Clin Oncol.* 2006;24:3150—3156.   https://doi.org/10.1200/JCO.2005.04.5856.

73. Scarfò I, Ormhøj M, Frigault MJ, et al. Anti-CD37 chimeric antigen receptor T-cells are active against B- and T-cell lymphomas. *Blood.* 2018;132:1495—1506. https://doi.org/10.1182/blood-2018-04-842708.

74. Horwitz SM, Advani RH, Bartlett NL, et al. Objective responses in relapsed T-cell lymphomas with single-agent brentuximab vedotin. *Blood.* 2014;123:3095—3100. https://doi.org/10.1182/blood-2013-12-542142.

75. Ramos CA, Ballard B, Zhang H, et al. Clinical and immunological responses after CD30-specific chimeric antigen receptor-redirected lymphocytes. *J Clin Invest.* 2017;127:3462—3471. https://doi.org/10.1172/JCI94306.

76. Wang C-M, Wu Z-Q, Wang Y, et al. Autologous T-cells expressing CD30 chimeric antigen receptors for relapsed or refractory Hodgkin lymphoma: an open-label phase I

trial. *Clin Cancer Res.* 2017;23:1156—1166. https://doi.org/10.1158/1078-0432.CCR-16-1365.

77. Mamonkin M, Rouce RH, Tashiro H, Brenner MK. A T-cell—directed chimeric antigen receptor for the selective treatment of T-cell malignancies. *Blood.* 2015;126:983—992. https://doi.org/10.1182/blood-2015-02-629527.

78. Eyquem J, Mansilla-Soto J, Giavridis T, et al. Targeting a CAR to the TRAC locus with CRISPR/Cas9 enhances tumour rejection. *Nature.* 2017;543:113—117. https://doi.org/10.1038/nature21405.

79. MacLeod DT, Antony J, Martin AJ, et al. Integration of a CD19 CAR into the TCR alpha chain locus streamlines production of allogeneic gene-edited CAR T-cells. *Mol Ther.* 2017;25:949—961. https://doi.org/10.1016/j.ymthe.2017.02.005.

80. Ren J, Liu X, Fang C, Jiang S, June CH, Zhao Y. Multiplex genome editing to generate universal CAR T-cells resistant to PD1 inhibition. *Clin Cancer Res.* 2017;23:2255—2266. https://doi.org/10.1158/1078-0432.CCR-16-1300.

81. Gerby B, Clappier E, Armstrong F, et al. Expression of CD34 and CD7 on human T-cell acute lymphoblastic leukemia discriminates functionally heterogeneous cell populations. *Leukemia.* 2011;25:1249—1258. https://doi.org/10.1038/leu.2011.93.

82. Cox CV, Martin HM, Kearns PR, Virgo P, Evely RS, Blair A. Characterization of a progenitor cell population in childhood T-cell acute lymphoblastic leukemia. *Blood.* 2007;109:674—682. https://doi.org/10.1182/blood-2006-06-030445.

83. Gomes-Silva D, Srinivasan M, Sharma S, et al. CD7-edited T-cells expressing a CD7-specific CAR for the therapy of T-cell malignancies. *Blood.* 2017;130:285—296. https://doi.org/10.1182/blood-2017-01-761320.

84. Gomes-Silva D, Atilla E, Atilla PA, et al. CD7 CAR T-cells for the therapy of acute myeloid leukemia. *Mol Ther.* 2019;27:272—280. https://doi.org/10.1016/j.ymthe.2018.10.001.

85. Fleischer LC, Raikar SS, Moot R, Knight KA, Doering CB, Spencer HT. Engineering CD5-targeted chimeric antigen receptors and edited T-cells for the treatment of T-cell leukemia. *Blood.* 2017;130:1914.

86. Pinz K, Liu H, Golightly M, et al. Preclinical targeting of human T-cell malignancies using CD4-specific chimeric antigen receptor (CAR)-engineered T-cells. *Leukemia.* 2016;30:701—707. https://doi.org/10.1038/leu.2015.311.

87. Glienke W, Esser R, Priesner C, et al. Advantages and applications of CAR-expressing natural killer cells. *Front Pharmacol.* 2015;6. https://doi.org/10.3389/fphar.2015.00021.

88. Pinz KG, Yakaboski E, Jares A, et al. Targeting T-cell malignancies using anti-CD4 CAR NK-92 cells. *Oncotarget.* 2017;8:112783—112796. https://doi.org/10.18632/oncotarget.22626.

89. Pinto NR, Applebaum MA, Volchenboum SL, et al. Advances in risk classification and treatment strategies for neuroblastoma. *J Clin Oncol.* 2015;33:3008—3017. https://doi.org/10.1200/JCO.2014.59.4648.

90. Neuroblastoma Treatment (PDQ(R)): Health Professional version, in: PDQ Cancer Information Summaries, Bethesda (MD). 2002. https://www.ncbi.nlm.nih.gov/pubmed/26389190.

91. Schulz G, Cheresh DA, Varki NM, Yu A, Staffileno LK, Reisfeld RA. Detection of ganglioside GD2 in tumor tissues and sera of neuroblastoma patients. *Cancer Res.* 1984;44:5914—5920.

92. Yu AL, Gilman AL, Ozkaynak MF, et al. Anti-GD2 antibody with GM-CSF, interleukin-2, and isotretinoin for neuroblastoma. *N Engl J Med.* 2010;363:1324—1334. https://doi.org/10.1056/NEJMoa0911123.

93. Ozkaynak MF, Gilman AL, London WB, et al. A comprehensive safety trial of chimeric antibody 14.18 with GM-CSF, IL-2, and isotretinoin in high-risk neuroblastoma patients following myeloablative therapy: children's oncology group study ANBL0931. *Front Immunol.* 2018;9:1355. https://doi.org/10.3389/fimmu.2018.01355.

94. Rossig C, Bollard CM, Nuchtern JG, Merchant DA, Brenner MK. Targeting of G(D2)-positive tumor cells by human T lymphocytes engineered to express chimeric T-cell receptor genes. *Int J Cancer.* 2001;94:228—236.

95. Louis CU, Savoldo B, Dotti G, et al. Antitumor activity and long-term fate of chimeric antigen receptor-positive T-cells in patients with neuroblastoma. *Blood.* 2011;118:6050—6056. https://doi.org/10.1182/blood-2011-05-354449.

96. Pule MA, Savoldo B, Myers GD, et al. Virus-specific T-cells engineered to coexpress tumor-specific receptors: persistence and antitumor activity in individuals with neuroblastoma. *Nat Med.* 2008;14:1264—1270. https://doi.org/10.1038/nm.1882.

97. Yang Y, Kohler ME, Chien CD, et al. TCR engagement negatively affects CD8 but not CD4 CAR T-cell expansion and leukemic clearance. *Sci Transl Med.* 2017;9. https://doi.org/10.1126/scitranslmed.aag1209.

98. Hombach AA, Abken H. Costimulation by chimeric antigen receptors revisited the T-cell antitumor response benefits from combined CD28-OX40 signalling. *Int J Cancer.* 2011;129:2935—2944. https://doi.org/10.1002/ijc.25960.

99. Pule MA, Straathof KC, Dotti G, Heslop HE, Rooney CM, Brenner MK. A chimeric T-cell antigen receptor that augments cytokine release and supports clonal expansion of primary human T-cells. *Mol Ther.* 2005;12:933—941. https://doi.org/10.1016/j.ymthe.2005.04.016.

100. Heczey A, Louis CU, Savoldo B, et al. CAR T-cells administered in combination with lymphodepletion and PD-1 inhibition to patients with neuroblastoma. *Mol Ther.* 2017;25:2214—2224. https://doi.org/10.1016/j.ymthe.2017.05.012.

101. Long AH, Haso WM, Shern JF, et al. 4-1BB costimulation ameliorates T-cell exhaustion induced by tonic signaling of chimeric antigen receptors. *Nat Med.* 2015;21:581—590. https://doi.org/10.1038/nm.3838.

102. Quintarelli C, Orlando D, Boffa I, et al. Choice of costimulatory domains and of cytokines determines CAR T-cell activity in neuroblastoma. *Oncoimmunology*. 2018;7: e1433518. https://doi.org/10.1080/2162402X.2018.1433518.

103. Nakamura K, Tanaka Y, Shitara K, Hanai N. Construction of humanized anti-ganglioside monoclonal antibodies with potent immune effector functions. *Cancer Immunol Immunother*. 2001;50:275–284.

104. Thomas S, Straathof K, Himoudi N, Anderson J, Pule M. An optimized GD2-targeting retroviral cassette for more potent and safer cellular therapy of neuroblastoma and other cancers. *PLoS One*. 2016;11: e0152196. https://doi.org/10.1371/journal.pone.0152196.

105. Straathof K, Flutter B, Wallace R, et al. Abstract CT145: a Cancer Research UK phase I trial of anti-GD2 chimeric antigen receptor (CAR) transduced T-cells (1RG-CART) in patients with relapsed or refractory neuroblastoma. *Cancer Res*. 2018;78:CT145. https://doi.org/10.1158/1538-7445.AM2018-CT145.

106. Yang L, Ma X, Liu Y-C, et al. Chimeric antigen receptor 4SCAR-GD2-modified T-cells targeting high-risk and recurrent neuroblastoma: a phase II multi-center trial in China. *Blood*. 2017;130:3335.

107. Richman SA, Nunez-Cruz S, Moghimi B, et al. High-affinity GD2-specific CAR T-cells induce fatal encephalitis in a preclinical neuroblastoma model. *Cancer Immunol Res*. 2018;6:36–46. https://doi.org/10.1158/2326-6066.CIR-17-0211.

108. Hoefnagel CA, Rutgers M, Buitenhuis CK, et al. A comparison of targeting of neuroblastoma with mIBG and anti L1-CAM antibody mAb chCE7: therapeutic efficacy in a neuroblastoma xenograft model and imaging of neuroblastoma patients. *Eur J Nucl Med*. 2001; 28:359–368.

109. Gavert N, Conacci-Sorrell M, Gast D, et al. L1, a novel target of beta-catenin signaling, transforms cells and is expressed at the invasive front of colon cancers. *J Cell Biol*. 2005;168:633–642. https://doi.org/10.1083/jcb.200408051.

110. Izumoto S, Ohnishi T, Arita N, Hiraga S, Taki T, Hayakawa T. Gene expression of neural cell adhesion molecule L1 in malignant gliomas and biological significance of L1 in glioma invasion. *Cancer Res*. 1996;56: 1440–1444.

111. Thies A, Schachner M, Moll I, et al. Overexpression of the cell adhesion molecule L1 is associated with metastasis in cutaneous malignant melanoma. *Eur J Cancer*. 2002;38: 1708–1716.

112. Arlt MJ, Novak-Hofer I, Gast D, et al. Efficient inhibition of intra-peritoneal tumor growth and dissemination of human ovarian carcinoma cells in nude mice by anti-L1-cell adhesion molecule monoclonal antibody treatment. *Cancer Res*. 2006;66:936–943. https://doi.org/10.1158/0008-5472.CAN-05-1818.

113. Euer NI, Kaul S, Deissler H, Mobus VJ, Zeillinger R, Weidle UH. Identification of L1CAM, Jagged2 and Neuromedin U as ovarian cancer-associated antigens. *Oncol Rep*. 2005;13:375–387.

114. Fogel M, Gutwein P, Mechtersheimer S, et al. L1 expression as a predictor of progression and survival in patients with uterine and ovarian carcinomas. *Lancet*. 2003;362: 869–875. https://doi.org/10.1016/S0140-6736(03)14342-5.

115. Calvo A, Xiao N, Kang J, et al. Alterations in gene expression profiles during prostate cancer progression: functional correlations to tumorigenicity and down-regulation of selenoprotein-P in mouse and human tumors. *Cancer Res*. 2002;62:5325–5335.

116. Allory Y, Matsuoka Y, Bazille C, Christensen EI, Ronco P, Debiec H. The L1 cell adhesion molecule is induced in renal cancer cells and correlates with metastasis in clear cell carcinomas. *Clin Cancer Res*. 2005;11:1190–1197.

117. Gast D, Riedle S, Riedle S, et al. L1 augments cell migration and tumor growth but not beta3 integrin expression in ovarian carcinomas. *Int J Cancer*. 2005;115:658–665. https://doi.org/10.1002/ijc.20869.

118. Mechtersheimer S, Gutwein P, Agmon-Levin N, et al. Ectodomain shedding of L1 adhesion molecule promotes cell migration by autocrine binding to integrins. *J Cell Biol*. 2001;155:661–673. https://doi.org/10.1083/jcb.200101099.

119. Montgomery AM, Becker JC, Siu CH, et al. Human neural cell adhesion molecule L1 and rat homologue NILE are ligands for integrin alpha v beta 3. *J Cell Biol*. 1996;132: 475–485.

120. Silletti S, Yebra M, Perez B, Cirulli V, McMahon M, Montgomery AM. Extracellular signal-regulated kinase (ERK)-dependent gene expression contributes to L1 cell adhesion molecule-dependent motility and invasion. *J Biol Chem*. 2004;279:28880–28888. https://doi.org/10.1074/jbc.M404075200.

121. Park JR, Digiusto DL, Slovak M, et al. Adoptive transfer of chimeric antigen receptor re-directed cytolytic T lymphocyte clones in patients with neuroblastoma. *Mol Ther*. 2007;15: 825–833. https://doi.org/10.1038/sj.mt.6300104.

122. Gonzalez S, Naranjo A, Serrano LM, Chang WC, Wright CL, Jensen MC. Genetic engineering of cytolytic T lymphocytes for adoptive T-cell therapy of neuroblastoma. *J Gene Med*. 2004;6:704–711. https://doi.org/10.1002/jgm.489.

123. Schonmann SM, Iyer J, Laeng H, Gerber HA, Kaser H, Blaser K. Production and characterization of monoclonal antibodies against human neuroblastoma. *Int J Cancer*. 1986;37:255–262.

124. Meli ML, Carrel F, Waibel R, et al. Anti-neuroblastoma antibody chCE7 binds to an isoform of L1-CAM present in renal carcinoma cells. *Int J Cancer*. 1999;83:401–408.

125. Iwahara T, Fujimoto J, Wen D, et al. Molecular characterization of ALK, a receptor tyrosine kinase expressed specifically in the nervous system. *Oncogene*. 1997;14: 439–449. https://doi.org/10.1038/sj.onc.1200849.

126. Chiarle R, Voena C, Ambrogio C, Piva R, Inghirami G. The anaplastic lymphoma kinase in the pathogenesis of

cancer. *Nat Rev Cancer.* 2008;8:11−23. https://doi.org/10.1038/nrc2291.

127. Mosse YP, Laudenslager M, Longo L, et al. Identification of ALK as a major familial neuroblastoma predisposition gene. *Nature.* 2008;455:930−935. https://doi.org/10.1038/nature07261.

128. Chen Y, Takita J, Choi YL, et al. Oncogenic mutations of ALK kinase in neuroblastoma. *Nature.* 2008;455:971−974. https://doi.org/10.1038/nature07399.

129. George RE, Sanda T, Hanna M, et al. Activating mutations in ALK provide a therapeutic target in neuroblastoma. *Nature.* 2008;455:975−978. https://doi.org/10.1038/nature07397.

130. De Brouwer S, De Preter K, Kumps C, et al. Meta-analysis of neuroblastomas reveals a skewed ALK mutation spectrum in tumors with MYCN amplification. *Clin Cancer Res.* 2010;16:4353−4362. https://doi.org/10.1158/1078-0432.CCR-09-2660.

131. Moog-Lutz C, Degoutin J, Gouzi JY, et al. Activation and inhibition of anaplastic lymphoma kinase receptor tyrosine kinase by monoclonal antibodies and absence of agonist activity of pleiotrophin. *J Biol Chem.* 2005;280:26039−26048. https://doi.org/10.1074/jbc.M501972200.

132. Walker AJ, Majzner RG, Zhang L, et al. Tumor antigen and receptor densities regulate efficacy of a chimeric antigen receptor targeting anaplastic lymphoma kinase. *Mol Ther.* 2017;25:2189−2201. https://doi.org/10.1016/j.ymthe.2017.06.008.

133. Baral A, Ye HX, Jiang PC, Yao Y, Mao Y. B7-H3 and B7-H1 expression in cerebral spinal fluid and tumor tissue correlates with the malignancy grade of glioma patients. *Oncol Lett.* 2014;8:1195−1201. https://doi.org/10.3892/ol.2014.2268.

134. Gregorio A, Corrias MV, Castriconi R, et al. Small round blue cell tumours: diagnostic and prognostic usefulness of the expression of B7-H3 surface molecule. *Histopathology.* 2008;53:73−80. https://doi.org/10.1111/j.1365-2559.2008.03070.x.

135. Zhou Z, Luther N, Ibrahim GM, et al. B7-H3, a potential therapeutic target, is expressed in diffuse intrinsic pontine glioma. *J Neuro Oncol.* 2013;111:257−264. https://doi.org/10.1007/s11060-012-1021-2.

136. Zhao JL, Chen FL, Zhou Q, et al. B7-H3 protein expression in a murine model of osteosarcoma. *Oncol Lett.* 2016;12:383−386. https://doi.org/10.3892/ol.2016.4675.

137. Ye Z, Zheng Z, Li X, et al. B7-H3 overexpression predicts poor survival of cancer patients: a meta-analysis. *Cell Physiol Biochem.* 2016;39:1568−1580. https://doi.org/10.1159/000447859.

138. Picarda E, Ohaegbulam KC, Zang X. Molecular pathways: targeting B7-H3 (CD276) for human cancer immunotherapy. *Clin Cancer Res.* 2016;22:3425−3431. https://doi.org/10.1158/1078-0432.CCR-15-2428.

139. Powderly J, Cote G, Flaherty K, et al. Interim results of an ongoing Phase I, dose escalation study of MGA271 (Fc-optimized humanized anti-B7-H3 monoclonal antibody) in patients with refractory B7-H3-expressing neoplasms or neoplasms whose vasculature expresses B7-H3. *J Immunother Cancer.* 2015;3:O8. https://doi.org/10.1186/2051-1426-3-S2-O8.

140. Kramer K, Kushner BH, Modak S, et al. Compartmental intrathecal radioimmunotherapy: results for treatment for metastatic CNS neuroblastoma. *J Neuro Oncol.* 2010;97:409−418. https://doi.org/10.1007/s11060-009-0038-7.

141. Kramer K, Pandit-Taskar N, Humm JL, et al. A phase II study of radioimmunotherapy with intraventricular (131) I-3F8 for medulloblastoma. *Pediatr Blood Cancer.* 2018:65. https://doi.org/10.1002/pbc.26754.

142. Du H, Hirabayashi K, Ahn S, et al. Antitumor responses in the absence of toxicity in solid tumors by targeting B7-H3 via chimeric antigen receptor T-cells. *Cancer Cell.* 2019;35:221−237.e8. https://doi.org/10.1016/j.ccell.2019.01.002.

143. Filmus J, Capurro M, Rast J, Glypicans. *Genome Biol.* 2008;9:224. https://doi.org/10.1186/gb-2008-9-5-224.

144. Ivins JK, Litwack ED, Kumbasar A, Stipp CS, Lander AD. Cerebroglycan, a developmentally regulated cell-surface heparan sulfate proteoglycan, is expressed on developing axons and growth cones. *Dev Biol.* 1997;184:320−332. https://doi.org/10.1006/dbio.1997.8532.

145. Stipp CS, Litwack ED, Lander AD. Cerebroglycan: an integral membrane heparan sulfate proteoglycan that is unique to the developing nervous system and expressed specifically during neuronal differentiation. *J Cell Biol.* 1994;124:149−160.

146. Bosse KR, Raman P, Zhu Z, et al. Identification of GPC2 as an oncoprotein and candidate immunotherapeutic target in high-risk neuroblastoma. *Cancer Cell.* 2017;32:295−309.e12. https://doi.org/10.1016/j.ccell.2017.08.003.

147. Li N, Fu H, Hewitt SM, Dimitrov DS, Ho M. Therapeutically targeting glypican-2 via single-domain antibody-based chimeric antigen receptors and immunotoxins in neuroblastoma. *Proc Natl Acad Sci U S A.* 2017;114:E6623−E6631. https://doi.org/10.1073/pnas.1706055114.

148. Zeromski J, Nyczak E, Dyszkiewicz W. Significance of cell adhesion molecules, CD56/NCAM in particular, in human tumor growth and spreading. *Folia Histochem Cytobiol.* 2001;39(Suppl 2):36−37.

149. Shah MH, Lorigan P, O'Brien ME, et al. Phase I study of IMGN901, a CD56-targeting antibody-drug conjugate, in patients with CD56-positive solid tumors. *Invest New Drugs.* 2016;34:290−299. https://doi.org/10.1007/s10637-016-0336-9.

150. Crossland DL, Denning WL, Ang S, et al. Antitumor activity of CD56-chimeric antigen receptor T-cells in neuroblastoma and SCLC models. *Oncogene.* 2018;37:3686−3697. https://doi.org/10.1038/s41388-018-0187-2.

151. Ou JY, Spraker-Perlman H, Dietz AC, Smits-Seemann RR, Kaul S, Kirchhoff AC. Conditional survival of pediatric, adolescent, and young adult soft tissue sarcoma and

bone tumor patients. *Cancer Epidemiol.* 2017;50: 150—157. https://doi.org/10.1016/j.canep.2017.08.015.

152. Kailayangiri S, Altvater B, Meltzer J, et al. The ganglioside antigen G(D2) is surface-expressed in Ewing sarcoma and allows for MHC-independent immune targeting. *Br J Cancer.* 2012;106:1123—1133. https://doi.org/10.1038/bjc.2012.57.

153. Roth M, Linkowski M, Tarim J, et al. Ganglioside GD2 as a therapeutic target for antibody-mediated therapy in patients with osteosarcoma. *Cancer.* 2014;120:548—554. https://doi.org/10.1002/cncr.28461.

154. Long AH, Highfill SL, Cui Y, et al. Reduction of MDSCs with all-trans retinoic acid improves CAR therapy efficacy for sarcomas. *Cancer Immunol Res.* 2016;4:869—880. https://doi.org/10.1158/2326-6066.CIR-15-0230.

155. Ahmed N, Salsman VS, Yvon E, et al. Immunotherapy for osteosarcoma: genetic modification of T-cells overcomes low levels of tumor antigen expression. *Mol Ther.* 2009; 17:1779—1787. https://doi.org/10.1038/mt.2009.133.

156. Morgan RA, Yang JC, Kitano M, Dudley ME, Laurencot CM, Rosenberg SA. Case report of a serious adverse event following the administration of T-cells transduced with a chimeric antigen receptor recognizing ERBB2. *Mol Ther.* 2010;18:843—851. https://doi.org/10.1038/mt.2010.24.

157. Ahmed N, Brawley VS, Hegde M, et al. Human epidermal growth factor receptor 2 (HER2) -specific chimeric antigen receptor-modified T-cells for the immunotherapy of HER2-positive sarcoma. *J Clin Oncol.* 2015;33: 1688—1696. https://doi.org/10.1200/JCO.2014.58.0225.

158. Gardner RA, Finney O, Annesley C, et al. Intent-to-treat leukemia remission by CD19 CAR T-cells of defined formulation and dose in children and young adults. *Blood.* 2017;129:3322—3331. https://doi.org/10.1182/blood-2017-02-769208.

159. Ross JF, Chaudhuri PK, Ratnam M. Differential regulation of folate receptor isoforms in normal and malignant tissues in vivo and in established cell lines. Physiologic and Clinical Implications. *Cancer.* 1994; 73:2432—2443.

160. Yang R, Kolb EA, Qin J, et al. The folate receptor alpha is frequently overexpressed in osteosarcoma samples and plays a role in the uptake of the physiologic substrate 5-methyltetrahydrofolate. *Clin Cancer Res.* 2007;13: 2557—2567. https://doi.org/10.1158/1078-0432.CCR-06-1343.

161. De Jesus E, Keating JJ, Kularatne SA, et al. Comparison of folate receptor targeted optical contrast agents for intraoperative molecular imaging. *Int J Mol Imaging.* 2015; 2015:469047. https://doi.org/10.1155/2015/469047.

162. Lu YJ, Chu H, Wheeler LW, et al. Preclinical evaluation of bispecific adaptor molecule controlled folate receptor CAR-T-cell therapy with special focus on pediatric malignancies. *Front Oncol.* 2019;9. https://doi.org/10.3389/fonc.2019.00151.

163. Ganti R, Skapek SX, Zhang J, et al. Expression and genomic status of EGFR and ErbB-2 in alveolar and embryonal rhabdomyosarcoma. *Mod Pathol.* 2006;19: 1213—1220. https://doi.org/10.1038/modpathol.3800636.

164. Ho R, Minturn JE, Hishiki T, et al. Proliferation of human neuroblastomas mediated by the epidermal growth factor receptor. *Cancer Res.* 2005;65:9868—9875. https://doi.org/10.1158/0008-5472.CAN-04-2426.

165. Mendelsohn J, Baselga J. The EGF receptor family as targets for cancer therapy. *Oncogene.* 2000;19:6550—6565. https://doi.org/10.1038/sj.onc.1204082.

166. Hynes NE, Lane HA. ERBB receptors and cancer: the complexity of targeted inhibitors. *Nat Rev Cancer.* 2005; 5:341—354. https://doi.org/10.1038/nrc1609.

167. Mendelsohn J, Baselga J. Epidermal growth factor receptor targeting in cancer. *Semin Oncol.* 2006;33:369—385. https://doi.org/10.1053/j.seminoncol.2006.04.003.

168. Li T, Perez-Soler R. Skin toxicities associated with epidermal growth factor receptor inhibitors. *Target Oncol.* 2009;4:107—119. https://doi.org/10.1007/s11523-009-0114-0.

169. Luwor RB, Johns TG, Murone C, et al. Monoclonal antibody 806 inhibits the growth of tumor xenografts expressing either the de2-7 or amplified epidermal growth factor receptor (EGFR) but not wild-type EGFR. *Cancer Res.* 2001;61:5355—5361.

170. Li D, Ji H, Zaghlul S, et al. Therapeutic anti-EGFR antibody 806 generates responses in murine de novo EGFR mutant-dependent lung carcinomas. *J Clin Invest.* 2007; 117:346—352. https://doi.org/10.1172/JCI30446.

171. Reilly EB, Phillips AC, Buchanan FG, et al. Characterization of ABT-806, a humanized tumor-specific anti-EGFR monoclonal antibody. *Mol Cancer Ther.* 2015;14: 1141—1151. https://doi.org/10.1158/1535-7163.MCT-14-0820.

172. Scott AM, Lee FT, Tebbutt N, et al. A phase I clinical trial with monoclonal antibody ch806 targeting transitional state and mutant epidermal growth factor receptors. *Proc Natl Acad Sci U S A.* 2007;104:4071—4076. https://doi.org/10.1073/pnas.0611693104.

173. Cleary JM, Reardon DA, Azad N, et al. A phase 1 study of ABT-806 in subjects with advanced solid tumors. *Invest New Drugs.* 2015;33:671—678. https://doi.org/10.1007/s10637-015-0234-6.

174. Huang X, Park H, Greene J, et al. IGF1R- and ROR1-specific CAR T-cells as a potential therapy for high risk sarcomas. *PLoS One.* 2015;10:e0133152. https://doi.org/10.1371/journal.pone.0133152.

175. Plummer M, de Martel C, Vignat J, Ferlay J, Bray F, Franceschi S. Global burden of cancers attributable to infections in 2012: a synthetic analysis. *The Lancet Glob Health.* 2016;4:e609—e616. https://doi.org/10.1016/S2214-109X(16)30143-7.

176. Jin BY, Campbell TE, Draper LM, et al. Engineered T-cells targeting E7 mediate regression of human papillomavirus cancers in a murine model. *JCI Insight.* 2018;3. https://doi.org/10.1172/jci.insight.99488.

177. Stevanović S, Pasetto A, Helman SR, et al. Landscape of immunogenic tumor antigens in successful

immunotherapy of virally induced epithelial cancer. *Science*. 2017;356:200–205. https://doi.org/10.1126/science.aak9510.

178. Tzannou I, Papadopoulou A, Naik S, et al. Off-the-Shelf virus-specific T-cells to treat BK virus, human herpesvirus 6, cytomegalovirus, Epstein-Barr virus, and adenovirus infections after allogeneic hematopoietic stem-cell transplantation. *J Clin Oncol*. 2017;35:3547–3557. https://doi.org/10.1200/JCO.2017.73.0655.

179. Cherkassky L, Morello A, Villena-Vargas J, et al. Human CAR T-cells with cell-intrinsic PD-1 checkpoint blockade resist tumor-mediated inhibition. *J Clin Investig*. 2016;126:3130–3144. https://doi.org/10.1172/JCI83092.

180. Morello A, Sadelain M, Adusumilli PS. Mesothelin-targeted CARs: driving T-cells to solid tumors. *Cancer Discov*. 2016;6:133–146. https://doi.org/10.1158/2159-8290.CD-15-0583.

181. Beatty GL, Haas AR, Maus MV, et al. Mesothelin-specific chimeric antigen receptor mRNA-engineered T-cells induce anti-tumor activity in solid malignancies. *Cancer Immunol Res*. 2014;2:112–120. https://doi.org/10.1158/2326-6066.CIR-13-0170.

182. Cao L, Yu Y, Thomas A, et al. Megakaryocyte potentiating factor as a predictive biomarker for therapies against malignant mesothelioma. *JCO Precis Oncol*. 2018;(2018). https://doi.org/10.1200/PO.17.00282.

183. Zhang Y-F, Phung Y, Gao W, et al. New high affinity monoclonal antibodies recognize non-overlapping epitopes on mesothelin for monitoring and treating mesothelioma. *Sci Rep*. 2015;5:9928. https://doi.org/10.1038/srep09928.

184. Kaneko O, Gong L, Zhang J, et al. A binding domain on mesothelin for CA125/MUC16. *J Biol Chem*. 2009;284:3739–3749. https://doi.org/10.1074/jbc.M806776200.

185. Thayaparan T, Petrovic RM, Achkova DY, et al. CAR T-cell immunotherapy of MET-expressing malignant mesothelioma. *Oncoimmunology*. 2017;6:e1363137. https://doi.org/10.1080/2162402X.2017.1363137.

186. Sharma S, Barry M, Gallagher DJ, Kell M, Sacchini V. An overview of triple negative breast cancer for surgical oncologists. *Surg Oncol*. 2015;24:276–283. https://doi.org/10.1016/j.suronc.2015.06.007.

187. Vergote IB, Marth C, Coleman RL. Role of the folate receptor in ovarian cancer treatment: evidence, mechanism, and clinical implications. *Cancer Metastasis Rev*. 2015;34:41–52. https://doi.org/10.1007/s10555-014-9539-8.

188. Kelley KMM, Rowan BG, Ratnam M. Modulation of the folate receptor alpha gene by the estrogen receptor: mechanism and implications in tumor targeting. *Cancer Res*. 2003;63:2820–2828.

189. Song D-G, Ye Q, Poussin M, Chacon JA, Figini M, Powell DJ. Effective adoptive immunotherapy of triple-negative breast cancer by folate receptor-alpha redirected CAR T-cells is influenced by surface antigen expression level. *J Hematol Oncol*. 2016;9. https://doi.org/10.1186/s13045-016-0285-y.

190. Biberacher V, Decker T, Oelsner M, et al. The cytotoxicity of anti-CD22 immunotoxin is enhanced by bryostatin 1

in B-cell lymphomas through CD22 upregulation and PKC- II depletion. *Haematologica*. 2012;97:771–779. https://doi.org/10.3324/haematol.2011.049155.

191. Nanda A, Carson-Walter EB, Seaman S, et al. TEM8 interacts with the cleaved C5 domain of collagen α3(VI). *Cancer Res*. 2004;64:817–820. https://doi.org/10.1158/0008-5472.CAN-03-2408.

192. Byrd TT, Fousek K, Pignata A, et al. TEM8/ANTXR1-Specific CAR T-cells as a targeted therapy for triple-negative breast cancer. *Cancer Res*. 2018;78:489–500. https://doi.org/10.1158/0008-5472.CAN-16-1911.

193. Chen D, Bhat-Nakshatri P, Goswami C, Badve S, Nakshatri H. ANTXR1, a stem cell-enriched functional biomarker, connects collagen signaling to cancer stem-like cells and metastasis in breast cancer. *Cancer Res*. 2013;73:5821–5833. https://doi.org/10.1158/0008-5472.CAN-13-1080.

194. Davies G, Rmali KA, Watkins G, Mansel RE, Mason MD, Jiang WG. Elevated levels of tumour endothelial marker-8 in human breast cancer and its clinical significance. *Int J Oncol*. 2006;29:1311–1317.

195. Vlad AM, Kettel JC, Alajez NM, Carlos CA, Finn OJ. MUC1 immunobiology: from discovery to clinical applications. In: *Advances in Immunology*. Elsevier; 2004:249–293. https://doi.org/10.1016/S0065-2776(04)82006-6.

196. Wilkie S, Picco G, Foster J, et al. Retargeting of human T-cells to tumor-associated MUC1: the evolution of a chimeric antigen receptor. *J Immunol*. 2008;180:4901–4909.

197. Posey AD, Schwab RD, Boesteanu AC, et al. Engineered CAR T-cells targeting the cancer-associated Tn-glycoform of the membrane mucin MUC1 control adenocarcinoma. *Immunity*. 2016;44:1444–1454. https://doi.org/10.1016/j.immuni.2016.05.014.

198. Schmittgen TD, Teske S, Vessella RL, True LD, Zakrajsek BA. Expression of prostate specific membrane antigen and three alternatively spliced variants of PSMA in prostate cancer patients. *Int J Cancer*. 2003;107:323–329. https://doi.org/10.1002/ijc.11402.

199. Su SL, Huang IP, Fair WR, Powell CT, Heston WD. Alternatively spliced variants of prostate-specific membrane antigen RNA: ratio of expression as a potential measurement of progression. *Cancer Res*. 1995;55:1441–1443.

200. Kloss CC, Lee J, Zhang A, et al. Dominant-negative TGF-β receptor enhances PSMA-targeted human CAR T-cell proliferation and augments prostate cancer eradication. *Mol Ther*. 2018;26:1855–1866. https://doi.org/10.1016/j.ymthe.2018.05.003.

201. Serganova I, Moroz E, Cohen I, et al. Enhancement of PSMA-directed CAR adoptive immunotherapy by PD-1/PD-L1 blockade. *Mol Ther Oncolytics*. 2017;4:41–54. https://doi.org/10.1016/j.omto.2016.11.005.

202. Santoro SP, Kim S, Motz GT, et al. T-cells bearing a chimeric antigen receptor against prostate-specific membrane antigen mediate vascular disruption and result in

tumor regression. *Cancer Immunol Res.* 2015;3:68–84. https://doi.org/10.1158/2326-6066.CIR-14-0192.

203. Reiter RE, Gu Z, Watabe T, et al. Prostate stem cell antigen: a cell surface marker overexpressed in prostate cancer. *Proc Natl Acad Sci U S A.* 1998;95:1735–1740.

204. Gu Z, Thomas G, Yamashiro J, et al. Prostate stem cell antigen (PSCA) expression increases with high gleason score, advanced stage and bone metastasis in prostate cancer. *Oncogene.* 2000;19:1288–1296. https://doi.org/10.1038/sj.onc.1203426.

205. Heinrich M-C, Göbel C, Kluth M, et al. PSCA expression is associated with favorable tumor features and reduced PSA recurrence in operated prostate cancer. *BMC Canc.* 2018; 18:612. https://doi.org/10.1186/s12885-018-4547-7.

206. Priceman SJ, Gerdts EA, Tilakawardane D, et al. Co-stimulatory signaling determines tumor antigen sensitivity and persistence of CAR T-cells targeting PSCA+ metastatic prostate cancer. *Oncoimmunology.* 2018;7: e1380764. https://doi.org/10.1080/2162402X.2017.1380764.

207. Becht E, de Reyniès A, Giraldo NA, et al. Immune and stromal classification of colorectal cancer is associated with molecular subtypes and relevant for precision immunotherapy. *Clin Cancer Res.* 2016;22:4057–4066. https://doi.org/10.1158/1078-0432.CCR-15-2879.

208. Dienstmann R, Salazar R, Tabernero J. The evolution of our molecular understanding of colorectal cancer: what we are doing now, what the future holds, and how tumor profiling is just the beginning. *Am Soc Clin Oncol Educ Book.* 2014;34:91–99. https://doi.org/10.14694/EdBook_AM.2014.34.91.

209. Overman MJ, McDermott R, Leach JL, et al. Nivolumab in patients with metastatic DNA mismatch repair-deficient or microsatellite instability-high colorectal cancer (CheckMate 142): an open-label, multicentre, phase 2 study. *Lancet Oncol.* 2017;18:1182–1191. https://doi.org/10.1016/S1470-2045(17)30422-9.

210. Magee MS, Abraham TS, Baybutt TR, et al. Human GUCY2C-targeted chimeric antigen receptor (CAR)-Expressing T-cells eliminate colorectal cancer metastases. *Cancer Immunol Res.* 2018;6:509–516. https://doi.org/10.1158/2326-6066.CIR-16-0362.

211. Birbe R, Palazzo JP, Walters R, Weinberg D, Schulz S, Waldman SA. Guanylyl cyclase C is a marker of intestinal metaplasia, dysplasia, and adenocarcinoma of the gastrointestinal tract. *Hum Pathol.* 2005;36:170–179. https://doi.org/10.1016/j.humpath.2004.12.002.

212. Carrithers SL, Barber MT, Biswas S, et al. Guanylyl cyclase C is a selective marker for metastatic colorectal tumors in human extraintestinal tissues. *Proc Natl Acad Sci U S A.* 1996;93:14827–14832.

213. Sia D, Villanueva A, Friedman SL, Llovet JM. Liver cancer cell of origin, molecular class, and effects on patient prognosis. *Gastroenterology.* 2017;152:745–761. https://doi.org/10.1053/j.gastro.2016.11.048.

214. Xu F, Jin T, Zhu Y, Dai C. Immune checkpoint therapy in liver cancer. *J Exp Clin Cancer Res.* 2018;37:110. https://doi.org/10.1186/s13046-018-0777-4.

215. Zhang Y-F, Ho M. Humanization of high-affinity antibodies targeting glypican-3 in hepatocellular carcinoma. *Sci Rep.* 2016;6:33878. https://doi.org/10.1038/srep33878.

216. Ishiguro T, Sano Y, Komatsu S, et al. An anti–glypican 3/CD3 bispecific T-cell–redirecting antibody for treatment of solid tumors. *Sci Transl Med.* 2017;9:eaal4291. https://doi.org/10.1126/scitranslmed.aal4291.

217. Jiang Z, Jiang X, Chen S, et al. Anti-GPC3-CAR T-cells suppress the growth of tumor cells in patient-derived xenografts of hepatocellular carcinoma. *Front Immunol.* 2017; 7. https://doi.org/10.3389/fimmu.2016.00690.

218. Pan Z, Di S, Shi B, et al. Increased antitumor activities of glypican-3-specific chimeric antigen receptor-modified T-cells by coexpression of a soluble PD1–CH3 fusion protein. *Cancer Immunol Immunother.* 2018;67: 1621–1634. https://doi.org/10.1007/s00262-018-2221-1.

219. Thistlethwaite FC, Gilham DE, Guest RD, et al. The clinical efficacy of first-generation carcinoembryonic antigen (CEACAM5)-specific CAR T-cells is limited by poor persistence and transient pre-conditioning-dependent respiratory toxicity. *Cancer Immunol Immunother.* 2017; 66:1425–1436. https://doi.org/10.1007/s00262-017-2034-7.

220. Holzinger A, Abken H. CAR T-cells targeting solid tumors: carcinoembryonic antigen (CEA) proves to be a safe target. *Cancer Immunol Immunother.* 2017;66: 1505–1507. https://doi.org/10.1007/s00262-017-2045-4.

221. Wang F, Meng W, Wang B, Qiao L. Helicobacter pylori-induced gastric inflammation and gastric cancer. *Cancer Lett.* 2014;345:196–202. https://doi.org/10.1016/j.canlet.2013.08.016.

222. Brandt S, Kwok T, Hartig R, Konig W, Backert S. NF- B activation and potentiation of proinflammatory responses by the Helicobacter pylori CagA protein. *Proc Natl Acad Sci.* 2005;102:9300–9305. https://doi.org/10.1073/pnas.0409873102.

223. Kim M, Pyo S, Kang CH, et al. Folate receptor 1 (FOLR1) targeted chimeric antigen receptor (CAR) T-cells for the treatment of gastric cancer. *PLoS One.* 2018;13: e0198347. https://doi.org/10.1371/journal.pone.0198347.

224. Kim DP, Kus KJB, Ruiz E. Basal cell carcinoma review. *Hematol Oncol Clin N Am.* 2019;33:13–24. https://doi.org/10.1016/j.hoc.2018.09.004.

225. Waldman A, Schmults C. Cutaneous squamous cell carcinoma. *Hematol Oncol Clin N Am.* 2019;33:1–12. https://doi.org/10.1016/j.hoc.2018.08.001.

226. Trodello C, Higgins S, Ahadiat O, et al. Cetuximab as a component of multimodality treatment of high-risk cutaneous squamous cell carcinoma: a retrospective analysis from a single tertiary academic medical center. *Dermatol Surg.* 2019;45:254–267. https://doi.org/10.1097/DSS.0000000000001755.

227. Coradini D, Casarsa C, Oriana S. Epithelial cell polarity and tumorigenesis: new perspectives for cancer detection

and treatment. *Acta Pharmacol Sin.* 2011;32:552−564. https://doi.org/10.1038/aps.2011.20.

228. Wu H, Lotan R, Menter D, Lippman SM, Xu XC. Expression of E-cadherin is associated with squamous differentiation in squamous cell carcinomas. *Anticancer Res.* 2000;20:1385−1390.

229. Desmouliere A, Guyot C, Gabbiani G. The stroma reaction myofibroblast: a key player in the control of tumor cell behavior. *Int J Dev Biol.* 2004;48:509−517. https://doi.org/10.1387/ijdb.041802ad.

230. Kalluri R, Zeisberg M. Fibroblasts in cancer. *Nat Rev Cancer.* 2006;6:392−401. https://doi.org/10.1038/nrc1877.

231. Tran E, Chinnasamy D, Yu Z, et al. Immune targeting of fibroblast activation protein triggers recognition of multipotent bone marrow stromal cells and cachexia. *J Exp Med.* 2013;210:1125−1135. https://doi.org/10.1084/jem.20130110.

232. Jia D, Liu Z, Deng N, et al. A COL11A1-correlated pancancer gene signature of activated fibroblasts for the prioritization of therapeutic targets. *Cancer Lett.* 2016;382:203−214. https://doi.org/10.1016/j.canlet.2016.09.001.

233. Kawase A, Ishii G, Nagai K, et al. Podoplanin expression by cancer associated fibroblasts predicts poor prognosis of lung adenocarcinoma. *Int J Cancer.* 2008;123:1053−1059. https://doi.org/10.1002/ijc.23611.

234. Shiina S, Ohno M, Ohka F, et al. CAR T-cells targeting podoplanin reduce orthotopic glioblastomas in mouse brains. *Cancer Immunol Res.* 2016;4:259−268. https://doi.org/10.1158/2326-6066.CIR-15-0060.

235. Ilieva KM, Cheung A, Mele S, et al. Chondroitin sulfate proteoglycan 4 and its potential as an antibody immunotherapy target across different tumor types. *Front Immunol.* 2018;8:1911. https://doi.org/10.3389/fimmu.2017.01911.

236. Bocca P, Di Carlo E, Caruana I, et al. Bevacizumab-mediated tumor vasculature remodelling improves tumor infiltration and antitumor efficacy of GD2-CAR T-cells in a human neuroblastoma preclinical model. *Oncoimmunology.* 2018;7:e1378843. https://doi.org/10.1080/2162402X.2017.1378843.

237. Chinnasamy D, Yu Z, Theoret MR, et al. Gene therapy using genetically modified lymphocytes targeting VEGFR-2 inhibits the growth of vascularized syngenic tumors in mice. *J Clin Investig.* 2010;120:3953−3968. https://doi.org/10.1172/JCI43490.

238. Wang W, Ma Y, Li J, et al. Specificity redirection by CAR with human VEGFR-1 affinity endows T lymphocytes with tumor-killing ability and anti-angiogenic potency. *Gene Ther.* 2013;20:970−978. https://doi.org/10.1038/gt.2013.19.

239. Highfill SL, Cui Y, Giles AJ, et al. Disruption of CXCR2-mediated MDSC tumor trafficking enhances anti-PD1 efficacy. *Sci Transl Med.* 2014;6:237ra67. https://doi.org/10.1126/scitranslmed.3007974.

240. Burga RA, Thorn M, Point GR, et al. Liver myeloid-derived suppressor cells expand in response to liver metastases in mice and inhibit the anti-tumor efficacy of anti-CEA CAR-T. *Cancer Immunol Immunother.* 2015;64:817−829. https://doi.org/10.1007/s00262-015-1692-6.

241. Bajgain P, Tawinwung S, D'Elia L, et al. CAR T-cell therapy for breast cancer: harnessing the tumor milieu to drive T-cell activation. *J Immunother Cancer.* 2018;6:34. https://doi.org/10.1186/s40425-018-0347-5.

242. Okano M, Konno M, Kano Y, et al. Human colorectal CD24+ cancer stem cells are susceptible to epithelial-mesenchymal transition. *Int J Oncol.* 2014;45:575−580. https://doi.org/10.3892/ijo.2014.2462.

243. Klapdor R, Wang S, Morgan M, et al. Characterization of a novel third-generation anti-CD24-CAR against ovarian cancer. *Int J Mol Sci.* 2019;20:660. https://doi.org/10.3390/ijms20030660.

244. Zöller M. CD44: can a cancer-initiating cell profit from an abundantly expressed molecule? *Nat Rev Cancer.* 2011;11:254−267. https://doi.org/10.1038/nrc3023.

245. Neu S, Geiselhart A, Sproll M, et al. Expression of CD44 isoforms by highly enriched CD34-positive cells in cord blood, bone marrow and leukaphereses. *Bone Marrow Transplant.* 1997;20:593−598. https://doi.org/10.1038/sj.bmt.1700940.

246. Casucci M, Nicolis di Robilant B, Falcone L, et al. CD44v6-targeted T-cells mediate potent antitumor effects against acute myeloid leukemia and multiple myeloma. *Blood.* 2013;122:3461−3472. https://doi.org/10.1182/blood-2013-04-493361.

247. Hekele A, Dall P, Moritz D, et al. Growth retardation of tumors by adoptive transfer of cytotoxic T lymphocytes reprogrammed by CD44v6-specific scFv:zeta-chimera. *Int J Cancer.* 1996;68:232−238. https://doi.org/10.1002/(SICI)1097-0215(19961009)68:2<232::AID-IJC16>3.0.CO;2-C.

248. Wang Y, Chen M, Wu Z, et al. CD133-directed CAR T-cells for advanced metastasis malignancies: A phase I trial. *Oncoimmunology.* 2018;7:e1440169. https://doi.org/10.1080/2162402X.2018.1440169.

249. Feng K, Guo Y, Liu Y, et al. Cocktail treatment with EGFR-specific and CD133-specific chimeric antigen receptor-modified T-cells in a patient with advanced cholangiocarcinoma. *J Hematol Oncol.* 2017;10:4. https://doi.org/10.1186/s13045-016-0378-7.

CHAPTER 12

CAR T-Cell Therapy for CNS Malignancies

KHALED SANBER, MD, PHD • SUJITH K. JOSEPH, PHD • NABIL AHMED, MD, MPH

INTRODUCTION

Central nervous system (CNS) tumors are a diverse group of neoplasms that have been classified by the World Health Organization (WHO) based on their cells of origin. Malignant gliomas arise from glial cells or their progenitors and account for around 80% of all malignant primary CNS tumors.[1] In adults, glioblastoma (GBM) is the most common and aggressive variant. The most common malignant CNS tumor in children is medulloblastoma, which arises from neuronal progenitors and accounts for around 20% of cases.[2]

Malignant CNS tumors are generally associated with poor prognosis and poor quality of life due to the neurological deficits and cognitive decline associated with the disease and its treatment, including surgical resection and radiotherapy. Primary GBM is associated with dismal outcomes, with a 5-year overall survival of 2%–4% despite current standard-of-care treatment.[3] Since the efficacy of currently available therapies against recurrent GBM is suboptimal, patients and their clinicians are strongly encouraged to consider clinical trials. Although conventional therapies for primary medulloblastoma have better clinical responses with a 5-year overall survival of 65%–80%, recurrent disease is highly resistant to salvage therapy.[2] Other less common CNS malignancies, such as diffuse intrinsic pontine glioma (DIPG)[4] and recurrent ependymoma,[5] have limited treatment options and are similarly associated with poor prognoses.

Immunotherapy using monoclonal antibodies that block inhibitory receptors lead to durable responses in multiple cancer types including solid malignancies,[6] resulting in a paradigm shift in the field of cancer therapy. Now, these novel therapies have been approved by the Food and Drug Administration (FDA) for the treatment of a growing list of solid malignancies including melanoma, non–small-cell lung cancer (NSCLC), renal cell carcinoma, urothelial cancer, and head and neck squamous cell carcinoma. Pembrolizumab, an anti-PD1 blocking antibody, has also been FDA approved for microsatellite instability (MSI)–high or mismatch repair (MMR)–deficient solid tumors of any histology, as they characteristically have a high mutational burden.

For CNS malignancies, treatment with anti-PD1 blocking antibody nivolumab led to durable responses in two siblings with recurrent GBM caused by germline biallelic MMR deficiency.[7] Multiple ongoing clinical trials are actively investigating the use of checkpoint blockade to treat other CNS malignancies,[8,9] but despite promising preclinical data, success to date has been limited.[10–13] Multiple barriers may curtail the success of this approach in the CNS, including the erratic bioavailability of monoclonal antibodies, the highly suppressive tumor microenvironment (TME) of some CNS malignancies like GBM,[14] and the compensatory upregulation of nontargeted inhibitory receptors on T-cells following monotherapy with immune checkpoint blockers.[15] Thus, novel approaches are needed to treat these aggressive tumors and improve clinical outcomes.

Adoptive transfer of autologous T-cells genetically engineered to express chimeric antigen receptors (CARs) is one particularly promising approach for the treatment of CNS malignancies.[16,17] CARs consist of an extracellular single-chain variable fragment (scFv) directed against a particular tumor-associated antigen (TAA), a transmembrane domain, and an intracellular signaling domain(s). First-generation CARs only carry the CD3 ζ signaling domain. Later iterations of CARs incorporated additional costimulatory signaling domains (most commonly those derived from CD28 and/or 4-1BB molecules): second-generation CARs have one costimulatory domain, and third-generation CARs have two costimulatory domains.[18] The addition of costimulatory signals significantly improved the efficacy and durability of CAR T-cell antitumor activity.[19]

The FDA approved the use of second-generation CAR T-cells directed against CD19 for the treatment of B-cell hematological malignancies following remarkable responses in multiple clinical trials.[20−22] However, solid malignancies pose multiple unique barriers to endogenous as well as genetically engineered T-cell responses. To begin with, malignant tumors exhibit significant inter- and intratumoral heterogeneity. The former can limit the number of patients that can benefit from CAR T-cells directed against a particular TAA, whereas the latter may facilitate the escape of clones that do not express the targeted antigen.[23] For brain tumors, the blood−brain barrier (BBB) also represents a unique (but not insurmountable) obstacle to CAR T-cells that can limit their physical access to tumor cells.[24,25] The sequestration of T-cells within the bone marrow in patients with GBM and glioma mouse models has been recently described as another barrier to T-cell−based therapies of CNS malignancies.[26] Additionally, CAR T-cells that reach the tumor bed face a highly immune-suppressive TME with multiple immune and metabolic checkpoints that hinder their expansion, persistence, and antitumor activity.[14]

CHIMERIC ANTIGEN RECEPTOR T-CELLS FOR CENTRAL NERVOUS SYSTEM MALIGNANCIES: CLINICAL EXPERIENCE TO DATE

Pioneering clinical trials using CAR T-cells to treat CNS malignancies have focused on GBM, which is particularly aggressive and resistant to conventional therapies (Table 12.1). Preclinical studies have also tested CAR T-cells in animal models of medulloblastoma,[27,28] ependymoma,[29] and DIPG.[30] Based on lessons learned from the early trials targeting GBM, as well as the ever-growing body of preclinical data, ongoing trials have included patients with other types of CNS malignancies (Table 12.2). In the following sections, we first summarize the data obtained from the published clinical trials targeting CNS malignancies. We then highlight the successes attained thus far, as well as the remaining obstacles facing the field.

Summary of Published Chimeric Antigen Receptor T-Cell Clinical Trials Targeting Central Nervous System Malignancies

Early reports of clinical trials utilizing second-generation CAR T-cells for the treatment of GBM have been published[31−33] (Table 12.1). Multiple other trials targeting GBM and other primary CNS malignancies are currently ongoing (Table 12.2). As it is important to use the available clinical data to highlight the successes and identify the major obstacles facing the field to guide the design of future preclinical and clinical studies, we summarize each of the published studies in the following sections.

Clinical trials targeting IL-13R∝2

In a phase 1 trial targeting recurrent/progressive GBM, Brown and colleagues used CAR T-cells against IL-13R∝2[34] (see Section Interleukin-13 receptor alpha 2). In this trial, a first-generation CAR with the CD3ζ signaling domain, but no costimulatory domain, was expressed in T-cells using electroporation.

Patients were enrolled after the initial diagnosis of GBM, and peripheral blood mononuclear cells (PBMCs) were collected by leukapheresis to manufacture the CAR T-cell product. After tumor recurrence, patients underwent surgical resection of the tumor with placement of a Rickham catheter. Tumor tissue was then tested for the expression of the target antigen, which had notable intra- and interpatient heterogeneity. The three patients whose tumor tested positive for IL-13R∝2 expression subsequently received 11 (1/3 patients) or 12 (2/3 patients) intracavitary doses of CAR T-cells at 2-week intervals. An intrapatient dose escalation strategy was employed for the first three doses (1×10^7, 5×10^7, and then 1×10^8 CAR+ T-cells), and the highest dose was then used for all subsequent doses. Patients were evaluated using brain MRI at week 3 and week 6 after the first infusion.

In this trial, there was only transient antitumor activity that was mostly localized to the site of CAR T-cell infusion. The disease progressed in all patients resulting in a mean overall survival of 11 months after relapse.[34] The use of a less effective first-generation CAR lacking a costimulatory signal[35] and the relatively long ex vivo manipulation process, which can affect the quality and potency of manufactured CAR T-cells,[36] may partially explain the apparent lack of efficacy. Moreover, trafficking of the infused CAR T-cells following intracavitary delivery appeared to be limited as new lesions developed at distal sites. Of note, there was evidence of a reduction in expression of IL-13R∝2 in a postinfusion tumor biopsy that was available for one patient who underwent resection for tumor recurrence.[34] Although this might be considered as evidence of antitumor activity, it also raises concern over the potential for antigen escape.

TABLE 12.1
Published Clinical Trials Targeting Primary CNS Malignancies.

Center		Baylor College of Medicine	City of Hope Medical Center		University of Pennsylvania
NCT		NCT01109095.[31]	NCT00730613.[34]	NCT02208362.[33]	NCT02209937.[32]
Patient characteristics	• Number of patients • Age range (yr) • Number of failed lines of treatment	• 17 (7 pediatric, 10 adult) • 10–17, 30–69 • 1 (7 pts)–8	• 3 (adult) • 36–57 • 1–2	• 1 (adult) • 50 • 1	• 10 (adult) • 45–76 • 2–4
Target tumor		Progressive or recurrent GBM	Recurrent GBM	Recurrent GBM MGMT nonmethylated	Recurrent GBM MGMT nonmethylated
Target antigen	• Target Ag • Expression assay	• HER-2 • IHC	• IL13-Rα2 • IHC, PCR	• IL13-Rα2 • IHC, PCR	• EGFRvIII • NGS-based assay (RNA)
CAR	• Endodomain • Vector • % transduced	• CD28 • GRV • 18%–67%	• N/A (1st generation) • DNA EP • N/A (drug selection)	• 4-1BB • SIN LVV • 64%–81%	• 4-1BB • SIN LVV • 4.8%–25.6%
Lymphodepletion		No	No	No	No
Administration	• Route • Dose • Number of doses	• IV • 1–100 × 10^6 CAR + cells/m^2 • 1 dose: 11 pts 2 doses: 4 pts 3 or 6 doses: 1 pt each	• IC • 1–10 × 10^7 CAR + cells • 11–12	• IC-IVT • 2–10 × 10^6 CAR + cells • 21	• IV • 1.75–5 × 10^8 CAR + cells • 1
Toxicity	• DLT • Systemic CRS • Grade 3 or 4 AEs	• No • No • Lymphopenia, neutropenia, fatigue, weakness, HA, cerebral edema, hydrocephalus, hyponatremia	• No • No • HA, tongue deviation + shuffling gait	• No • No • No	• No • No • Weakness, cerebral edema, seizures, HA, ICH, LV dysfunction
Efficacy	• Response criteria • Median OS • PFS • SD • PR/CR	• RECIST[64] • 11.1 mo • 3.5 mo • 7 with 3 long-term (24–29 mo) • 1 PR (9.2 mo → SD)	• N/A • 11 mo • N/A • None • None	• RANO[45] • 11 mo • N/A • N/A • CR (7.5 mo → PD)	• RANO[45] • 8 mo • N/A • 1 SD (3 mo) → alive at 33 mo[b] • None

AE, adverse event; Ag, antigen; CRS, cytokine release syndrome; DLT, dose-limiting toxicity; DNA, deoxyribonucleotide; EGFRvIII, epidermal growth factor receptor variant III; EP, electroporation; GBM, glioblastoma; HA, headache; HER-2, human epidermal growth factor receptor-2; ICH, intracranial hypertension; IHC, immunohistochemistry; IL-13Rα2, interleukin-13 receptor α2; IC, intracavitary; IV, intravenous; IVT, intraventricular; LV, left ventricle; LVV, lentiviral vector; mo, month; N/A, not applicable; NCT, national clinical trial; NGS, next-generation sequencing; OS, overall survival; PCR, polymerase chain reaction; PFS, progression-free survival; PR, partial response; pts, patients; RNA, ribonucleotide; SD, stable disease; SIN, self-inactivating; yr, year.

TABLE 12.2
Unpublished Clinical Trials Targeting Primary CNS Malignancies.

Sponsor	NCT[a]	Target Tumor	Target Antigen	Route of Admin	LymphoDepletion	Phase
Baylor College of Medicine	NCT02442297	Recurrent or refractory CNS tumors (or metastatic tumors)	HER-2	Intracranial	N/A	I
City of Hope Medical Center	NCT02208362	Recurrent or refractory malignant glioma	IL-13Rα 2	Intratumoral/IC/ IVC/	N/A	I
City of Hope Medical Center	NCT03389230	Recurrent or refractory malignant glioma	HER-2	Intratumoral/IC/ IVC/	N/A	I
National Cancer Institute (NCI)	NCT01454596.[a]	Recurrent malignant glioma	EGFRvIII	IV + aldesleukin (on day 1–5 postinfusion)	Yes: Flu/Cy	I/II
University of Washington	NCT03500991	Multiple CNS tumors*	HER-2	Arm A: IC, Arm B: IVC	N/A	I
University of Washington	NCT03638167	Multiple CNS tumors*	EGFR806	Arm A: IC, Arm B: IVC	N/A	I
Duke University	NCT03283631	Recurrent GBM	EGFRvIII	Intratumoral	N/A	I[b]
Duke University	NCT02664363	Newly diagnosed GBM	EGFRvIII	IV Note: CAR T-cell infusions initiated after SOC therapy with TMZ and XRT	Yes: TMZ	I
Beijing Sanbo Brain Hospital	NCT02844062	Recurrent GBM	EGFRvIII	IV	Yes: Flu/Cy	I
Xuanwu Hospital, Beijing	NCT03423992	Recurrent malignant glioma	EGFRvIII, IL-13Rα2, HER-2, CD133, EphA2, GD2	Not specified	Not specified	I
Shenzhen Geno-Immune Medical Institute	NCT03170141	GBM	EGFRvIII. CAR T-cells also produce immune checkpoint inhibitor	IC/IV	Yes: Flu/Cy	I/II

CNS, central nervous system; EGFRvIII, epidermal growth factor receptor variant III; EPhA2, Ephrin type A receptor 2; Flu/Cy, fludarabine/ cyclophosphamide; GD2, disialoganglioside Il3(NeuAc)2GgOse3Cer; IC, intracavitary; IV, intravenous; IVT, intraventricular; Flu/Cy, fludarabine/ cyclophosphamide; HER-2, human epidermal growth factor receptor-2; TMZ, temozolomide; XRT, radiotherapy.
Notes:Trials targeting malignancies that are metastatic to the brain are not included: NCT03696030.
Trials with a malignant brain tumor arm are not included: NCT02839954, NCT02617134, NCT02713984, NCT02541370.
*Multiple CNS tumors: glioma, ependymoma, medulloblastoma, germ cell tumor, atypical teratoid/rhabdoid tumor, primitive neuroectodermal tumor, choroid plexus carcinoma, pineoblastoma.
[a] Completed but not published.
[b] Suspended.

In a follow-up clinical trial, Brown et al. used a self-inactivating lentiviral vector to transduce enriched central memory T-cells with a second-generation anti-IL-13R∝2 CAR incorporating the 4-1BB costimulatory domain. A brief report detailing the treatment and response of a single patient treated as part of this trial was published recently.[33] This patient had recurrent GBM with leptomeningeal spread documented around 6 months after standard-of-care therapy. Before the initiation of CAR T-cell infusions, three of five detectable tumor sites were resected, and a Rickham catheter was placed at one of these tumor sites. The patient then received a total of six scheduled intracavitary doses of CAR T-cells (dose 1: 2×10^6 CAR+ T-cells, doses 2–6: 10×10^6 CAR+ T-cells). Despite stabilization of the tumor at the infusion site, the other tumor sites continued to progress, and new lesions developed at distant sites, again suggesting these CAR T-cells were unable to traffic to distal sites following intracavitary infusion. A second intraventricular catheter was therefore placed in this patient, who went on to receive 10 additional intraventricular doses of CAR T-cells (doses 7–16: 10×10^6 CAR+ T-cells).

The patient responded to CAR T-cell therapy with a gradual decrease in the size of all tumor lesions that had been detected prior to initiation of intraventricular CAR T-cell infusions. He was also successfully tapered off of systemic dexamethasone. These lesions eventually became undetectable by MRI/PET CT and did not recur. However, the tumor recurred at four new sites at around 7.5 months (228 days) after the first CAR T-cell infusion. Notably, there were no dose-limiting toxicities (DLTs) and no grade 3 or 4 adverse events recorded during treatment. However, the concomitant administration of supportive/symptomatic therapies, including dexamethasone (tapered dose ≤ 4 mg per day), divalproex (7500 mg twice daily), and acetaminophen, may have reduced the risk for adverse events and DLTs.

Furthermore, in this patient, all detectable GBM lesions (including a spinal lesion) decreased in size after the start of intraventricular CAR T-cell infusions, suggesting that this route improved the trafficking of the infused cells compared with intracavitary delivery.[33] Moreover, the elimination of tumor lesions that have a nonuniform expression of IL-13R∝2 (as detected by immunohistochemistry [IHC]) is encouraging. However, whether this represents a "bystander" effect of activated CAR T-cells in the TME or the recruitment of the endogenous immune system is unclear.

Despite these encouraging observations, this case report also highlighted notable limitations of CAR T-cell therapies. Importantly, CAR T-cells failed to expand significantly following intraventricular administration, and their persistence was limited (detectable in the cerebrospinal fluid [CSF] for up to 7 days postinfusion). Multiple factors may have contributed to these observations including the concomitant administration of low-dose dexamethasone, the route of administration, and the highly immune-suppressive TME of GBM. Lastly, a decrease in IL-13R∝2 expression was noted in the tumor that recurred following CAR T-cell infusion, raising concerns about the possibility of antigen escape after targeting a single TAA.

Clinical trial targeting human epidermal growth factor receptor-2

Another phase 1 clinical trial conducted by Ahmed et al. targeted the human epidermal growth factor receptor-2 (HER-2) (see Section Human epidermal growth factor receptor 2) to treat recurrent or progressive GBM.[31] In this trial, autologous virus-specific T-cells (VSTs) were transduced with a gamma-retroviral vector encoding a second-generation anti-HER-2 CAR with the CD28 endodomain. VSTs reactive against viral antigens derived from cytomegalovirus (CMV), Epstein-Barr virus (EBV), or adenovirus were used in an effort to coopt the natural T-cell receptor (TCR)–mediated signaling and improve CAR T-cell functionality and longevity. The HER2 VSTs were delivered intravenously (IV), as prior clinical trials had demonstrated T-cell trafficking to the CNS.[37,38]

A total of 17 patients (10 adults and 7 children) with recurrent GBM were treated, and 16 were evaluable as one patient was excluded from analysis because they received chemotherapy within 6 weeks from T-cell infusion. Patients received one or more IV infusions of autologous HER2-CAR VSTs at five dose levels ($1–100 \times 10^6$ HER2-CAR+ VSTs; with a cohort size of three patients per dose level). This dose-escalation strategy starting at a relatively low dose of 1×10^6 cells/m^2 was designed to address concerns for possible off-target adverse events. These concerns were fueled by a report of a patient who suffered lethal cytokine release syndrome (CRS) with multiorgan failure and possible on-target/off-tumor toxicity due to reactivity against lung epithelial cells after intravenous infusion of a high dose (1×10^{10} cells) of anti-HER2 CAR T-cells that incorporated the scFv derived from trastuzumab.[39,40] Ahmed et al., however, utilized a CAR with an scFv derived from the FRP5 antibody that targets a more distal epitope compared with trastuzumab.[41,42] FRP5-derived HER2 CAR T-cells were shown to be safe in a recent dose-escalation phase 1 trial targeting sarcoma.[43] Importantly, no dose-limiting adverse events were noted in this trial, but one patient had grade 4 cerebral edema, two had grade 3 headaches, and one had grade 3 hydrocephalus[31] (Table 12.1), highlighting the need for close monitoring of patients receiving CAR T-cell therapies for local, CNS-related side effects.

All patients were evaluated with a baseline brain MRI prior to initiation of CAR T-cell infusions and a repeat MRI at 6 weeks postinfusion. The RECIST criteria were used to evaluate radiographic responses.[44] Patients who had evidence of response were eligible to receive up to six additional doses of T-cells at 6- to 12-week intervals at the same dose level (Table 12.1). In this study, the median overall survival was 11.1 months from the first infusion and 24.5 months from diagnosis.

Notable responses were documented in this trial, including a 17-year-old patient who received two doses at 1×10^6 cells/m^2 and had a partial response (PR) that lasted 9.2 months after the first infusion and survived for a total 26.9 months from that date. Seven patients had stable disease (SD) lasting 8 weeks to 29 months postinfusion, and three of these patients were alive at study conclusion (with SD lasting 24, 28.8, and 29 months). Although eight patients were considered to have progressive disease (PD) based on their follow-up MRIs, six survived for more than 6 months postinfusion. These patients were classified as having progressive disease based on the RECIST criteria, but the radiographic changes noted may have presented local inflammation owing to local T-cell expansion and activation, a phenomenon referred to as "pseudoprogression" in other immunotherapy trials. Since the end of this trial, criteria used for radiologic assessment of tumor responses in immunotherapy trials have been modified by multiple groups in an attempt to improve accuracy.[45–47]

Additionally, HER2 VST levels in the peripheral blood were assessed serially by qPCR, with levels peaking at 3 hours in 15 of 17 patients and declining thereafter. This rapid peak and subsequent gradual decline suggests that the autologous HER2 VSTs had limited in vivo expansion. Although the persistence of HER2 VSTs was limited in the majority of patients, the cells were detectable in the peripheral blood up to 12 months after the initial infusion in two out of six patients evaluated after receiving multiple infusions (see Section Chimeric Antigen Receptor T-Cell Pharmacokinetics in the Setting of Central Nervous System Malignancies). Of note, whether VSTs are more effective than nonselected T-cell populations remains an open question. Although CMV seropositivity was part of the inclusion criteria, only five patients had pp65-positive GBM (as assessed by IHC); of these patients, two had SD and three had PD.

Another interesting observation from this study is that patients who had received salvage therapies prior to trial enrollment had shorter median survival. Although these patients might have had more aggressive tumors prompting the use of salvage therapies, exposure to these potentially cytotoxic agents may have also led to T-cell defects that compromised the quality of the autologous CAR T-cell product. Such adverse effects following multiple cytotoxic chemotherapy cycles have been recently described in a cohort of pediatric patients with a range of different malignancies.

Clinical trial targeting epidermal growth factor receptor variant III

O'Rourke et al. conducted a clinical trial treating 10 adult patients with recurrent/progressive GBM with a single IV dose of autologous anti-EGFRvIII (epidermal growth factor receptor variant III) CAR T-cells[32] (see Section Epidermal growth factor receptor variant III). T-cells were transduced with a lentiviral vector to express a second-generation anti-EGFRvIII CAR incorporating a 4-1BB costimulatory domain. Patients with newly diagnosed or recurrent/progressive GBM were tested for EGFRvIII expression using an RNA-based next-generation sequencing assay. Those who tested positive and met the other eligibility criteria underwent leukapheresis for PBMC collection and storage. Any subsequent evidence of disease progression triggered CAR T-cell manufacturing.

Patients were evaluated with a baseline brain MRI followed by a single IV infusion of $1.75–5 \times 10^8$ CAR+ T-cells. Of the 10 patients treated, six were evaluated with a repeat brain MRI at week 4 postinfusion. Five of these patients had SD and one had PD based on the RANO criteria. Given the complexity of the radiographic findings noted postinfusion, the authors focused subsequent analyses on the CAR T-cell engraftment and trafficking to the tumor, as well as their subsequent effects on the TME.

CAR T-cells were detectable (by flow cytometry and qPCR) in the peripheral blood of all patients, with peak levels seen at around 1–2 weeks postinfusion. However, the detection level declined thereafter, and CAR T-cells were no longer detectable in the peripheral blood by day 30 postinfusion in all patients. To test whether CAR T-cells were able to successfully traffic to the tumor site within the CNS, the authors determined the levels of CAR T-cells in postinfusion tumor biopsies whenever available. In all four patients who underwent surgical resection within 2 weeks postinfusion, CAR T-cells were detectable. In contrast, they were detectable in only one of three patients who underwent resection at later time points.

Further testing on the biopsies obtained from the four patients who underwent early resection provided insight into potentially important changes within the TME post-CAR T-cell infusion. Patchy lymphocyte infiltrates consisting of a mix of CD8+ and CD8− cells were noted, and a greater percentage of CD8+ Ki67+ cells were also detected postinfusion, indicating a proliferating cell population. However, there was a concomitant increase in the percentage of CD3+ T-cells expressing regulatory T-cell (T$_{reg}$) markers postinfusion. Other markers of immune suppression in the TME (including IL-10, indoleamine 2,3-deoxygenase [IDO1], and programmed death ligand 1 [PD-L1]) also were upregulated postinfusion, and many of these factors are known to be upregulated by IFNγ, an effector cytokine secreted by activated T-cells.[48,49] In contrast, the changes were not as dramatic in biopsies obtained at later time points (more than 2 weeks postinfusion).

The authors also analyzed the TCR repertoire of the CAR T-cell product and the tumor-infiltrating lymphocytes (TILs) in the tumor biopsy samples obtained pre- and postinfusion. A minority of TCRs detectable in the infusion product were also detected in the postinfusion biopsy, suggesting limited trafficking of peripherally infused cells to the tumor site. However, the detected T-cells represented a relatively large proportion of postinfusion TILs. Additionally, the postinfusion TCR repertoire of TILs was broader than their preinfusion TCR repertoire, indicating the possibility of epitope spreading; however, no further analyses were available to support this at the time of publication. Of note, the percentage of TILs with a regulatory phenotype also rose postinfusion, and this may represent a component of the immune evasion mechanisms employed by solid tumors in response to local CAR T-cell activation.

Importantly, the investigators also examined the effects of CAR T-cell infusion on the expression of the target antigen. In five of seven patients tested, the EGFR-vIII mRNA expression levels (assessed by qPCR) decreased. The remaining two patients had stable expression levels. Of these, one patient had a spatially heterogeneous expression of EGFRvIII mRNA, whereas the other had poor CAR T-cell engraftment and early progression. The reduction in EGFRvIII level may reflect the activity of anti-EGFRvIII CAR T-cells, but it also raises concerns over the risk for antigen escape following CAR T-cell therapies targeting a single antigen, especially in malignancies that exhibit significant intratumoral antigen heterogeneity.[50–52]

Chimeric Antigen Receptor T-Cells for Central Nervous System Malignancies: Successes and Obstacles

In the published trials, CAR T-cell manufacturing was feasible, and adequate doses of autologous CAR T-cells were successfully prepared for heavily pretreated patients.[31–33] However, early collection of T-cells for CAR T-cell manufacturing may still be advantageous to improve the quality of the T-cell product and minimize the defects that can accumulate in T-cells following multiple cycles of chemotherapy.[53,54] Early T-cell collection may also minimize the multifactorial, cancer-related T-cell dysfunction noted in patients with advanced malignancies.[55,56]

The two trials conducted by Ahmed et al. and O'Rourke et al. add to the growing body of evidence that supports a revised view of the CNS as a site that is in dynamic communication with the peripheral immune system rather than a classically immune-privileged site.[24,37,38] Both trials provide indirect evidence of T-cell trafficking to the CNS since intravenously administered CAR T-cells resulted in objective responses in patients with GBM.[31,32] Although CAR T-cell trafficking from the peripheral blood to the tumor site in the CNS is likely suboptimal, O'Rourke et al. provided immunohistochemical evidence that CAR T-cells can reach the tumor site following IV administration.[32] However, it should be noted that CAR T-cell trafficking may have occurred at sites where the blood-brain barrier may have been compromised by tumors and/or prior surgeries. Furthermore, intraventricular delivery of anti-IL-13R∝2 CAR T-cells appeared to allow more efficient trafficking within the CNS compared to intracavitary delivery.[33,34] Of note, alternative methods of monitoring CAR T-cell kinetics and trafficking through various imaging techniques are actively being developed and may offer more comprehensive insights into the unique kinetics of these cellular therapies if utilized in future trials.[57,58]

It has also been proposed that CAR T-cell–mediated antitumor activity may induce an inflammatory response at the tumor site, which may exert an adjuvant-like effect and help trigger more effective endogenous immune responses. The three published trials offer preliminary indirect evidence supporting a possible role for the endogenous immune system in mediating the antitumor activity. In particular, the TCR repertoire (as determined by sequencing of the TCR Vβ chain) expanded postinfusion in all three patients tested in the study conducted by O'Rourke et al.[32] Moreover, clinical responses in some of the patients in the trial conducted by Ahmed et al. appeared to outlast the CAR T-cells, which became undetectable within a few weeks postinfusion.[31] Additionally, tumor lesions with a heterogeneous expression of the target antigen were eliminated after the infusion of CAR T-cells in the patient treated by Brown et al.[33] However, more direct evidence of epitope spreading is needed to confirm the involvement of the endogenous immune system in mediating clinical responses in CAR T-cell clinical trials, and correlative studies aimed at elucidating such mechanisms should be incorporated in future trial designs.

Another important observation is that there were no dose-limiting adverse events reported in the three published trials (Table 12.1). However, CNS side effects were noted in all three trials including headaches, seizures, cerebral edema, hydrocephalus, focal weakness, and, in one patient, intracerebral hemorrhage.[31–33] These studies highlight the need for close neurological monitoring of patients with CNS malignancies who are treated with CAR T-cells, as some of these side effects can have life-threatening consequences, including, but not limited to, increased intracranial pressure (ICP) and brain herniation syndromes if left untreated.

These early clinical trials highlight several obstacles. In particular, CAR T-cells had limited expansion and persistence in the peripheral blood,[31,32] CSF,[33] and at the tumor site,[32] which may be partly due to the immune-suppressive TME of GBM[14,59,60] (see Section Brain Tumor Microenvironment and Chimeric Antigen Receptor T-Cell Function). The TME may also undergo dynamic changes in response to CAR T-cell infiltration and activation, leading to the upregulation of multiple immune-suppressive mechanisms, as evidenced by the increase in the number of CD4+ CD25+ Foxp3+ T_{regs} and the rise in the levels of expression of multiple inhibitory molecules/markers (such as PD-L1, IDO, and IL-10) postinfusion.[32,48,49] These changes may limit any further expansion, persistence and function of CAR T-cells at the TME. Since many of these mechanisms are induced/upregulated by cytokines released by activated CAR T-cells, such as IFNγ, this phenomenon is likely to be relevant to the application of T-cell–based therapies to the treatment of solid malignancies in general. Indeed, local inhibitory mechanisms within the TME have been implicated in inhibiting CAR T-cells in preclinical models of solid malignancies.[60] Engineering CAR T-cells to become less susceptible to inhibition/exhaustion is, therefore, an active area of research (reviewed in Ref. 61). Repeated infusions of CAR T-cells may offer another simple strategy to partly overcome this obstacle. Indeed, patients who received multiple infusions[31,33] had more pronounced and longer-lasting responses compared with those who received a single CAR T-cell infusion[32] in the early trials targeting GBM. However, the caveat that selection bias may have influenced this observation should be highlighted, since patients who showed an initial response were eligible to receive repeat infusions.[31] Another strategy that can improve the expansion and persistence of CAR T-cells is the use of preinfusion lymphodepleting regimens (see Section Chimeric Antigen Receptor T-Cell Pharmacokinetics in the Setting of Central Nervous System Malignancies). This approach is being tested in ongoing clinical trials of CAR T-cells targeting CNS malignancies (Table 12.2).

Another significant mechanism that can potentially impede the durability of CAR T-cell activity is antigen escape. This has led to tumor relapse in patients treated with anti-CD19 CAR T-cells as recurring tumor cells had lost or downregulated the target antigen/epitope through various mechanisms (reviewed in Ref. 62). In the study conducted by O'Rourke et al., five of seven patients who underwent postinfusion resection showed a reduction in EGFRvIII expression. Similarly, a decrease in IL-13R∝2 expression level was noted in one patient for whom tumor tissue was analyzed before and after first-generation CAR T-cell infusion.[32] The risk of antigen escape is particularly relevant to solid malignancies with significant intratumoral antigenic heterogeneity and may be partly offset by targeting multiple TAAs simultaneously.[50–52]

As noted in other immunotherapy trials, the radiographic assessment of tumor responses in CAR T-cell trials targeting GBM may be complicated by transient increases in two-dimensional tumor measurements that may be partly due to the inflammation induced by CAR T-cell activation at the tumor site, a phenomenon referred to as "pseudoprogression."[63] Thus, these changes may be inaccurately interpreted as evidence of disease progression. As previously mentioned, recent updates in the criteria used for the assessment of tumor responses in immunotherapy trials targeting solid malignancies have attempted to address some of these issues to facilitate the proper classification of patient responses,[45–47] and this remains an area of active research (see Section Combinatorial Therapies: Aiding Chimeric Antigen Receptor T-Cells to Improve Clinical Responses).

TARGETING BRAIN TUMOR ANTIGENS

Conventionally, the brain was considered an "immune-privileged" location.[64] This notion included inadequate immune infiltration due to the presence of the BBB, as well as poor antigen presentation[65,66] owing to the absence of draining lymphatics. The BBB is a semipermeable barrier made of endothelial cells, end feet of astrocytes and pericytes on a thick basement membrane. The barrier helps prevent circulating blood from mixing with the CSF in the CNS. Along with regulating the entry of large solutes and ionic molecules, the BBB and glia limitans also tightly control lymphocyte entry into the brain parenchyma, only allowing activated T-cells to enter.[67,68] Additionally, the brain parenchyma lacks a conventional lymphatic system and thus relies more on the glial-associated lymphatic pathway,[69] or glymphatic system, where limited exchange between the interstitial fluid in the parenchyma and the CSF draining into the dural, cervical, and nasal lymphatics carries tumor antigens and immune cells to the nearest secondary or tertiary lymphoid organs.[70] However, recent studies revealed that tumor antigens and immune cells present in the CSF of ventricular and subdural spaces drain efficiently to the peripheral lymphatics.[70–74] Thus, though no longer considered immune privileged,[75] the CNS still poses a major challenge to the adaptive arm of the immune system in terms of effective antigen presentation and initiating a systemic immune response against CNS tumors.[76–79]

The success of CAR T-cell therapy for CNS tumors depends not only on the design of the CAR itself and manufacture of T-cell products, as discussed earlier, but also on the selection of an appropriate target antigen. Target antigens must have expression that is unique to the tumor to prevent "on-target, off-tumor" toxicities. Alternatively, molecules that have acquired mutations that lead to their recognition as neoantigens by the immune system also make for promising CAR T-cell targets. A scarcity of surface-expressed neoantigens in brain tumors makes targeting tumor-specific antigens by CAR T-cells using antibody-derived scFv or mutein a challenge. Additionally, CNS tumors such as GBM have cellular and molecular heterogeneity[80–83] that makes targeting a single antigen difficult. In spite of these limitations, multiple tumor antigens have been investigated preclinically and clinically as targets for CAR T-cell therapy against CNS malignancies.

Central Nervous System Tumor-Associated Targets in Clinical Trials
Epidermal growth factor receptor variant III
EGFRvIII is the first and only neoantigen to date used as a CAR T-cell target to treat brain tumors, primarily GBM. Amplification of the *EGFR* gene is the most frequent genetic change associated with GBM, common in the classic or receptor tyrosine kinase type 2 molecular subtype of isocitrate dehydrogenase (IDH) wild-type GBM.[84–87] The EGFR-amplified GBM also expresses the tumor-specific deletion variant (EGFRvIII), present in 25%–33% of all patients with GBM. First identified by Sugawa and colleagues, variant III of EGFR is a truncated protein formed by identical splicing of exon 1 to exon 8 as a consequence of a deletion-rearrangement of the amplified gene.[88,89] This rearrangement results in the loss of 801 coding bases (exons 2–7) and creation of a new codon for glycine at the novel splice site in their corresponding transcripts, leading to a neoantigenic epitope that is not present in any normal tissues. The truncated receptor protein lacks major parts of the extracellular domain, and while unable to bind its ligands,[90] it remains constitutively active,[91–93] leading to proliferation of tumor cells. The prognostic role of EGFRvIII positivity in EGFR-amplified primary and recurrent GBMs has been controversial,[94–97] with earlier studies associating both prolonged and poorer overall survival to EGFRvIII positivity. A recent study by Felsberg et al. at German Glioma Network reported that EGFRvIII was not prognostic in EGFR-amplified GBM in their cohort.[98] Additionally, this group reported changes in EGFRvIII expression levels at recurrence, thus recommending repeated biopsy for EGFRvIII status for recurrent GBM patients receiving EGFRvIII-targeted therapies. Apart from GBM, EGFRvIII has been previously reported in pediatric DIPGs.[99]

The discovery of monoclonal antibody (mAb) 806 and development of other antibodies such as mAb139 that specifically inhibited the growth of tumor xenografts expressing either the EGFRvIII or amplified EGFR, but not wild-type EGFR, initiated immunotherapeutic targeting of EGFR-amplified GBM.[100–103] The first CAR molecule, also referred to as chimeric immune receptor targeting EGFRvIII, was developed by Bullain and colleagues at Massachusetts General Hospital, Boston.[104] Subsequently, investigators at the National Cancer Institute developed the first EGFRvIII targeted CAR T-cells based on mAb139.[105] Their studies demonstrated specific recognition and antitumor activity against glioma stem cell lines and glioma cell lines expressing mutant EGFRvIII without reactivity to wild-type EGFR. Developing further on established preclinical data for EGFRvIII-targeted CAR T-cells, Johnson and colleagues rationally tested and characterized a battery of humanized anti-EGFRvIII CAR T-cells derived from murine mAb139 scFvs.[106,107] The team's first-in-human study of intravenous delivery of a single dose of autologous EGFRvIII CAR T-cells against recurrent GBM (NCT02209376) demonstrated safety without any DLTs,[32] and other findings from this study are summarized in Summary of Published Chimeric Antigen

Receptor T-Cell Clinical Trials Targeting Central Nervous System Malignancies section. There are currently multiple active trials for EGFRvIII-targeted CAR T-cells recruiting patients at the National Cancer Institute and the Duke Cancer Institute (NCT03283631), the Abramson Cancer Center of the University of Pennsylvania (NCT03726515), and the Beijing Sanbo Brain Hospital in China (NCT02844062).

Human epidermal growth factor receptor 2

Human epidermal growth factor receptor 2 (HER-2, also known as receptor tyrosine-protein kinase erbB-2, CD340, or protooncogene Neu) is a 185-kDa protein receptor with tyrosine kinase activity and extensive homology to EGFR. When present in tumors, HER-2 acts as the preferred heterodimerization partner for other ErbB receptors and a potent signal amplifier.[108] In tumors of the CNS, especially GBM, HER-2 expression is associated with poor prognosis.[109] HER-2 is not expressed in the normal adult brain,[110] and in brain tumors, its expression is associated with increased cell proliferation,[111,112] metastasis, and the inhibition of apoptosis. Glial tumors expressing HER-2 are also less differentiated.[113] Gilbertson and colleagues identified HER-2 expression in 83.6% of childhood medulloblastoma in their cohort[114] and demonstrated that HER-2 signaling results in aggressive disease behavior in ependymoma by promoting tumor cell proliferation.[115] Though not directly demonstrated, atypical teratoid/rhabdoid tumor (ATRT) responds to inhibition of ErbB2-EGFR pathway by the small molecule inhibitor lapatinib.[116] Thus, HER-2 is an attractive candidate for immunotherapy-based approaches against CNS tumors.

Unlike many epithelial tumors including breast,[117] ovarian,[118] or gastric[119] cancer, amplification of HER-2 is not observed in CNS tumors.[120] Therefore, therapy with monoclonal antibody, trastuzumab (4D5), is ineffective in these tumors. Ahmed and colleagues at Baylor College of Medicine first demonstrated the antitumor efficacy of HER-2-targeted CAR T-cells based on the FRP5 mAb in preclinical models of medulloblastoma and GBM,[27,121] and the latter study used patient-derived GBM cells and GBM stem cells. The team then completed a first-in-man clinical trial for patients with progressive or recurrent GBM using HER-2 CARs grafted on CMV-specific T-cells (NCT01109095).[31] The results of this trial are detailed in Summary of Published Chimeric Antigen Receptor T-Cell Clinical Trials Targeting Central Nervous System Malignancies section. Encouraged by the safety profile of this trial, in which T-cells were delivered systemically, the team is currently testing whether intracranial delivery of HER-2 CAR T-cells either to resection cavities or to the ventricular space will improve their trafficking and antitumor activity (NCT02442297). Another widely used HER-2 CAR for CNS tumors is based on the scFv from trastuzumab mAb (4D5). CAR T-cells using this scFv are currently being evaluated in clinical trials at City of Hope Medical Center in California (NCT03696030 and NCT03389230), Seattle Children's Hospital (NCT03500991), and Xuanwu Hospital, Beijing, China (NCT03423992).

Interleukin-13 receptor alpha 2

Interleukin-13 receptor alpha 2 (IL-13Rα2) is a GBM-associated protein that is overexpressed on up to 78% of tumors. Due to its negligible expression in the normal brain,[122] IL13Rα2 is a promising candidate for targeted therapy. IL13Rα2 is an isolated receptor that binds IL-13 only and, unlike the widespread IL13Rα1 receptor, does not form a heterodimer with IL4R.[123] Since the receptor lacks a signaling domain and has only a short cytoplasmic tail and a high affinity for the cytokine, it was initially thought to be a "decoy" receptor sequestering IL-13 and thus neutralizing its effect. In fact, IL-13Rα2 blocks IL-13-driven STAT6 signaling by binding IL-13 with high affinity.[124,125] One recent study suggested that the IL-13/IL-13Rα2 axis is important in mediating signal transduction by increasing expression of AP-1 transcription factors in IL-13Rα2-positive, but not in IL-13Rα2-negative, glioma cell lines.[126] Along with poor survival prognosis in GBM, IL-13Rα2 gene expression is reported to be associated with GBM resistance to temozolomide (TMZ) chemotherapy.[127] The presence of IL-13Rα2 has also been described in pediatric cancers such as medulloblastoma and ependymoma.[128,129] Recently, IL-13Rα2 has been shown to act in cooperation with EGFRvIII signaling to promote proliferation of GBM cells.[130]

The initial iterations of CAR T-cells targeting IL-13Rα2 were based on membrane-tethered IL-13 as binding exodomains and termed as "IL-13-zetakine."[131] The substitution of an amino acid (E13Y) improved the specificity of the zetakine CAR to IL-13α2 and reduced its activity against targets expressing IL-13Rα1.[132] The IL13 (E13Y)-zetakine CAR entered phase 1 trial at the City of Hope Medical Center (NCT02208362) and has demonstrated safety and objective responses after intracavitary or intratumoral administration.[33,34] Later, an IL-13 mutein CAR was designed with two IL-13 mutations (E13K and K105R) and showed potent antitumor activity in xenograft models of GBM but recognized IL-13Rα1.[133] Kong et al. also designed a zetakine CAR based on mutated IL13 extracellular domain (E13K and R109K) linked to intracellular signaling elements of the CD28 costimulatory molecule and CD3ζ.[134] The IL-13 mutation enhanced the selectivity of CAR recognition of IL13Rα2 receptor compared with the IL13Rα1 receptor or the composite IL13Ra1/IL4Ra receptor. Recently, Krenciute and colleagues developed a series of IL13Rα2 CARs based on the scFv 47 and demonstrated that T-cells transduced with the CAR constructs bearing a short hinge showed the best antitumor activity in preclinical models of GBM.[135] This study was followed by scFv-based IL13Rα2-specific CARs from groups at the University of Pennsylvania[136] and City of Hope Medical Center.[137] Another clinical trial testing the safety of IL13Rα2-directed CAR T-cells is ongoing at Xuanwu Hospital, Beijing, China (NCT03423992).

CD133

CD133, also known as AC133 and prominin-1, is a 97-kDa pentaspanning transmembrane glycoprotein that is expressed on cells with a stem-like phenotype. Indeed, CD133 has been used as a cell surface marker[138] to isolate cancer stem cells from various solid tumors, including neoplasms of the brain. The marker was first used to describe cancer stem cells in pediatric tissue samples of medulloblastoma and glioma.[139] Singh et al. found that CD133-expressing tissues could regenerate a heterogeneous tumor, attributable to the increased capacity for self-renewal observed in clinically aggressive medulloblastoma.[139] Zhu and Niedermann at the University Hospital Freiburg, Germany, developed CARs targeting the AC133 epitope of CD133 and demonstrated antitumor activity against GBM stem cells in an orthotopic tumor model.[140] Recently, a team from the Chinese PLA General Hospital reported on the phase 1 trial of CD133-directed CAR T-cells for advanced metastatic malignancies,[141] but this trial did not accrue patients with CNS tumors (NCT02541370). Currently, one active clinical trial is reported at Xuanwu Hospital (NCT03423992) using CD133-directed CAR T-cells for malignant glioma.

Disialoganglioside II3(NeuAc)2GgOse3Cer

Disialoganglioside II3(NeuAc)2GgOse3Cer (GD2) is commonly overexpressed in pediatric and adult solid tumors, including neuroblastoma, glioma, retinoblastoma, most sarcomas, small-cell lung cancer, and melanoma. Traylor and Hogan first observed elevated proportions of gangliosides including GD2 in human gliomas compared with normal brain tissue.[142] Later, another group demonstrated the reactivity of GD2-

specific mAb DMAb-20 in 16 of 20 (80%) malignant glioma and 5 of 5 medulloblastoma cell lines.[143] Mount et al. observed that GD2 was expressed at high levels on patient-derived DIPG cultures and was conserved as a surface marker across DIPG patients and other histone H3 K27M (H3K27M)−mutated diffuse midline gliomas (DMGs).[30] Furthermore, Mount and colleagues showed that T-cells grafted with GD2-specific CARs derived from 14g2a mAb scFv and delivered systemically had potent antitumor efficacy against xenograft models H3K27M-mutant DMGs and DIPG. A randomized, open-label combined phase 1 and 2 trial for GD2 CAR T-cells was completed at Fuda Cancer Hospital, China (NCT03252171), but the study outcomes have not yet been reported. An active clinical trial with GD-2 CAR T-cells is ongoing at Xuanwu Hospital (NCT03423992).

Central Nervous System Tumor-Associated Targets Under Preclinical Investigation
Ephrin type-A receptor 2

Ephrin type-A receptor 2 (EphA2) is a tyrosine kinase receptor binding membrane-bound ephrin-A family ligand residing on adjacent cells and leads to contact-dependent bidirectional signaling. EphA2 was found to be elevated in approximately 90% of GBM specimens and cell lines but is not elevated in normal brain.[144] Increased EphA2 expression was also correlated with worse disease outcome in GBM patients.[145] Based on these studies, EphA2 has been tested as a target for CAR T-cell therapy against GBM. EphA2 endows glioma stem cells with an invasive phenotype in cooperation with Akt signaling and has been shown to regulate glioma stem cell properties, which may lead to the adverse outcomes observed.[146] Preclinical studies using adoptive transfer of EphA2-CAR-T-cells based on scFv of humanized EphA2 monoclonal antibody 4H5 resulted in the regression of glioma xenografts.[147,148]

CD70

CD70 (also known as CD27L, TNFSF7) is a cytokine that belongs to the tumor necrosis factor (TNF) ligand family and is the ligand for CD27. CD70 is normally surface expressed on activated T and B lymphocytes; however, it is also aberrantly expressed in a subset of CNS tumors (8.8% of high-grade gliomas) exhibiting moderate-to-strong immunoreactivity and enriched for the IDH wild-type GBM variants gliosarcoma and epithelioid GBM.[149] In a recent study, researchers identified 35% of primary GBMs and 69% of recurrent GBMs expressed CD70.[150] This report also demonstrated antiglioma activity of CD70-directed CAR T-cells in xenograft mouse models, where the CAR was based on the CD27 truncated extracellular domain model developed by Wang and colleagues at the NCI.[151]

B7-H3

B7-H3, also referred to as CD276, is a type I transmembrane glycoprotein that is part of the B7-CD28 family. Modak and Cheung from Memorial Sloan-Kettering Cancer Center in New York used the monoclonal antibody 8H9 to find expression of B7-H3 in multiple brain tumors including GBM, oligodendroglioma, astrocytoma, meningioma, schwannoma, medulloblastoma, neurofibroma, neuronoglial tumor, ependymoma, and pineoblastoma.[152] Later, Zhou et al. confirmed widespread expression of B7-H3 in DIPG.[153] B7-H3 and B7-H1 expression in the CSF and tumor tissue also correlated with malignancy grade in glioma patients.[154] In a recent report, CAR T-cells designed with the preferentially tumor B7-H3-binding antibody MGA271 demonstrated antitumor activity against primary medulloblastoma models, among other solid tumors.[155]

Chondroitin sulfate proteoglycan 4

Chondroitin sulfate proteoglycan 4 (CSPG4), also known as neuron glia-2 (NG2), high-molecular-weight melanoma-associated antigen (HMW-MAA) or melanoma proteoglycan (MPG), is a 300-kDa transmembrane chondroitin sulfate proteoglycan aberrantly expressed by several solid tumors. Chekenya et al. reported expression of CSPG4 on tumor neovasculature in human malignant brain tumors.[156,157] Furthermore, the authors demonstrated that CSPG4 promotes drug resistance through integrin-activated PI3K/Akt signaling. Another report from the NCI showed that CSPG4 is expressed on GBM cancer stem cells.[158] The team developed CSPG4-specific CAR molecules based on murine mAb 225 and demonstrated that anti-CSPG4 CAR T-cells recognized and killed these stem cells. Another CSPG4-specific CAR was later developed from the anti-CSPG4 mAb 763.74, and T-cells transduced with these CARs demonstrated activity against primary GBM neurospheres.[159]

Podoplanin

Podoplanin (PDPN) is a type I integral membrane glycoprotein with mucin-like character that is expressed in the lymphatic endothelium. PDPN is overexpressed in some solid tumors, especially the mesenchymal type of GBM and malignant astrocytic tumors. In a study reported by Mishima and colleagues, 25.6% of anaplastic astrocytomas and 47.0% of GBMs expressed PDPN on the tumor cell surface.[160] However, PDPN expression was not observed in diffuse astrocytoma. Preclinical evaluation of PDPN CAR T-cells, based on the NZ-1 scFv, demonstrated antitumor activity both in vitro and in an intracranial glioma xenograft model of GBM.[161]

CHIMERIC ANTIGEN RECEPTOR T-CELL PHARMACOKINETICS IN THE SETTING OF CENTRAL NERVOUS SYSTEM MALIGNANCIES

The kinetics of pharmacologic agents including cellular therapies likely influence their antitumor activity and associated toxicities. Therefore, an understanding of CAR T-cell kinetics is essential for their safe and effective clinical application. The pharmacokinetics of CAR T-cell therapies are governed by unique rules that differ from those governing more traditional molecular or biologic drugs. After being infused, CAR T-cells are expected to traffic to the tumor site, bind their target antigen, and undergo CAR-mediated activation and proliferation. Furthermore, T-cells must maintain CAR transgene expression and the ability to acquire/exert effector functions. Thus, a multitude of factors determine the kinetics of these novel cell-based therapies, including the following:

i. CAR design: number[33,34,162,163]/nature[19] of costimulatory domains utilized, tonic signaling,[30,164] CAR avidity to target antigen.

ii. T-cell product: T-cell phenotype,[165,166] ex vivo manipulation.[36]

iii. Other treatments: preinfusion lymphodepletion,[167] combinatorial therapies including immune checkpoint inhibition.[168]

iv. Dose: number of infused CAR T-cells.[169]

v. Route of administration.[28,31–33]

vi. Disease-related factors: tumor site/accessibility, disease burden,[162] immunosuppression (systemic and within TME), and target antigen expression level.

The most valuable information regarding the in vivo kinetics of CAR T-cells is derived from correlative studies conducted as part of early clinical trials. Most of these studies tracked CAR T-cells with quantitative polymerase chain reaction (qPCR) and/or flow cytometry. qPCR is more sensitive, but flow cytometry confirms CAR protein expression on the cell surface. A recent analysis of anti-CD19 CAR T-cells in trials targeting pediatric and adult acute lymphoblastic leukemia (ALL) and chronic lymphocytic leukemia (CLL) demonstrated greater expansion in responding patients.[170] A similar phenomenon was seen in patients with multiple myeloma treated with anti-BCMA CAR T-cells.[169] In patients with CLL, complete or partial responders also appeared to have longer CAR T-cell persistence compared with nonresponders.[170]

In terms of CAR T-cell design, one recent study involving the simultaneous infusion of second-generation (carrying the CD28 costimulatory domain) and third-generation (carrying the CD28 and 4-1BB costimulatory domains) anti-CD19 CAR T-cells to patients with non-Hodgkin's lymphoma suggested that third-generation CAR T-cells may offer an advantage in patients with low disease burden.[162] These factors are also likely to be important determinants of CAR T-cell kinetics and clinical responses in patients with solid tumors.

Other factors, including the route of administration, accessibility to the tumor site, and systemic/local immunosuppression, are likely to represent additional barriers to achieving optimal CAR T-cell kinetics in the setting of solid malignancies and particularly CNS malignancies. Experience to date in clinical trials targeting GBM has demonstrated limited expansion and persistence of second-generation CAR T-cells, reinforcing the unique challenges facing immunotherapies for these tumors. Nevertheless, important observations related to CAR T-cell kinetics can be gleaned from these early trials.

The three trials reported so far, coupled with preclinical studies, demonstrate that intracranial administration may offer improved bioavailability and facilitate the use of lower doses of CAR T-cells compared with intravenous administration[28,31,33] (Table 12.1). Moreover, in the patient treated by Brown et al., intraventricular administration of CAR T-cells resulted in regression of multiple lesions, including a distant spinal metastatic lesion, suggesting that it may enable better trafficking of CAR T-cells within the CNS compared with intracavitary delivery, which resulted only in stabilization of the local lesion at the site of delivery. In this patient, CAR T-cell levels in the CSF generally peaked at day 1 or 2 postinfusion, declined rapidly after that, and were detectable at a maximum of 7 days following intraventricular infusion.[33] These results highlight the limited expansion and persistence of CAR T-cells in the CSF following local delivery. It should be noted, however, that the concomitant administration of dexamethasone in this patient may have contributed to the limited expansion and persistence of the infused T-cells. Importantly, whether long-term immune responses can be elicited in the unique immune environment of the CNS following intracranial administration of CAR T-cells remains unknown.

CAR T-cell kinetics following systemic delivery also demonstrated limited expansion. Anti-HER-2 CAR VSTs carrying a CD28 costimulatory domain peaked at 3 hours postinfusion in 15 of 17 patients treated, implying a failure to expand. In the other two patients treated in this trial, T-cells peaked between 1 and 2 weeks.[31] Anti-EGFRvIII CAR T-cells carrying the 4-1BB costimulatory domain demonstrated slightly better expansion, with peak levels noted at 1−2 weeks postinfusion in all 10 patients treated.[32] However, peak levels were lower than those observed with anti-CD19 CAR T-cells carrying a similar second-generation 4-1BBζ CAR delivered via lentiviral vector transduction. This disparity may reflect the limited antigen exposure of CAR T-cells in the peripheral blood of patients with CNS malignancies and/or increased trafficking to the tumor site. However, the latter is unlikely to play a major role in limiting peripheral expansion, especially since TCR repertoire analysis revealed that only a minority (<5%) of T-cells detectable in the anti-EGFRvIII CAR T-cell product was also detectable at the tumor site even when biopsies were obtained within 2 weeks after infusion. Furthermore, EGFRvIII CAR T-cells were undetectable by day 30 postinfusion.[32] In contrast, HER2 CAR VSTs were detectable for longer periods, up to 6 weeks postinfusion in 7 of 15 patients tested (46%). Levels of detectable CAR VSTs gradually declined thereafter, with only two of six patients (33%) showing detectable levels at 12 months with repeat infusions.[31] Of note, in the trial conducted by Ahmed et al., the administration of multiple doses of CAR VSTs appeared to partly offset the cells' limited expansion and persistence.

Valuable insight into CAR T-cell trafficking to the CNS and kinetics at the tumor site was afforded by postinfusion surgical resection in 7 of 10 patients treated by O'Rourke and colleagues. Four of these seven patients underwent resection within 2 weeks postinfusion, and CAR T-cells were detectable in the tumor tissue from all four patients. In contrast, CAR T-cells were detectable (by qPCR but not IHC) in only one of three patients who underwent resection at later time points. Moreover, Ki67 IHC staining in postinfusion tumor biopsies showed evidence of local CAR T-cell proliferation at the tumor site.[32]

Aside from the administration of multiple CAR T-cell doses, other strategies may be used to improve CAR T-cell engraftment, expansion, and persistence. Combining CAR T-cell therapy with other strategies that block immune checkpoints like programmed cell death-1 (PD-1) may also improve the kinetics and antitumor activity of CAR T-cells.[171,172] Co-opting homeostatic cytokine signaling, such as that of IL-15[173] or IL-7,[174] may also have a favorable effect on CAR T-cell kinetics.

Furthermore, the use of lymphodepleting chemotherapy improved the persistence and antitumor activity of adoptively transferred T-cells in TIL-based immunotherapy trials,[175] as well as in CAR T-cell–based therapies targeting hematologic malignancies.[176] Additionally, a preinfusion lymphodepleting chemotherapeutic regimen resulted in improved CAR T-cell expansion and encouraging objective clinical responses in patients with advanced sarcoma[167] and neuroblastoma,[177] although the latter trial also utilized a PD-1 blocking antibody. For CNS malignancies, lymphodepletion with total body irradiation (TBI)[106] or TMZ[178] prior to anti-EGFRvIII CAR T-cell infusion resulted in improved antitumor activity and longer survival in an immune-competent mouse model of GBM. None of the published clinical trials targeting CNS malignancies utilized lymphodepleting chemotherapy prior to CAR T-cell infusion. Following encouraging results in preclinical models of GBM that utilized preinfusion lymphodepleting regimens,[106,178] results from ongoing clinical trials of CAR T-cell–based therapies (Table 12.2) are awaited to evaluate the effect of preinfusion chemotherapeutic regimens on cellular kinetics and clinical responses in patients with CNS malignancies. Lymphodepletion is thought to facilitate CAR T-cell engraftment and subsequent persistence and expansion through multiple mechanisms, including the elimination of endogenous nonmodified T-cells that may compete with the infused CAR T-cells for the limited supply of γ-chain cytokines (such as IL-7, IL-15, and IL-21), elimination of T_{regs}, and activation of antigen-presenting cells at the tumor site following tumor cell death.[179] Lymphodepleting chemotherapeutic regimens may also facilitate the translocation of gut microflora, resulting in the induction of cytokine production that can support T-cell expansion.[180]

Of note, vigilant monitoring for adverse events is warranted whenever novel strategies aimed at improving CAR T-cell kinetics are tested, especially in patients with high disease burden. In the patient treated by Brown and colleagues, adverse events appeared to correlate with the peak of inflammatory cytokines in CSF. Therefore, particular attention should be paid for possible localized CRS within the CNS, as well as for neurological side effects that may result from local inflammation induced by the activated and expanding CAR T-cells within the limited intracranial space as seen in early clinical trials (Table 12.1).

BRAIN TUMOR MICROENVIRONMENT AND CHIMERIC ANTIGEN RECEPTOR T-CELL FUNCTION

The TME of malignant brain tumors such as GBM consists of a heterogeneous population of cells including immune cells, endothelial cells, and tissue-resident cells such as glial and neuronal cells.[14] Through complex cross-talk with these cell populations, malignant cells are able to create a highly immune-suppressive microenvironment that supports their growth and facilitates immune evasion. Thus, mechanisms that normally regulate T-cell activity and limit immune-mediated damage to local tissues are co-opted by the TME of solid malignancies and can inhibit endogenous and engineered tumor-specific T-cells such as CAR T-cells. These mechanisms may also cause T-cells to enter a dysfunctional state that hampers cell-mediated immune responses against the tumor (reviewed in Ref. 56).

T-cell dysfunction in cancer is thought to involve a broad spectrum of states characterized by the progressive loss of proliferative capacity, effector function, and memory potential (reviewed in Ref. 55). These states share some transcriptional and molecular features with exhausted (studied in animal models of chronic viral infection) and self-tolerant T-cells and appear to be driven primarily by persistent antigen stimulation. However, they also exhibit unique characteristics that may be influenced by the immune-suppressive TME. Importantly, this process of T-cell dysfunction is thought to begin early during tumorigenesis and is associated with progressive metabolic and epigenetic changes.[181–184] Cancer-induced T-cell dysfunction may partly explain the observation that tumors can progress despite the presence of detectable tumor-specific T-cells that target antigens expressed by malignant cells.[185] Similar to endogenous and vaccine-induced tumor-reactive TILs, genetically engineered CAR T-cells infiltrating tumors are likely to be susceptible to the local immune-suppressive mechanisms at the TME. Indeed, tumor-infiltrating CAR T-cells have been shown to become functionally impaired in a mouse model of mesothelioma, and this effect was reversible by culturing the tumor-infiltrating CAR T-cells in fresh culture medium ex vivo.[60]

To begin with, both malignant cells and immune cells recruited to the TME express inhibitory ligands that engage their cognate receptors on T-cells. Inhibitory cytokines are also released by various cell types in the TME, including T_{regs} and myeloid cells such as tumor-associated macrophages (TAMs) and myeloid-derived suppressor cells (MDSCs). Furthermore, the high metabolic activity of malignant cells depletes nutrients that are essential for proper T-cell function. TAMs/MDSCs can secrete enzymes, like IDO-1, that contribute to local nutrient depletion. Various products of metabolic pathways can also have direct immune-suppressive effects. In addition to that, physical barriers imposed by the local stroma and necrotic tissue as well as the BBB can further limit T-cell access to CNS malignancies and modulate their activity. Furthermore, the chronic antigen stimulation of CAR T-cells can lead to T-cell dysfunction/exhaustion, leading to a state similar to that seen after chronic antigen stimulation through TCRs in cancer models.[182] This results in a distinct transcriptional profile[186,187] as well as metabolic[181] and epigenetic changes that may not be readily reversible by immune checkpoint blockade.[188] In this section, we discuss in more detail the mechanisms by which various factors in the TME of CNS malignancies can hinder CAR T cell-based immunotherapies. We also discuss emerging approaches that are being utilized to counteract this TME-mediated inhibition.

Immune Checkpoints
Inhibition of T-cells by immune cells in the tumor microenvironment
Myeloid cells: tumor-associated macrophages and myeloid-derived suppressor cells. TAMs are a major component of high-grade gliomas in which they represent the most abundant immune cell type and may constitute up to 30% of the tumor mass,[189–191] and some studies have suggested that the degree of TAM infiltration may correlate with histologic grade and patient outcomes.[192] Multiple chemokines are involved in recruiting macrophages to the TME of high-grade gliomas including CCL2 and CSF-1.[189] Recently, osteopontin has also been implicated in TAM recruitment to the GBM microenvironment.[193] Once in the TME of high-grade gliomas, TAMs can be polarized toward an immune suppressive phenotype. This polarization is likely driven by multiple factors including hypoxia,[194] lactic acid,[195] IL-4,[196] CSF-1,[197] and periostin198.

TAMs and MDSCs also infiltrate other malignant brain tumors to varying degrees. For example, TAMs have been detected in various medulloblastoma subgroups and are more abundant in the Sonic Hedgehog (SHH) subgroup.[199] Multiple studies have also documented the accumulation of MDSCs in the peripheral blood of patients with GBM[200] as well as at the tumor site[201] where they can suppress T-cell function.

TAMs and MDSCs within the TME can exert important immune suppressive and protumoral effects through multiple mechanisms. They secrete growth factors that support glioma stem cell survival as well as abnormal angiogenesis.[189] They also secrete metalloproteases that may promote glioma invasiveness.[189] In addition to functioning as ineffective antigen-presenting cells,[202] TAMs and MDSCs can suppress endogenous as well as adoptively transferred, engineered T-cells by producing multiple suppressive cytokines that recruit and promote the differentiation of T_{regs} including IL-4, IL-10, and transforming growth factor β (TGF-β).[203] Furthermore, arginase-1 (Arg1) and indoleamine 2,3-deoxygenase (IDO) production by TAMs contribute to L-arginine and L-tryptophan/cysteine depletion, respectively, which can subsequently impair T-cell proliferation and function.[204–206] TAMs can also upregulate the expression of inhibitory ligands such as PD-L1/PD-L2 as well as B7-1/2 that bind inhibitory receptors on T-cells.[203] Blocking this interaction has been implicated as a major mechanism through which anti-PD-1/PD-L1 antibodies exert their therapeutic effect.[207,208] The upregulation of death ligands such as FasL can promote T-cell apoptosis by engaging their cognate receptors.[203,209]

The anti-GBM activity seen in preclinical models following treatment with therapies that repolarize or deplete TAMs/MDSCs, for example using CSF1R inhibition, highlights the role of these cells in tumor growth and immune evasion.[197,210] Although a phase 2 clinical trial of a small molecule inhibitor of CSF1R and KIT (PLX3397) did not result in objective responses in patients with GBM,[211] PLX3397 is being evaluated in combination with temozolamide in an ongoing phase 2 trial (NCT01349036). Moreover, preclinical studies have suggested a possible role for the PI3K pathway in mediating resistance to CSF1R inhibition.[210] Synergistic effects of targeting TAMs/MDSCs in combination with other immune therapies are also being actively investigated in preclinical models of CNS tumors including GBM.[212,213]

It has been postulated that targeting immune suppressive myeloid cells may improve CAR T-cell therapies. A recent study tested nanoparticles loaded with an MDSC antagonist and a natural killer T-cell (NKT) agonist to modulate the TME prior to CAR T-cell infusion in a genetically engineered immune-competent mouse model of human GBM. In this model, a second-generation CAR with a CD28 signaling endodomain was tested. Adjuvant therapy with TME-modulating nanoparticles lead to a 12-fold increase in CAR T-cell expansion at the tumor site compared with CAR T-cell infusion alone, improving tumor control and increasing the overall survival in dual-treated mice. Similar results were also obtained in a breast cancer mouse model.[214] Other studies used different strategies to target MDSCs in combination with CAR T-cell therapies directed against non-CNS solid malignancies in mouse models.[215,216] These interventions lead to reductions in intratumoral MDSCs and improved antitumor activity.

Regulatory T-cells. Regulatory T-cells (T_{regs}) are present in the TME of multiple CNS malignancies including malignant gliomas and medulloblastoma,[217,218] and T_{reg} accumulation in malignant gliomas appears to correlate with their WHO grade.[219,220] Furthermore, in the clinical trial conducted by O'Rourke et al., tumor biopsies obtained after CAR T-cell infusion showed a notable increase in T_{reg} infiltration,[32] which can potentially dampen the antitumor effects of the infused CAR T-cells.

T_{regs} can be recruited to the TME of brain tumors by multiple chemokines including CCL2 produced by glioma cells and TAMs[221], and multiple factors within the TME can promote T_{reg} differentiation including IL10 and TGF-β.[222] IDO activity within the TME also leads to tryptophan depletion and kynurenine production, both of which can increase T_{reg} recruitment and activation.[48,223]

In turn, T_{regs} can exert direct immune-suppressive effects that can limit CAR T-cell function.[224,225] They secrete multiple inhibitory cytokines including IL-10 and TGF-β and consume important proliferative and homeostatic cytokines in the local microenvironment. They also express CD73 and CD39, which are surface-expressed molecules with enzymatic activities that convert ATP to adenosine. The latter can suppress effector T-cells by binding the adenosine A2 receptor (A_2AR), and blocking this interaction enhanced the antitumor activity of CAR T-cells in a breast cancer mouse model.[226] T_{regs} also express multiple inhibitory receptors including CTLA-4 and LAG-3, which can block the maturation of dendritic cells and limit their capacity for antigen presentation.[224] Although CAR T-cells bypass the need for antigen presentation, these defects impair endogenous T-cell responses and may limit epitope spreading. Importantly, the depletion of tumor-infiltrating T_{regs} has been shown to improve control of multiple established solid tumors in animal models.[227] In light of the above, it would be interesting

to test if combining CAR T-cells with T_{reg}-targeting therapies can improve outcomes in patients with CNS malignancies.

Inhibition of T-cells by nonimmune cells in the tumor microenvironment

Non-immune cells present in the TME of malignant brain tumors can also exert direct or indirect immune-suppressive effects on T-cells. Tumor cells express inhibitory ligands such as PD-L1/PD-L2 that can be upregulated by interferon gamma (IFNγ) and can engage their cognate inhibitory receptors on CAR T-cells.[228] Moreover, tumor cells are key players in building up an immune suppressive microenvironment through the production of inhibitory cytokines and chemokines that recruit regulatory immune cells.[229] In addition to representing an essential component of the BBB that can limit cellular trafficking and drug delivery to CNS malignancies, endothelial cells can also secrete multiple factors that can support the glioma stem cell population and/or recruit other cells such as TAMs to the TME.[14,193]

Metabolic Checkpoints

It is increasingly recognized that T-cells have different metabolic demands and dependencies that are tailored to their differentiation state and function. For example, naïve T-cells (T_N) are mainly quiescent and depend on fatty acid oxidation (FAO) and oxidative phosphorylation (OXPHOS) to meet their relatively limited metabolic and ATP demands in this resting state. Upon encountering their cognate antigen, T_N cells become activated and undergo multiple rounds of proliferation and differentiate into effector cells. To meet the bioenergetic demands of this phase, activated T-cells undergo profound metabolic changes including the upregulation of glucose uptake, aerobic glycolysis, and anabolic pathways. The upregulation of glycolysis may be essential for optimal T-cell effector function as the engagement of GAPDH relieves its posttranscriptional inhibition of IFNγ production[230] and provides reducing intermediates (NADH, NADPH) as well as substrates for the production of nucleotides (through the pentose phosphate pathway), which are essential for the anabolic metabolism of activated T-cells. During this phase, T-cells differentiate and progressively acquire various effector or memory functions that are influenced primarily by the costimulatory signals and cytokines present in the surrounding milieu.

Upon elimination of their target, effector T-cells rapidly die, and a small memory population persists.

These memory T-cells are largely dependent on lipid-based metabolism (involving a seemingly "futile" cycle of fatty acid synthesis from extracellular glucose followed by FAO) and OXPHOS that is supported by a high mitochondrial mass.[231] OXPHOS not only supports the long-term survival of memory T-cells by utilizing "less efficient" metabolites for energy production but also facilitates the rapid recall responses when these cells re-encounter their cognate antigen.[232] Moreover, memory T-cells retain the capacity to rapidly upregulate aerobic glycolysis to meet the metabolic demands during rapid recall responses.[233,234]

Thus, tumor-specific T-cells that encounter their target antigen in the TME and undergo rapid activation require an adequate supply of nutrients and ATP to meet their metabolic demands. However, the solid TME features multiple hostile metabolic conditions including nutrient depletion and the accumulation of toxic/suppressive metabolites that can profoundly limit the activation of endogenous TILs as well as engineered CAR T-cells that infiltrate solid tumors. Additionally, cellular machinery needed to utilize some metabolites may be repressed in dysfunctional TILs.[235] Chronic antigen stimulation may also lead to metabolic changes that alter the metabolic dependencies of T-cells and contribute to T-cell dysfunction.[181] In this section, we highlight the key metabolic challenges that face CAR T-cells in the TME of CNS tumors.

Nutrient depletion

Glucose and amino acid depletion. Rapidly proliferating malignant cells undergo profound metabolic reprogramming to meet their high metabolic demands. The subsequent consumption of nutrients locally in the microenvironment of solid tumors can often result in their depletion. In particular, malignant cells preferentially use glycolysis (rather than the more efficient OXPHOS) as their primary source of energy even in the presence of oxygen (a phenomenon known as the Warburg effect). They also upregulate various anabolic pathways to support their dysregulated proliferation.[236,237] Thus, they consume local nutrient supplies and outcompete other cells in the TME for glucose, amino acids,[238] and fatty acids[239] (glioma metabolism is reviewed in Refs 237,240). Enzymes secreted by tumor cells and TAMs/MDSCs, which are prominent in the TME of high-grade gliomas, can further contribute to nutrient depletion. For example, inducible nitric oxide synthase and arginase metabolize arginine,[241] whereas IDO converts tryptophan to kynurenines.[48] Thus, tumor-infiltrating T-cells face fierce competition over various nutrients including glucose, amino acids

(such as glutamine, arginine and tryptophan), and fatty acids, which are required for optimal effector T-cell function and proliferation as well as memory T-cell rapid recall responses.

A harsh metabolic environment depleted of multiple metabolites can impair T-cell activation, proliferation, and effector function. For example, glucose depletion can decrease phosphoenolpyruvate production and subsequently impair Ca^{2+}-NFAT signaling in T-cells. This impaired signaling reduced the anti-tumor activity of TILs in a melanoma mouse model.[242] Decreased L-arginine uptake and intracellular levels can also negatively affect T-cell survival, whereas complete depletion of L-arginine from culture medium impairs T-cell proliferation.[243] Similarly, glutamine depletion in culture medium leads to decreased T-cell proliferation and effector cytokine production.[244] In contrast, high intracellular arginine levels promote oxidative phosphorylation in T-cells and their differentiation into central memory-like T-cells. This improved T-cell-mediated anti-tumor activity in a melanoma mouse model.[204]

Manipulating the metabolic machinery of T-cells through gene editing/gene transfer techniques may allow them to overcome some of the metabolic challenges in the TME. For example, PKC1 overexpression can increase phosphoenolpyruvate production and improve T-cell effector functions. Similar strategies may be used to alter the metabolic fitness of CAR T-cells and improve their antitumor activity within the TME.

Fatty acid metabolism and mitochondrial dysfunction. Malignant cells also compete for fatty acids in the TME. For example, GBM cells have been found to upregulate fatty acid uptake under hypoxic conditions, and lipid stored in these cells may help protect them against reactive oxygen species (ROS) during hypoxia-reoxygenation events.[239] Reduced fatty acid availability in the glucose-depleted TME may adversely affect less differentiated T-cell populations (such as naïve and central memory T-cells [T_{CM}]).[245] Memory T-cells also appear to be highly dependent on fatty acid metabolism and mitochondrial function,[231] and disturbances in these pathways may adversely affect endogenously and possibly engineered T-cell–mediated antitumor responses. TILs have been found to have a reduced mitochondrial mass and a decreased capacity for oxidative phosphorylation compared with peripheral blood T-cells. In a melanoma mouse model, PGC1α overexpression improved mitochondrial function and tumor control by adoptively transferred tumor-reactive T-cells.[246] In another study utilizing a mouse model of chronic viral infection, the modulation of the mTORC2 pathway enhanced memory differentiation of T-cells and improved their recall responses.[247] These cells were found to have a higher capacity for mitochondrial oxidative phosphorylation and increased FAO. Strategies aimed at improving oxidative phosphorylation and mitochondrial metabolism in CAR T-cells may also enhance the efficacy and durability of their antitumor activity.

Hypoxia. Hypoxia affects T-cells directly and indirectly through its effects on other cells in the TME. As outlined in Regulatory T-cells section, hypoxia upregulates CD39 and CD73 expression in various cells in the TME and thereby increases adenosine-mediated T-cell inhibition. Furthermore, hypoxia-mediated upregulation of PD-L1 on tumor cells and MDSCs[248,249] can suppress T-cells by engaging the PD-1 receptors on their surface. Lactic acid production also increases under hypoxic conditions and can further suppress T-cells. On the other hand, the direct effects of hypoxia on T-cells appear to depend on the T-cell phenotype. Although naïve (T_N) and central memory T-cells (T_{CM}) are inhibited under hypoxic conditions, effector memory (T_{EM}) and terminal effector T-cells (T_{TE}) exhibit enhanced proliferation and effector function.[250,251] Interestingly, when CAR T-cells were cocultured with tumor cells, they showed improved cytotoxic activity under hypoxic conditions.[250] However, in in vivo tumor models, the reduced T-cell infiltration and survival in hypoxic tumor areas may outweigh any enhancement in T-cell effector functions.[194] In this case, the overall effect of hypoxia on TME is likely to be detrimental to endogenous and/or engineered T-cell–mediated immune responses. This is supported by recent studies in which the modulation of the hypoxic TME improved T-cell infiltration and the antitumor activity when combined with immune checkpoint inhibition.[252,253] Whether such an intervention can improve CAR T-cell function against solid malignancies remains to be answered.

Metabolic by-products
Acidosis and lactate. Malignant cells and activated CAR T-cells can produce lactate and, thereby, increase the acidity of the TME. Lactate can directly impair T-cell activation by decreasing NFAT signaling and decreasing IFNγ production.[254] Furthermore, lactate has been shown to inhibit T-cell motility as well as CD8+ T-cell cytotoxic activity.[255] Additionally, lactate

can indirectly contribute to T-cell dysfunction within the TME by promoting TAM differentiation toward a more immune-suppressive (M2) phenotype as well as upregulating arginase expression.[195]

Potassium. Cell death in the TME leads to the release of potassium ions and increases the extracellular potassium concentration, which subsequently results in an increase in the intracellular concentration of potassium in T-cells and leads to protein phosphatase 2A–mediated (PP2A) inhibition of the Akt-mTOR pathway.[256] Of note, overexpression of the Kv1.3 potassium channel (which is involved in potassium efflux) in tumor-specific T-cells resulted in improved tumor control in vivo in a melanoma mouse model.[256] In contrast, inhibition of the Kv1.3 channel can impair T-cell function.[257] Future studies should elucidate whether the modulation of intracellular potassium concentration in CAR T-cells can enhance their activity against solid malignancies.

Adenosine. Necrotic and apoptotic cells in the TME release ATP into the extracellular environment where it is converted to AMP by CD39 endonucleotidase activity. CD73 endonucleotidase activity subsequently converts AMP into adenosine. Both CD39 and CD73 are expressed on tumor cells as well as T_{regs} and endothelial cells and can be upregulated by hypoxia through a HIF1α-mediated mechanism (reviewed in Ref. 258). Furthermore, CD73 upregulation has been associated with a worse prognosis in patients with GBM.[259] A2AR is the dominant adenosine receptor on T-cells, and its ligation leads to increased intracellular cAMP concentration, which activates PKA and inhibits proximal TCR signaling by activating Csk[260] and results in decreased production of effector cytokines, particularly IL-2.[261] Furthermore, cAMP can block IL2 signaling via p27kip1 activation.[262,263] Notably, A2AR knockout in CAR T-cells resulted in increased effector cytokine production and improved antitumor activity in a mouse model of triple-negative breast cancer.[226]

Indoleamine-2,3-dioxygenase: tryptophan depletion and kynurenine production
IDO is an IFNγ-inducible enzyme that metabolizes tryptophan into kynurenine and downstream metabolites. The resultant tryptophan depletion activates GCN2, which can impair T-cell proliferation and promote CD4+ T-cell differentiation into T_{regs}.[48] Kynurenine and its downstream products can also directly inhibit T-cell proliferation[264] and promote T_{reg} differentiation. Notably, patient-derived GBM cells have been

found to express IDO, and high IDO mRNA expression levels have been associated with poor prognosis.[223,265]

Moreover, combinatorial IDO and dual immune checkpoint blockade (PD-1 and CTLA-4) resulted in improved tumor control in a GBM mouse model.[266] Thus, IDO expression in brain tumors including GBM may be upregulated in response to CAR T-cell activation (and subsequent IFNγ secretion) as noted in the trial conducted by O'Rourke and colleagues and may attenuate CAR T-cell activity.[32] Interestingly, IDO inhibition using 1-methyl-tryptophan improved antitumor activity of CAR T-cells in a lymphoma mouse model.[205] Therefore, combining IDO targeting with CAR T-cell therapy may improve their anti-tumor activity in the setting of CNS malignancies.

RATIONAL ENGINEERING OF CHIMERIC ANTIGEN RECEPTOR MOLECULES

In 1859, George Bissell and Edwin Drake drilled a hole into the ground and in so doing established the first oil field that fueled a world already primed for the industrial revolution. Similarly, in 1993, Gideon "Gidi" Gross and Zelig Eshhar, published their story about a synthetic molecule that tapped into the evolutionary complexity of T-cells. This molecule, which later served as a prototype for CARs, allowed T-cells to recognize and mount an adaptable and amplifiable immune response against specific targets.[267] Their design exploited the versatility and customizability of the humoral immune system (the variable light and heavy chains) as well as the ability of the ζ-chain of the TCR to initiate the signaling cascades that lead to T-cell activation. Multiple scientists further improved the CAR design, most notably the Sadelain group,[268] culminating in FDA approval of CD19-targeting CAR T-cells for the treatment of refractory B-cell leukemia/lymphoma.

However, replicating the success of CAR T-cells in other malignancies, especially solid cancers, requires new approaches to tackle the challenges facing the field including the antigenic heterogeneity of solid malignancies and the paucity of tumor-specific surface molecules that are not expressed on normal tissues. Additional roadblocks include limited CAR T-cell expansion and persistence in vivo, as well as the suboptimal CAR T-cell trafficking to the tumor site and the multitude of suppressive mechanisms T-cells face within the TME. To overcome the myriad of obstacles faced by CAR T-cells in solid tumors, a rational approach to CAR design should be adopted. While the field is young, in this section, we share our

perspective on rational CAR engineering including design tools and technologies that could refine these chimeric molecules and incorporate various elements of the human immune system to overcome the complexities of difficult-to-cure brain tumors.

Target Molecules in Solid Cancers: The Case for Defining an Antigenic Profile

Primary tumors exhibit antigen expression patterns that vary intratumorally as well as across patients. In contrast to lymphoreticular malignancies, the variability in antigen expression between patients harboring the same histologic tumor type is substantial. Moreover, there is considerable spatial variability within individual tumor lesions and between different lesions in the same patient.

Under the stress of conventional or targeted therapies, solid tumors develop alternative tumor antigen expression patterns. *Antigen escape*, especially seen after targeted therapies, has been demonstrated in solid cancers[50–52] as well as in lymphoreticular malignancies (reviewed in Ref. 269). The tumor employs various mechanisms that result in the downregulation of the target antigen or its modification in a manner that allows them to evade the effects of the targeted therapy (reviewed in Ref. 62).

Conversely, tumor cell death induced by targeted therapies may result in the release of nontargeted antigens within an inflamed environment, which can promote the reinstatement, augmentation, or de novo induction of an immune response against non-targeted (neo)antigens. This phenomenon has been termed "antigen spreading" and represents a favorable occurrence that could be exploited to create more effective cellular immunotherapies.[270–272]

Thus, there may be no one ideal target molecule for a solid tumor. The de novo heterogeneity of solid cancers and their capacity to dynamically adapt under the selection pressure of various therapies call for adopting a broader definition of targetable antigenic profiles that more accurately reflect the complex antigenic landscape of solid tumors. This notion is further supported by the realization that both antigen escape and spreading can occur simultaneously during treatment, adding to the complexity of a dynamic antigenic profile. Tumor antigenic profiles can be defined using data from antigen expression patterns derived from treatment-naïve and treatment-resistant human cancers using high-dimensional technologies such as mass cytometry[273] and/or multiplexed ion beam imaging (MIBI).[274] Such profiles may fuel the development of more effective therapeutic strategies that take into account the heterogeneity and adaptability of the antigenic landscape of solid tumors and acknowledge the elusive nature of an ideal tumor-specific antigen.

Targeting Platforms and the Development of Chimeric Antigen Receptor Exodomains

The simple pooling of CAR T-cell products with different specificities offsets antigen escape. Pooled CAR T-cells better controlled tumors in preclinical models of GBM compared with CAR T-cells targeting a single antigen.[50] Grafting T-cells with multiple CAR molecules that have different specificities created bi- and trivalent CAR T-cells that exhibited more favorable additive activation dynamics, CAR immune synapse (CARIS) properties, and efficacy in preclinical models.[51,52]

Additionally, more sophisticated CAR T-cell products have been created (reviewed in Ref. 23). Some designs have used Boolean "or"[50] or "and"[275,276] logic in their operation to allow CAR T-cells to become fully activated when either one or both antigens are encountered on a target cell, respectively. Other CAR iterations utilize a Boolean "not" logic, whereby T-cells are activated only when one antigen is expressed on a target cell in the absence of a second antigen.[277] This approach is particularly useful to reduce on-target, off-tumor toxicities when a TAA is also expressed on normal tissues. Additionally, control switches can be included in CAR T-cell designs such that small molecules can be used to remotely control their activation/inactivation.

Tandem CAR molecules, which incorporate two different antigen recognition exodomains joined in tandem, have been described for solid[51] and, more recently, for resistant B lineage leukemia.[278] Clinical trials targeting leukemia using this approach are currently ongoing. These molecules broaden the repertoire of targetable tumors and may offer a synergistic advantage as evidenced by a burst-like increase in T-cell functionality when the two target antigens are encountered simultaneously. This synergy was attributed to the ability of tandem CARs to engage both target molecules simultaneously as revealed by subcellular CARIS imaging studies.[51] Interestingly, in silico modeling platforms, such as RosettaDock and FireDock, successfully predicted the functionality, or lack thereof, of these tandem CARs[51] and ought to be investigated more systematically to assess their utility as tools to guide the rational design of such complex molecules.

In conclusion, defining tumor antigen profiles will guide the design of multiplex CAR platforms that can efficiently target a broad repertoire of solid tumors

while mitigating antigen escape, reducing on-target off-tumor toxicities, and possibly taking advantage of the anticipated changes in antigen expression patterns.

The Devil Is in the Details: A Closer Look at Chimeric Antigen Receptor T-Cells

The formation and maturation of the CARIS upon encounter of its target antigen triggers a series of molecular events and signaling cascades that are thought to determine the efficacy of the antitumor (or cytotoxic) response. This burst of activity subsequently wanes, and the CARIS is disassembled, leading to the resolution of the encounter in a manner that is much less defined when compared with the TCR immune synapse. Studying the characteristics and dynamic changes associated with CARIS formation and dissolution at the subcellular level using techniques such as confocal microscopy[279] is intriguing. Indeed, an "imaging toolbox" has been described that allows the detailed examination of the CARIS dynamics including cytoskeletal rearrangements, microtubular organizing center polarization, and granule convergence/degranulation, which were previously described for NK cells. These processes can then be correlated to CAR T-cell functionality and antitumor activity.[51,279] Such efforts are still in their early stages but could represent significant tools that enable the refinement of CAR design by examining the effects of different modifications on the CARIS and CAR T-cell function. Thus, different exodomains with varying avidities to their target antigen, as well as various signaling endodomains, can be studied to better understand the mechanisms mediating their effects on the efficacy and durability of CAR T-cell antitumor activity.

The behavior of individual CAR T-cells is another major determinant of the performance of the bulk populations of CAR T-cells that are typically used therapeutically. Thus, sophisticated systems that assess the functionality of individual CAR T-cells can offer valuable insight into the quality of the CAR T-cell product and may be predictive of its antitumor function. For example, the time-lapse imaging microscopy in nanowell grids assay[280] allows for high-throughput evaluation of the dynamic interactions between fluorescent-labeled CAR T-cells and tumor cells that are coincubated in nanowells and imaged using time-lapse microscopy at a single-cell resolution. Assessment of the behavior of individual cells upon encounter of successive targets can give insight into their ability to function as "serial killers." Compilation of extensive data from tens of thousands of individual CAR T-cells can subsequently provide a candid assessment of the behaviors of various subsets constituting a CAR T-cell product. Such studies could guide the formulation of more efficacious cellular products in which individual T-cell subsets can be mixed in defined ratios.[281] Traditional bulk assays could then be designed and interpreted in conjunction with deeper assessments of the molecular, subcellular, and individual CAR T-cell characteristics as described earlier. Assessing CAR T-cell products systematically using such a "pipeline" of tests can help propel the field toward the rational design of CARs and CAR T-cells as opposed to empiric development of these highly promising therapeutic agents. This may, in turn, allow for more refined preclinical studies that would better reflect the performance of novel CAR T-cell products in the clinic.

Concluding Remarks on the Rational Design of Chimeric Antigen Receptor Molecules

The promising clinical development of CAR molecules for B precursor leukemia has demonstrated the massive potential of immunotherapy. Going forward, the ongoing characterization of the specific obstacles encountered in solid cancers, such as brain tumors, mandates a rational approach to the design and development of more advanced and effective CAR T-cell products. Thus, increasing our understanding of CARs is necessary for the development of molecules that can effectively redirect the immune system to target solid cancers. This line of research will require deep and high-throughput assays to answer complex basic, yet clinically relevant, questions. Efforts that incorporate multidisciplinary teams of biologists and bioinformaticians will be needed to develop new scientific concepts in the CAR field and refine more obsolete concepts.

DESIGNING CHIMERIC ANTIGEN RECEPTOR T-CELL CLINICAL TRIALS TARGETING CENTRAL NERVOUS SYSTEM MALIGNANCIES AND COMBINATORIAL THERAPIES

Early clinical trials of CAR T-cells directed against CNS malignancies have provided valuable evidence that CAR T-cells targeting carefully chosen, preclinically tested TAAs could induce clinically measurable antitumor responses. However, multiple barriers that can limit the activity of these novel cell-based therapies/tumor-reactive T-cells have been identified as well. To begin with, CAR T-cell trafficking to the tumor site and accessibility to malignant cells may be particularly limited in CNS malignancies. Moreover, CAR T-

cells infused without prior lymphodepletion in patients with solid malignancies have exhibited limited expansion and persistence. Tumor antigen heterogeneity and the risk of antigen escape, which have been documented in prior trials targeting B-cell malignancies and preclinical models of solid tumors, also warrant particular attention. Thus, the design of future clinical trial protocols should aim to address these unanswered questions to help advance the field and improve patient outcomes. In this section, we will propose a rational "blueprint" that may guide future phase 1/2 clinical trials of CAR T-cells targeting CNS malignancies.

Designing Chimeric Antigen Receptor T-Cell Clinical Trials Targeting Central Nervous System Malignancies

Various study designs can be employed in phase 1 trials where the primary objective traditionally involves the determination of the maximum tolerated dose. Model-based methods, such as the modified continual reassessment method (modified CRM), have been favored in recent years as they may reduce the risk of exposure to potentially toxic doses while allowing more accurate estimation of the maximum tolerated dose. They can also increase the number of patients treated with a therapeutic dose when compared with more conventional $3 + 3$ study design.[282,283] Such models allow investigators to start treating the first cohort of patients at the lowest safe dose level that may be predicted based on data obtained from animal models or prior clinical trials. Subsequent cohorts can then be treated at higher dose levels that are determined using data obtained from all previously treated patients with the aim of not exceeding the target rate of DLTs. Thus, the dose-toxicity model needs to be continuously updated by a statistician throughout the trial.[282]

A careful and streamlined patient selection process using prespecified inclusion criteria is critical for the success of clinical trials. Given the targeted nature of CAR T cell-based therapies and the limited access to tissue from CNS tumors, expression of the target antigen(s) on biopsied/resected tumor tissue at targetable levels should be evaluated using previously validated assays. For this purpose, protein-based assays would be preferred over RNA-based assays whenever available. Patients who test positive for the target antigen(s) would be eligible for collection of PBMCs (typically by apheresis) and initiation of the CAR T-cell manufacturing process if they meet the other inclusion criteria. These criteria typically include an acceptable performance status (evaluated using the Karnofsky/

Lansky score), adequate organ function, and a life expectancy that allows for adequate safety assessment (in addition to assessment of secondary endpoints) at the time of initiation of CAR T-cell infusion(s). A washout period of 4 weeks is also often employed prior to protocol initiation.

Patients for whom autologous CAR T-cell products are successfully manufactured can then undergo a baseline evaluation (including a brain MRI) before initiating CAR T-cell therapy. The CAR T-cell product is then infused at a prespecified dose as soon as possible after the diagnosis of recurrent disease. The remainder of the T-cell product can be kept in storage to be administered if the patient is eligible for repeat dosing.

Given the limited CAR T-cell expansion and survival especially in patients with solid malignancies to date, the administration of multiple CAR T-cell doses and/or the use of preinfusion lymphodepleting regimens should be considered (see Section Chimeric Antigen Receptor T-Cell Pharmacokinetics in the Setting of Central Nervous System Malignancies). The former may be facilitated by using a dose escalation study design or the continual reassessment method that would allow for the administration of multiple CAR T-cell infusions at the maximum tolerated dose.[31,283]

The administration of CAR T-cells soon after surgical resection may offer a valuable window of opportunity to treat patients in the setting of a relatively limited disease burden. Disease burden has been proposed as a critical factor in determining the efficacy of CAR T-cell therapies directed against hematological malignancies[22] and may similarly be important in the setting of solid malignancies. Moreover, surgical resection after CAR T-cell administration should be allowed if clinically indicated. Correlative studies performed on the resected tumor tissue may provide valuable insight into the CAR T-cell trafficking and kinetics as well as the dynamic effects of CAR T-cell activity on the local TME and target antigen expression levels.[32]

Another key aspect of clinical trial design is the determination of primary and secondary outcomes/endpoints. The primary outcome of phase 1 clinical trials typically involves the determination of the toxicity profile of the tested therapeutic agent and the maximum tolerated dose. Thus, treated patients should be monitored at regular intervals for possible adverse events including any signs of CRS (systemic or localized to the CNS), increased ICP, or neurological manifestations (such as focal neurological deficits or seizures; Table 12.1), which may warrant intervention with steroids or anti-IL6/anti-IL1 therapies.[284,285] Secondary outcomes of phase 1 trials have increasingly included measures of efficacy and/or drug pharmacokinetics and

pharmacodynamics to guide future phase 2 trials, as well as accelerate early drug development. Thus, clinically significant efficacy endpoints, such as progression-free survival and overall survival, are also increasingly included as secondary outcomes.

The evaluation of the tumor response to therapy in published CAR T-cell trials targeting GBM has typically included repeat imaging studies such as a brain MRI at 6 weeks post-CAR T-cell infusion. However, the interpretation of these studies can be complicated by the phenomenon of "pseudoprogression" in which a transient increase in tumor enhancement is seen on initial assessment that is not confirmed as tumor progression on subsequent evaluations.[45] One possible explanation for this phenomenon is CAR T-cell–induced inflammation at the tumor site. Therefore, T2-weighted/fluid-attenuated inversion recovery MRI sequences to measure the nonenhancing volume of tumors may be a more accurate way to evaluate responses in high-grade gliomas.[63] Repeat imaging to confirm radiographic progression also may more accurately assess tumor response to therapy especially when patients are clinically stable.[45]

In addition to evaluating tumor responses, noninvasive imaging modalities are being developed to facilitate monitoring of CAR T-cell kinetics and trafficking in patients.[57,58] Correlative studies performed on peripheral blood, CSF, and resected tumor tissue (if available) should also be included in the study design to evaluate CAR T-cell kinetics as well as possible mechanisms of resistance that may be triggered by CAR T-cell activity. Tumor tissue may be evaluated to determine the dynamics of target antigen expression levels and/or immune-regulatory mechanisms that may limit CAR T-cell activity as seen in prior trials.[32] Correlative studies should also monitor the endogenous humoral and cellular immune compartments for any evidence of antigen-spreading and antitumor immune responses that may be triggered by CAR T-cell activity.[286] Furthermore, analyses aimed at identifying biomarkers predictive of response and resistance should be conducted.[31] Quality of life assessments following treatment with CAR T-cells may also be warranted, given the detrimental neurological/cognitive consequences of CNS malignancies and conventional therapies.

Phase 1 clinical trials can be used to answer other important questions, including whether the choice of costimulatory endodomain(s) in second- or third-generation CAR T-cells can influence outcomes in patients with CNS malignancies. These questions may be addressed by trials designed with multiple parallel arms to test different CAR T-cell designs or combinations.[287] A recent study in patients with B-cell lymphoma in which second- and third-generation CAR T-cells were co-administered suggested that the latter may be advantageous in patients with lower disease burden.[162] A crossover study design involving interim analyses may also be used to evaluate other aspects of CAR T-cell therapies including routes of administration of the T-cells. Additionally, ongoing clinical trials are evaluating the use of lymphodepleting chemotherapeutic regimens to enhance CAR T-cell expansion and persistence (see Section Chimeric Antigen Receptor T-Cells for Central Nervous System Malignancies: Successes and Obstacles).

As more evidence accumulates on the safety and efficacy of CAR T-cell therapies directed against CNS and other solid malignancies, these cells may be used as first- or second-line treatment for aggressive tumors such as GBM for which there are no effective conventional therapies available. Such a strategy would facilitate the early collection of PBMCs, which can potentially improve the quality of the CAR T-cell product by limiting the T-cell dysfunction seen in patients with advanced malignancies including GBM[56,288,289] as well as in heavily pre-treated patients who typically receive multiple cycles of cytotoxic therapies.[31,54]

Combinatorial Therapies: Aiding Chimeric Antigen Receptor T-Cells to Improve Clinical Responses

CAR T-cells may be combined with other therapeutic modalities that may have synergistic effects or block adaptive resistance mechanisms that limit the antitumor activity of T-cells. Rational combination strategies that yield encouraging results in well-designed preclinical studies should also be tested in early phase 1 clinical trials. In the following text, we highlight promising CAR T-cell–based combinatorial strategies for the treatment of CNS malignancies.

Combining established chemotherapy/radiotherapy regimens with CAR T-cells is particularly feasible. Radiation therapy can also have immunomodulatory effects within the TME[290] and has led to improved outcomes in preclinical models of GBM when combined with immune checkpoint inhibition[291] or CAR T-cells.[292] In the latter study, radiation therapy improved CAR T-cell trafficking to the tumor site. A recent study also suggested that exposure of pancreatic tumor cell lines to radiotherapy may sensitize them to TRAIL-mediated killing by CAR T-cells in a target antigen-independent manner.[293] Moreover, radiotherapy may upregulate the expression of TAAs such as HER-2,[294] which may also be relevant to CNS malignancies where HER-2 is a potential target of CAR T-cell therapy.[27,121] Additionally, the use of lymphodepleting regimens can be combined with CAR T-cell therapy for CNS malignancies.

For example, in a GBM mouse model, lymphodepletion with TMZ prior to CAR T-cell infusion improved antitumor activity and survival rates.[178] Thus, a clinical trial testing a lymphodepleting TMZ regimen and anti-EGFRvIII CAR T-cells as first-line therapy in combination with the current standard of care has been initiated (NCT02664363; Table 12.2). Furthermore, CAR T-cells may be combined with other immunotherapies such as immune checkpoint inhibitors,[168,171,172,295,296] virotherapy,[297,298] and immune-modulating agents.[214,299,300] CAR T-cells may also be combined with metabolic modulation strategies to improve their antitumor activity.[205,226,266,301]

CONCLUSIONS

CAR T-cells are evolving into effective tools for targeting difficult-to-treat brain cancers. Pioneering clinical trials have provided evidence that CAR T-cells targeting TAAs can be safely administered locally or systemically. Additionally, these trials have provided encouraging evidence of antitumor activity in some patients with advanced GBM. A better understanding of the mechanisms that limit CAR T-cell expansion and proliferation as well as hinder their trafficking to brain tumors is important to improve the effectiveness of these therapies. Additionally, an improved profiling of brain tumor antigens may facilitate the development of multivalent CAR T-cell products that can better control tumors and reduce the risk of antigen escape. A more comprehensive characterization of the suppressive TME may also facilitate the rational engineering of CAR T-cells that can be administered as a single agent or in combination with other treatments to augment their antitumor activity. Therefore, preclinical studies and early clinical trials that are focused on these critical factors will be important to guide the development of improved CAR T-cell therapies for CNS tumors.

ABBREVIATIONS

A_2AR	adenosine A2 receptor
ALL	acute lymphoblastic leukemia
AMP	adenosine monophosphate
ATP	adenosine triphosphate
CAR	chimeric antigen receptor
CARIS	chimeric antigen receptor immune synapse
CLL	chronic lymphocytic leukemia
CNS	central nervous system
CRM	continual reassessment method
CRS	cytokine release syndrome
CSF-1	colony-stimulating factor-1
CTLA-4	cytotoxic T lymphocyte–associated protein-4

DNA	deoxyribonucleic acid
EphA	Ephrin type A receptor 2
FAO	fatty acid oxidation
FDA	Food and Drug Administration
GBM	glioblastoma
GLUT	glucose transporter
HER2	human epidermal growth factor receptor 2
HIF	hypoxia-inducible factor-1α
HNSCC	head and neck small-cell carcinoma
ICP	intracranial pressure
IDO	indoleamine 2,3-deoxygenase
IFNγ	interferon γ
IL13Rα	interleukin 13 receptor α
mAb	monoclonal antibody
MDSC	myeloid-derived suppressor cell
MHC	minor histocompatibility complex
MIBI	multiplexed ion beam imaging
MMR	mismatch repair
MRI	magnetic resonance imaging
MSI	microsatellite instability
NKT	natural killer T-cells
NSCLC	non–small-cell lung carcinoma
OXPHOS	oxidative phosphorylation
PBMC	peripheral blood mononuclear cell
PD-1	programmed cell death-1
PD-L1	programmed death ligand 1
PD-L2	programmed death ligand 2
PP2A	Protein phosphatase 2
RNA	ribonucleic acid
ROS	reactive oxygen species
ScFv	single-chain variable fragment
SLO	secondary lymphoid organ
TAA	tumor-associated antigen
TAM	tumor-associated macrophage
TBI	total body irradiation
TGF-β	transforming growth factor β
TIL	tumor-infiltrating lymphocyte
TME	tumor microenvironment
TMZ	temozolomide
T_{reg}	regulatory T-cell
VST	virus-specific T-cell
XRT	radiotherapy

ACKNOWLEDGMENT

We would like to thank Ms. Catherine Gillespie for the professional editing and proofreading of the chapter.

REFERENCES

1. Omuro A, DeAngelis LM. Glioblastoma and other malignant gliomas: a clinical review. *JAMA.* 2013;310(17): 1842–1850.
2. Martin AM, Raabe E, Eberhart C, Cohen KJ. Management of pediatric and adult patients with medulloblastoma. *Curr Treat Options Oncol.* 2014;15(4):581–594.
3. Stupp R, Taillibert S, Kanner AA, et al. Maintenance therapy with tumor-treating fields plus temozolomide vs temozolomide alone for glioblastoma: a randomized clinical trial. *JAMA.* 2015;314(23):2535–2543.
4. Jones C, Karajannis MA, Jones DTW, et al. Pediatric high-grade glioma: biologically and clinically in need of new thinking. *Neuro Oncol.* 2017;19(2):153–161.
5. Tsang DS, Burghen E, Klimo Jr P, Boop FA, Ellison DW, Merchant TE. Outcomes after reirradiation for recurrent pediatric intracranial ependymoma. *Int J Radiat Oncol Biol Phys.* 2018;100(2):507–515.
6. Wei SC, Duffy CR, Allison JP. Fundamental mechanisms of immune checkpoint blockade therapy. *Cancer Discov.* 2018;8(9):1069–1086.
7. Bouffet E, Larouche V, Campbell BB, et al. Immune checkpoint inhibition for hypermutant glioblastoma multiforme resulting from germline biallelic mismatch repair deficiency. *J Clin Oncol.* 2016;34(19): 2206–2211.
8. Simonelli M, Persico P, Perrino M, et al. Checkpoint inhibitors as treatment for malignant gliomas: "A long way to the top". *Cancer Treat Rev.* 2018;69:121–131.
9. Luksik AS, Maxwell R, Garzon-Muvdi T, Lim M. The role of immune checkpoint inhibition in the treatment of brain tumors. *Neurotherapeutics.* 2017;14(4):1049–1065.
10. Buerki RA, Chheda ZS, Okada H. Immunotherapy of primary brain tumors: facts and hopes. *Clin Cancer Res.* 2018;24(21):5198–5205.
11. Omuro A, Vlahovic G, Lim M, et al. Nivolumab with or without ipilimumab in patients with recurrent glioblastoma: results from exploratory phase I cohorts of CheckMate 143. *Neuro Oncol.* 2018;20(5):674–686.
12. Kurz SC, Cabrera LP, Hastie D, et al. PD-1 inhibition has only limited clinical benefit in patients with recurrent high-grade glioma. *Neurology.* 2018;91(14): e1355–e1359.
13. Reardon DA, Omuro A, Brandes AA, et al. OS10.3 randomized phase 3 study evaluating the efficacy and safety of nivolumab vs bevacizumab in patients with recurrent glioblastoma: CheckMate 143. *Neuro Oncol.* 2017; 19(suppl 3). iii21-iii.
14. Quail DF, Joyce JA. The microenvironmental landscape of brain tumors. *Cancer Cell.* 2017;31(3):326–341.
15. Koyama S, Akbay EA, Li YY, et al. Adaptive resistance to therapeutic PD-1 blockade is associated with upregulation of alternative immune checkpoints. *Nat Commun.* 2016;7:10501.
16. June CH, Sadelain M. Chimeric antigen receptor therapy. *N Engl J Med.* 2018;379(1):64–73.
17. Choi BD, Maus MV, June CH, Sampson JH. Immunotherapy for glioblastoma: adoptive T-cell strategies. *Clin Cancer Res.* 2019;25(7):2042–2048.
18. Sadelain M, Riviere I, Riddell S. Therapeutic T cell engineering. *Nature.* 2017;545(7655):423–431.

19. van der Stegen SJ, Hamieh M, Sadelain M. The pharmacology of second-generation chimeric antigen receptors. *Nat Rev Drug Discov.* 2015;14(7):499−509.

20. Neelapu SS, Locke FL, Bartlett NL, et al. Axicabtagene ciloleucel CAR T-cell therapy in refractory large B-cell lymphoma. *N Engl J Med.* 2017;377(26):2531−2544.

21. Schuster SJ, Svoboda J, Chong EA, et al. Chimeric antigen receptor T cells in refractory B-cell lymphomas. *N Engl J Med.* 2017;377(26):2545−2554.

22. Park JH, Riviere I, Gonen M, et al. Long-term follow-up of CD19 CAR therapy in acute lymphoblastic leukemia. *N Engl J Med.* 2018;378(5):449−459.

23. Navai SA, Ahmed N. Targeting the tumour profile using broad spectrum chimaeric antigen receptor T-cells. *Biochem Soc Trans.* 2016;44(2):391−396.

24. Louveau A, Harris TH, Kipnis J. Revisiting the mechanisms of CNS immune privilege. *Trends Immunol.* 2015;36(10):569−577.

25. Congdon KL, Sanchez-Perez LA, Sampson JH. Effective effectors: how T cells access and infiltrate the central nervous system. *Pharmacol Ther.* 2019;197:52−60.

26. Chongsathidkiet P, Jackson C, Koyama S, et al. Sequestration of T cells in bone marrow in the setting of glioblastoma and other intracranial tumors. *Nat Med.* 2018;24(9):1459−1468.

27. Ahmed N, Ratnayake M, Savoldo B, et al. Regression of experimental medulloblastoma following transfer of HER2-specific T cells. *Cancer Res.* 2007;67(12):5957−5964.

28. Nellan A, Rota C, Majzner R, et al. Durable regression of Medulloblastoma after regional and intravenous delivery of anti-HER2 chimeric antigen receptor T cells. *J Immunother Cancer.* 2018;6(1):30.

29. Donovan LK, Bielamowicz KJ, Manno A, Ahmed N, Taylor MD. Abstract A019: chimeric antigen receptors (CARs) as a low-impact treatment of pediatric ependymomas. *Cancer Immunol Res.* 2016;4(11 Supplement):A019.

30. Mount CW, Majzner RG, Sundaresh S, et al. Potent antitumor efficacy of anti-GD2 CAR T cells in H3-K27M(+) diffuse midline gliomas. *Nat Med.* 2018;24(5):572−579.

31. Ahmed N, Brawley V, Hegde M, et al. HER2-Specific chimeric antigen receptor-modified virus-specific T cells for progressive glioblastoma: a phase 1 dose-escalation trial. *JAMA Oncol.* 2017;3(8):1094−1101.

32. O'Rourke DM, Nasrallah MP, Desai A, et al. A single dose of peripherally infused EGFRvIII-directed CAR T cells mediates antigen loss and induces adaptive resistance in patients with recurrent glioblastoma. *Sci Transl Med.* 2017;9(399).

33. Brown CE, Alizadeh D, Starr R, et al. Regression of glioblastoma after chimeric antigen receptor T-cell therapy. *N Engl J Med.* 2016;375(26):2561−2569.

34. Brown CE, Badie B, Barish ME, et al. Bioactivity and safety of IL13Ralpha2-redirected chimeric antigen receptor CD8+ T cells in patients with recurrent glioblastoma. *Clin Cancer Res.* 2015;21(18):4062−4072.

35. Kowolik CM, Topp MS, Gonzalez S, et al. CD28 costimulation provided through a CD19-specific chimeric antigen receptor enhances in vivo persistence and antitumor efficacy of adoptively transferred T cells. *Cancer Res.* 2006;66(22):10995−11004.

36. Ghassemi S, Nunez-Cruz S, O'Connor RS, et al. Reducing ex vivo culture improves the antileukemic activity of chimeric antigen receptor (CAR) T cells. *Cancer Immunol Res.* 2018;6(9):1100−1109.

37. Hong JJ, Rosenberg SA, Dudley ME, et al. Successful treatment of melanoma brain metastases with adoptive cell therapy. *Clin Cancer Res.* 2010;16(19):4892−4898.

38. Maude SL, Frey N, Shaw PA, et al. Chimeric antigen receptor T cells for sustained remissions in leukemia. *N Engl J Med.* 2014;371(16):1507−1517.

39. Morgan RA, Yang JC, Kitano M, Dudley ME, Laurencot CM, Rosenberg SA. Case report of a serious adverse event following the administration of T cells transduced with a chimeric antigen receptor recognizing ERBB2. *Mol Ther.* 2010;18(4):843−851.

40. Lee DW, Gardner R, Porter DL, et al. Current concepts in the diagnosis and management of cytokine release syndrome. *Blood.* 2014;124(2):188−195.

41. Gerstmayer B, Altenschmidt U, Hoffmann M, Wels W. Costimulation of T cell proliferation by a chimeric B7-2 antibody fusion protein specifically targeted to cells expressing the erbB2 proto-oncogene. *J Immunol.* 1997;158(10):4584−4590.

42. Cho HS, Mason K, Ramyar KX, et al. Structure of the extracellular region of HER2 alone and in complex with the Herceptin Fab. *Nature.* 2003;421(6924):756−760.

43. Ahmed N, Brawley VS, Hegde M, et al. Human epidermal growth factor receptor 2 (HER2) -specific chimeric antigen receptor-modified T cells for the immunotherapy of HER2-positive sarcoma. *J Clin Oncol.* 2015;33(15):1688−1696.

44. Therasse P, Arbuck SG, Eisenhauer EA, et al. New guidelines to evaluate the response to treatment in solid tumors. European organization for research and treatment of cancer, national cancer institute of the United States, national cancer institute of Canada. *J Natl Cancer Inst.* 2000;92(3):205−216.

45. Okada H, Weller M, Huang R, et al. Immunotherapy response assessment in neuro-oncology: a report of the RANO working group. *Lancet Oncol.* 2015;16(15):e534−e542.

46. Seymour L, Bogaerts J, Perrone A, et al. iRECIST: guidelines for response criteria for use in trials testing immunotherapeutics. *Lancet Oncol.* 2017;18(3):e143−e152.

47. Hodi FS, Ballinger M, Lyons B, et al. Immune-modified response evaluation criteria in solid tumors (imRECIST): refining guidelines to assess the clinical benefit of cancer immunotherapy. *J Clin Oncol.* 2018;36(9):850−858.

48. Munn DH, Mellor AL. Ido in the tumor microenvironment: inflammation, counter-regulation, and tolerance. *Trends Immunol.* 2016;37(3):193−207.

49. Sun C, Mezzadra R, Schumacher TN. Regulation and function of the PD-L1 checkpoint. *Immunity.* 2018; 48(3):434—452.

50. Hegde M, Corder A, Chow KK, et al. Combinational targeting offsets antigen escape and enhances effector functions of adoptively transferred T cells in glioblastoma. *Mol Ther.* 2013;21(11):2087—2101.

51. Hegde M, Mukherjee M, Grada Z, et al. Tandem CAR T cells targeting HER2 and IL13Ralpha2 mitigate tumor antigen escape. *J Clin Investig.* 2016;126(8):3036—3052.

52. Bielamowicz K, Fousek K, Byrd TT, et al. Trivalent CAR T cells overcome interpatient antigenic variability in glioblastoma. *Neuro Oncol.* 2018;20(4):506—518.

53. Mackall CL, Fleisher TA, Brown MR, et al. Distinctions between CD8+ and CD4+ T-cell regenerative pathways result in prolonged T-cell subset imbalance after intensive chemotherapy. *Blood.* 1997;89(10):3700—3707.

54. Das RK, Vernau L, Grupp SA, Barrett DM. Naive T-cell deficits at diagnosis and after chemotherapy impair cell therapy potential in pediatric cancers. *Cancer Discov.* 2019; 9(4):492—499.

55. Thommen DS, Schumacher TN. T cell dysfunction in cancer. *Cancer Cell.* 2018;33(4):547—562.

56. Woroniecka KI, Rhodin KE, Chongsathidkiet P, Keith KA, Fecci PE. T-cell dysfunction in glioblastoma: applying a new framework. *Clin Cancer Res.* 2018;24(16): 3792—3802.

57. Keu KV, Witney TH, Yaghoubi S, et al. Reporter gene imaging of targeted T cell immunotherapy in recurrent glioma. *Sci Transl Med.* 2017;9(373).

58. Wang S, O'Rourke DM, Chawla S, et al. Multiparametric magnetic resonance imaging in the assessment of anti-EGFRvIII chimeric antigen receptor T cell therapy in patients with recurrent glioblastoma. *Br J Cancer.* 2019; 120(1):54—56.

59. Chen Z, Hambardzumyan D. Immune microenvironment in glioblastoma subtypes. *Front Immunol.* 2018;9: 1004.

60. Moon EK, Wang LC, Dolfi DV, et al. Multifactorial T-cell hypofunction that is reversible can limit the efficacy of chimeric antigen receptor-transduced human T cells in solid tumors. *Clin Cancer Res.* 2014;20(16):4262—4273.

61. Morgan MA, Schambach A. Engineering CAR-T cells for improved function against solid tumors. *Front Immunol.* 2018;9:2493.

62. Majzner RG, Mackall CL. Tumor antigen escape from CAR T-cell therapy. *Cancer Discov.* 2018;8(10): 1219—1226.

63. Wen PY, Macdonald DR, Reardon DA, et al. Updated response assessment criteria for high-grade gliomas: response assessment in neuro-oncology working group. *J Clin Oncol.* 2010;28(11):1963—1972.

64. Barker CF, Billingham RE. Immunologically privileged sites. *Adv Immunol.* 1977;25:1—54.

65. Medawar PB. Immunity to homologous grafted skin; the fate of skin homografts transplanted to the brain, to subcutaneous tissue, and to the anterior chamber of the eye. *Br J Exp Pathol.* 1948;29(1):58—69.

66. Matyszak MK, Perry VH. Demyelination in the central nervous system following a delayed-type hypersensitivity response to Bacillus Calmette-Guerin. *Neuroscience.* 1995; 64(4):967—977.

67. Engelhardt B. Regulation of immune cell entry into the central nervous system. *Results Probl Cell Differ.* 2006;43: 259—280.

68. Wilson EH, Weninger W, Hunter CA. Trafficking of immune cells in the central nervous system. *J Clin Investig.* 2010;120(5):1368—1379.

69. Iliff JJ, Wang M, Liao Y, et al. A paravascular pathway facilitates CSF flow through the brain parenchyma and the clearance of interstitial solutes, including amyloid beta. *Sci Transl Med.* 2012;4(147):147ra11.

70. Aspelund A, Antila S, Proulx ST, et al. A dural lymphatic vascular system that drains brain interstitial fluid and macromolecules. *J Exp Med.* 2015;212(7): 991—999.

71. Kida S, Pantazis A, Weller RO. CSF drains directly from the subarachnoid space into nasal lymphatics in the rat. Anatomy, histology and immunological significance. *Neuropathol Appl Neurobiol.* 1993;19(6):480—488.

72. Kaminski M, Bechmann I, Pohland M, Kiwit J, Nitsch R, Glumm J. Migration of monocytes after intracerebral injection at entorhinal cortex lesion site. *J Leukoc Biol.* 2012; 92(1):31—39.

73. Louveau A, Smirnov I, Keyes TJ, et al. Structural and functional features of central nervous system lymphatic vessels. *Nature.* 2015;523(7560):337—341.

74. Carare RO, Bernardes-Silva M, Newman TA, et al. Solutes, but not cells, drain from the brain parenchyma along basement membranes of capillaries and arteries: significance for cerebral amyloid angiopathy and neuroimmunology. *Neuropathol Appl Neurobiol.* 2008; 34(2):131—144.

75. Dunn GP, Okada H. Principles of immunology and its nuances in the central nervous system. *Neuro Oncol.* 2015;17(Suppl 7):vii3—vii8.

76. Okada H, Kalinski P, Ueda R, et al. Induction of CD8+ T-cell responses against novel glioma-associated antigen peptides and clinical activity by vaccinations with {alpha}-type 1 polarized dendritic cells and polyinosinic-polycytidylic acid stabilized by lysine and carboxymethylcellulose in patients with recurrent malignant glioma. *J Clin Oncol.* 2011;29(3):330—336.

77. Sampson JH, Heimberger AB, Archer GE, et al. Immunologic escape after prolonged progression-free survival with epidermal growth factor receptor variant III peptide vaccination in patients with newly diagnosed glioblastoma. *J Clin Oncol.* 2010;28(31):4722—4729.

78. Wheeler CJ, Black KL, Liu G, et al. Vaccination elicits correlated immune and clinical responses in glioblastoma multiforme patients. *Cancer Res.* 2008;68(14): 5955—5964.

79. Phuphanich S, Wheeler CJ, Rudnick JD, et al. Phase I trial of a multi-epitope-pulsed dendritic cell vaccine for patients with newly diagnosed glioblastoma. *Cancer Immunol Immunother.* 2013;62(1):125—135.

80. Szerlip NJ, Pedraza A, Chakravarty D, et al. Intratumoral heterogeneity of receptor tyrosine kinases EGFR and PDGFRA amplification in glioblastoma defines subpopulations with distinct growth factor response. *Proc Natl Acad Sci USA.* 2012;109(8):3041–3046.

81. Patel AP, Tirosh I, Trombetta JJ, et al. Single-cell RNA-seq highlights intratumoral heterogeneity in primary glioblastoma. *Science.* 2014;344(6190): 1396–1401.

82. Aum DJ, Kim DH, Beaumont TL, Leuthardt EC, Dunn GP, Kim AH. Molecular and cellular heterogeneity: the hallmark of glioblastoma. *Neurosurg Focus.* 2014;37(6):E11.

83. Brennan CW, Verhaak RG, McKenna A, et al. The somatic genomic landscape of glioblastoma. *Cell.* 2013;155(2): 462–477.

84. Libermann TA, Nusbaum HR, Razon N, et al. Amplification, enhanced expression and possible rearrangement of EGF receptor gene in primary human brain tumours of glial origin. *Nature.* 1985;313(5998):144–147.

85. Wong AJ, Bigner SH, Bigner DD, Kinzler KW, Hamilton SR, Vogelstein B. Increased expression of the epidermal growth factor receptor gene in malignant gliomas is invariably associated with gene amplification. *Proc Natl Acad Sci USA.* 1987;84(19):6899–6903.

86. Ekstrand AJ, James CD, Cavenee WK, Seliger B, Pettersson RF, Collins VP. Genes for epidermal growth factor receptor, transforming growth factor alpha, and epidermal growth factor and their expression in human gliomas in vivo. *Cancer Res.* 1991;51(8):2164–2172.

87. Sturm D, Witt H, Hovestadt V, et al. Hotspot mutations in H3F3A and IDH1 define distinct epigenetic and biological subgroups of glioblastoma. *Cancer Cell.* 2012; 22(4):425–437.

88. Ekstrand AJ, Sugawa N, James CD, Collins VP. Amplified and rearranged epidermal growth factor receptor genes in human glioblastomas reveal deletions of sequences encoding portions of the N- and/or C-terminal tails. *Proc Natl Acad Sci USA.* 1992;89(10):4309–4313.

89. Sugawa N, Ekstrand AJ, James CD, Collins VP. Identical splicing of aberrant epidermal growth factor receptor transcripts from amplified rearranged genes in human glioblastomas. *Proc Natl Acad Sci USA.* 1990;87(21): 8602–8606.

90. Moscatello DK, Montgomery RB, Sundareshan P, McDaniel H, Wong MY, Wong AJ. Transformational and altered signal transduction by a naturally occurring mutant EGF receptor. *Oncogene.* 1996;13(1):85–96.

91. Nishikawa R, Ji XD, Harmon RC, et al. A mutant epidermal growth factor receptor common in human glioma confers enhanced tumorigenicity. *Proc Natl Acad Sci USA.* 1994;91(16):7727–7731.

92. Fernandes H, Cohen S, Bishayee S. Glycosylation-induced conformational modification positively regulates receptor-receptor association: a study with an aberrant epidermal growth factor receptor (EGFRvIII/DeltaEGFR) expressed in cancer cells. *J Biol Chem.* 2001; 276(7):5375–5383.

93. Sugawa N, Yamamoto K, Ueda S, et al. Function of aberrant EGFR in malignant gliomas. *Brain Tumor Pathol.* 1998;15(1):53–57.

94. Shinojima N, Tada K, Shiraishi S, et al. Prognostic value of epidermal growth factor receptor in patients with glioblastoma multiforme. *Cancer Res.* 2003;63(20): 6962–6970.

95. Heimberger AB, Hlatky R, Suki D, et al. Prognostic effect of epidermal growth factor receptor and EGFRvIII in glioblastoma multiforme patients. *Clin Cancer Res.* 2005; 11(4):1462–1466.

96. Quan AL, Barnett GH, Lee SY, et al. Epidermal growth factor receptor amplification does not have prognostic significance in patients with glioblastoma multiforme. *Int J Radiat Oncol Biol Phys.* 2005;63(3):695–703.

97. Aldape KD, Ballman K, Furth A, et al. Immunohistochemical detection of EGFRvIII in high malignancy grade astrocytomas and evaluation of prognostic significance. *J Neuropathol Exp Neurol.* 2004;63(7):700–707.

98. Felsberg J, Hentschel B, Kaulich K, et al. Epidermal growth factor receptor variant III (EGFRvIII) positivity in EGFR-amplified glioblastomas: prognostic role and comparison between primary and recurrent tumors. *Clin Cancer Res.* 2017;23(22):6846–6855.

99. Li G, Mitra SS, Monje M, et al. Expression of epidermal growth factor variant III (EGFRvIII) in pediatric diffuse intrinsic pontine gliomas. *J Neuro Oncol.* 2012;108(3): 395–402.

100. Jungbluth AA, Stockert E, Huang HJ, et al. A monoclonal antibody recognizing human cancers with amplification/overexpression of the human epidermal growth factor receptor. *Proc Natl Acad Sci USA.* 2003;100(2):639–644.

101. Luwor RB, Johns TG, Murone C, et al. Monoclonal antibody 806 inhibits the growth of tumor xenografts expressing either the de2-7 or amplified epidermal growth factor receptor (EGFR) but not wild-type EGFR. *Cancer Res.* 2001;61(14):5355–5361.

102. Mishima K, Johns TG, Luwor RB, et al. Growth suppression of intracranial xenografted glioblastomas overexpressing mutant epidermal growth factor receptors by systemic administration of monoclonal antibody (mAb) 806, a novel monoclonal antibody directed to the receptor. *Cancer Res.* 2001;61(14):5349–5354.

103. inventors; Amgen Fremont Inc, assignee Weber R, Feng X, Foord O, et al. *Antibodies Directed to the Deletion Mutants of Epidermal Growth Factor Receptor and Uses Thereof.* 2005. United States.

104. Bullain SS, Sahin A, Szentirmai O, et al. Genetically engineered T cells to target EGFRvIII expressing glioblastoma. *J Neuro Oncol.* 2009;94(3):373–382.

105. Morgan RA, Johnson LA, Davis JL, et al. Recognition of glioma stem cells by genetically modified T cells targeting EGFRvIII and development of adoptive cell therapy for glioma. *Hum Gene Ther.* 2012;23(10):1043–1053.

106. Sampson JH, Choi BD, Sanchez-Perez L, et al. EGFRvIII mCAR-modified T-cell therapy cures mice with established intracerebral glioma and generates host immunity

against tumor-antigen loss. *Clin Cancer Res.* 2014;20(4):972–984.

107. Johnson LA, Scholler J, Ohkuri T, et al. Rational development and characterization of humanized anti-EGFR variant III chimeric antigen receptor T cells for glioblastoma. *Sci Transl Med.* 2015;7(275):275ra22.

108. Graus-Porta D, Beerli RR, Daly JM, Hynes NE. ErbB-2, the preferred heterodimerization partner of all ErbB receptors, is a mediator of lateral signaling. *EMBO J.* 1997;16(7):1647–1655.

109. Koka V, Potti A, Forseen SE, et al. Role of HER-2/neu overexpression and clinical determinants of early mortality in glioblastoma multiforme. *Am J Clin Oncol.* 2003;26(4):332–335.

110. Press MF, Cordon-Cardo C, Slamon DJ. Expression of the HER-2/neu proto-oncogene in normal human adult and fetal tissues. *Oncogene.* 1990;5(7):953–962.

111. Schlegel J, Merdes A, Stumm G, et al. Amplification of the epidermal-growth-factor-receptor gene correlates with different growth behaviour in human glioblastoma. *Int J Cancer.* 1994;56(1):72–77.

112. Hernan R, Fasheh R, Calabrese C, et al. ERBB2 upregulates S100A4 and several other prometastatic genes in medulloblastoma. *Cancer Res.* 2003;63(1):140–148.

113. Comprehensive genomic characterization defines human glioblastoma genes and core pathways. *Nature.* 2008;455(7216):1061–1068.

114. Gilbertson RJ, Pearson AD, Perry RH, Jaros E, Kelly PJ. Prognostic significance of the c-erbB-2 oncogene product in childhood medulloblastoma. *Br J Cancer.* 1995;71(3):473–477.

115. Gilbertson RJ, Bentley L, Hernan R, et al. ERBB receptor signaling promotes ependymoma cell proliferation and represents a potential novel therapeutic target for this disease. *Clin Cancer Res.* 2002;8(10):3054–3064.

116. Singh A, Lun X, Jayanthan A, et al. Profiling pathway-specific novel therapeutics in preclinical assessment for central nervous system atypical teratoid rhabdoid tumors (CNS ATRT): favorable activity of targeting EGFR- ErbB2 signaling with lapatinib. *Mol Oncol.* 2013;7(3):497–512.

117. Kallioniemi OP, Kallioniemi A, Kurisu W, et al. ERBB2 amplification in breast cancer analyzed by fluorescence in situ hybridization. *Proc Natl Acad Sci USA.* 1992;89(12):5321–5325.

118. Berchuck A, Kamel A, Whitaker R, et al. Overexpression of HER-2/neu is associated with poor survival in advanced epithelial ovarian cancer. *Cancer Res.* 1990;50(13):4087–4091.

119. Yonemura Y, Ninomiya I, Yamaguchi A, et al. Evaluation of immunoreactivity for erbB-2 protein as a marker of poor short term prognosis in gastric cancer. *Cancer Res.* 1991;51(3):1034–1038.

120. Schlegel J, Stumm G, Brandle K, et al. Amplification and differential expression of members of the erbB-gene family in human glioblastoma. *J Neuro Oncol.* 1994;22(3):201–207.

121. Ahmed N, Salsman VS, Kew Y, et al. HER2-specific T cells target primary glioblastoma stem cells and induce regression of autologous experimental tumors. *Clin Cancer Res.* 2010;16(2):474–485.

122. Debinski W, Gibo DM, Hulet SW, Connor JR, Gillespie GY. Receptor for interleukin 13 is a marker and therapeutic target for human high-grade gliomas. *Clin Cancer Res.* 1999;5(5):985–990.

123. Rahaman SO, Sharma P, Harbor PC, Aman MJ, Vogelbaum MA, Haque SJ. IL-13R(alpha)2, a decoy receptor for IL-13 acts as an inhibitor of IL-4-dependent signal transduction in glioblastoma cells. *Cancer Res.* 2002;62(4):1103–1109.

124. Arima K, Sato K, Tanaka G, et al. Characterization of the interaction between interleukin-13 and interleukin-13 receptors. *J Biol Chem.* 2005;280(26):24915–24922.

125. Krause S, Behrends J, Borowski A, et al. Blockade of interleukin-13-mediated cell activation by a novel inhibitory antibody to human IL-13 receptor alpha1. *Mol Immunol.* 2006;43(11):1799–1807.

126. Bhardwaj R, Suzuki A, Leland P, Joshi BH, Puri RK. Identification of a novel role of IL-13Ralpha2 in human Glioblastoma multiforme: interleukin-13 mediates signal transduction through AP-1 pathway. *J Transl Med.* 2018;16(1):369.

127. Han J, Puri RK. Analysis of the cancer genome atlas (TCGA) database identifies an inverse relationship between interleukin-13 receptor alpha1 and alpha2 gene expression and poor prognosis and drug resistance in subjects with glioblastoma multiforme. *J Neuro Oncol.* 2018;136(3):463–474.

128. Kawakami M, Kawakami K, Takahashi S, Abe M, Puri RK. Analysis of interleukin-13 receptor alpha2 expression in human pediatric brain tumors. *Cancer.* 2004;101(5):1036–1042.

129. Yeung JT, Hamilton RL, Okada H, Jakacki RI, Pollack IF. Increased expression of tumor-associated antigens in pediatric and adult ependymomas: implication for vaccine therapy. *J Neuro Oncol.* 2013;111(2):103–111.

130. Newman JP, Wang GY, Arima K, et al. Interleukin-13 receptor alpha 2 cooperates with EGFRvIII signaling to promote glioblastoma multiforme. *Nat Commun.* 2017;8(1):1913.

131. 672. Adoptive therapy evaluating human IL13-zetakine T cells engineered to target glioblastomas expressing IL13Rα2, a biomarker predicting poor prognosis. *Mol Ther.* 2012;20:S259–S260.

132. Kahlon KS, Brown C, Cooper LJ, Raubitschek A, Forman SJ, Jensen MC. Specific recognition and killing of glioblastoma multiforme by interleukin 13-zetakine redirected cytolytic T cells. *Cancer Res.* 2004;64(24):9160–9166.

133. Krebs S, Chow KK, Yi Z, et al. T cells redirected to interleukin-13Ralpha2 with interleukin-13 mutein–chimeric antigen receptors have anti-glioma activity but also recognize interleukin-13Ralpha1. *Cytotherapy.* 2014;16(8):1121–1131.

134. Kong S, Sengupta S, Tyler B, et al. Suppression of human glioma xenografts with second-generation IL13R-specific

chimeric antigen receptor-modified T cells. *Clin Cancer Res.* 2012;18(21):5949−5960.

135. Krenciute G, Krebs S, Torres D, et al. Characterization and functional analysis of scFv-based chimeric antigen receptors to redirect T cells to IL13Ralpha2-positive glioma. *Mol Ther.* 2016;24(2):354−363.

136. Yin Y, Boesteanu AC, Binder ZA, et al. Checkpoint blockade reverses anergy in IL-13ralpha2 humanized scfv-based CAR T cells to treat murine and canine gliomas. *Mol Ther Oncolytics.* 2018;11:20−38.

137. Brown CE, Aguilar B, Starr R, et al. Optimization of IL13Ralpha2-targeted chimeric antigen receptor T cells for improved anti-tumor efficacy against glioblastoma. *Mol Ther.* 2018;26(1):31−44.

138. Brescia P, Ortensi B, Fornasari L, Levi D, Broggi G, Pelicci G. CD133 is essential for glioblastoma stem cell maintenance. *Stem Cells.* 2013;31(5):857−869.

139. Singh SK, Hawkins C, Clarke ID, et al. Identification of human brain tumour initiating cells. *Nature.* 2004; 432(7015):396−401.

140. Zhu X, Prasad S, Gaedicke S, Hettich M, Firat E, Niedermann G. Patient-derived glioblastoma stem cells are killed by CD133-specific CAR T cells but induce the T cell aging marker CD57. *Oncotarget.* 2015;6(1): 171−184.

141. Wang Y, Chen M, Wu Z, et al. CD133-directed CAR T cells for advanced metastasis malignancies: A phase I trial. *OncoImmunology.* 2018;7(7):e1440169.

142. Traylor TD, Hogan EL. Gangliosides of human cerebral astrocytomas. *J Neurochem.* 1980;34(1):126−131.

143. Longee DC, Wikstrand CJ, Mansson JE, et al. Disialogan-glioside GD2 in human neuroectodermal tumor cell lines and gliomas. *Acta Neuropathol.* 1991;82(1):45−54.

144. Wykosky J, Gibo DM, Stanton C, Debinski W. EphA2 as a novel molecular marker and target in glioblastoma multiforme. *Mol Cancer Res.* 2005;3(10):541−551.

145. Wang LF, Fokas E, Bieker M, et al. Increased expression of EphA2 correlates with adverse outcome in primary and recurrent glioblastoma multiforme patients. *Oncol Rep.* 2008;19(1):151−156.

146. Miao H, Gale NW, Guo H, et al. EphA2 promotes infiltra-tive invasion of glioma stem cells in vivo through cross-talk with Akt and regulates stem cell properties. *Oncogene.* 2015;34(5):558−567.

147. Chow KK, Naik S, Kakarla S, et al. T cells redirected to EphA2 for the immunotherapy of glioblastoma. *Mol Ther.* 2013;21(3):629−637.

148. Yi Z, Prinzing BL, Cao F, Gottschalk S, Krenciute G. Opti-mizing EphA2-CAR T cells for the adoptive immuno-therapy of glioma. *Mol Ther Methods Clin Dev.* 2018;9: 70−80.

149. Pratt D, Pittaluga S, Palisoc M, et al. Expression of CD70 (CD27L) is associated with epithelioid and sarcomatous features in IDH-wild-type glioblastoma. *J Neuropathol Exp Neurol.* 2017;76(8):697−708.

150. Jin L, Ge H, Long Y, et al. CD70, a novel target of CAR T-cell therapy for gliomas. *Neuro Oncol.* 2018;20(1): 55−65.

151. Wang QJ, Yu Z, Hanada KI, et al. Preclinical evaluation of chimeric antigen receptors targeting CD70-expressing cancers. *Clin Cancer Res.* 2017;23(9):2267−2276.

152. Modak S, Kramer K, Gultekin SH, Guo HF, Cheung NK. Monoclonal antibody 8H9 targets a novel cell surface an-tigen expressed by a wide spectrum of human solid tumors. *Cancer Res.* 2001;61(10):4048−4054.

153. Zhou Z, Luther N, Ibrahim GM, et al. B7-H3, a potential therapeutic target, is expressed in diffuse intrinsic pontine glioma. *J Neuro Oncol.* 2013;111(3):257−264.

154. Baral A, Ye HX, Jiang PC, Yao Y, Mao Y. B7-H3 and B7-H1 expression in cerebral spinal fluid and tumor tissue corre-lates with the malignancy grade of glioma patients. *Oncol Lett.* 2014;8(3):1195−1201.

155. Majzner RG, Theruvath JL, Nellan A, et al. CAR T cells tar-geting B7-H3, a pan-cancer antigen, demonstrate potent preclinical activity against pediatric solid tumors and brain tumors. *Clin Cancer Res.* 2019;25(8):2560−2574.

156. Chekenya M, Enger PO, Thorsen F, et al. The glial precur-sor proteoglycan, NG2, is expressed on tumour neovascu-lature by vascular pericytes in human malignant brain tumours. *Neuropathol Appl Neurobiol.* 2002;28(5): 367−380.

157. Chekenya M, Krakstad C, Svendsen A, et al. The progen-itor cell marker NG2/MPG promotes chemoresistance by activation of integrin-dependent PI3K/Akt signaling. *Oncogene.* 2008;27(39):5182−5194.

158. Beard RE, Zheng Z, Lagisetty KH, et al. Multiple chimeric antigen receptors successfully target chondroitin sulfate proteoglycan 4 in several different cancer histologies and cancer stem cells. *J Immunother Cancer.* 2014;2:25.

159. Pellegatta S, Savoldo B, Di Ianni N, et al. Constitutive and TNFalpha-inducible expression of chondroitin sulfate proteoglycan 4 in glioblastoma and neurospheres: impli-cations for CAR-T cell therapy. *Sci Transl Med.* 2018; 10(430).

160. Mishima K, Kato Y, Kaneko MK, Nishikawa R, Hirose T, Matsutani M. Increased expression of podoplanin in ma-lignant astrocytic tumors as a novel molecular marker of malignant progression. *Acta Neuropathol.* 2006;111(5): 483−488.

161. Shiina S, Ohno M, Ohka F, et al. CAR T cells targeting podoplanin reduce orthotopic glioblastomas in mouse brains. *Cancer Immunol Res.* 2016;4(3):259−268.

162. Ramos CA, Rouce R, Robertson CS, et al. In vivo fate and activity of second- versus third-generation CD19-specific CAR-T cells in B cell non-hodgkin's lymphomas. *Mol Ther.* 2018;26(12):2727−2737.

163. Guedan S, Posey Jr AD, Shaw C, et al. Enhancing CAR T cell persistence through ICOS and 4-1BB costimulation. *JCI Insight.* 2018;3(1).

164. Gomes-Silva D, Mukherjee M, Srinivasan M, et al. Tonic 4-1BB costimulation in chimeric antigen receptors im-pedes T cell survival and is vector-dependent. *Cell Rep.* 2017;21(1):17−26.

165. Gattinoni L, Klebanoff CA, Restifo NP. Paths to stemness: building the ultimate antitumour T cell. *Nat Rev Cancer.* 2012;12(10):671−684.

166. Busch DH, Frassle SP, Sommermeyer D, Buchholz VR, Riddell SR. Role of memory T cell subsets for adoptive immunotherapy. *Semin Immunol.* 2016;28(1):28–34.

167. Hegde M, DeRenzo CC, Zhang H, et al. Expansion of HER2-CAR T cells after lymphodepletion and clinical responses in patients with advanced sarcoma. *J Clin Oncol.* 2017;35(15 suppl):10508.

168. Cherkassky L, Morello A, Villena-Vargas J, et al. Human CAR T cells with cell-intrinsic PD-1 checkpoint blockade resist tumor-mediated inhibition. *J Clin Investig.* 2016;126(8):3130–3144.

169. Ali SA, Shi V, Maric I, et al. T cells expressing an anti-B-cell maturation antigen chimeric antigen receptor cause remissions of multiple myeloma. *Blood.* 2016;128(13):1688–1700.

170. Mueller KT, Maude SL, Porter DL, et al. Cellular kinetics of CTL019 in relapsed/refractory B-cell acute lymphoblastic leukemia and chronic lymphocytic leukemia. *Blood.* 2017;130(21):2317–2325.

171. Ren J, Liu X, Fang C, Jiang S, June CH, Zhao Y. Multiplex genome editing to generate universal CAR T cells resistant to PD1 inhibition. *Clin Cancer Res.* 2017;23(9):2255–2266.

172. Liu X, Ranganathan R, Jiang S, et al. A chimeric switch-receptor targeting PD1 augments the efficacy of second-generation CAR T cells in advanced solid tumors. *Cancer Res.* 2016;76(6):1578–1590.

173. Hurton LV, Singh H, Najjar AM, et al. Tethered IL-15 augments antitumor activity and promotes a stem-cell memory subset in tumor-specific T cells. *Proc Natl Acad Sci USA.* 2016;113(48). E7788-e97.

174. Shum T, Omer B, Tashiro H, et al. Constitutive signaling from an engineered IL7 receptor promotes durable tumor elimination by tumor-redirected T cells. *Cancer Discov.* 2017;7(11):1238–1247.

175. Dudley ME, Wunderlich JR, Yang JC, et al. Adoptive cell transfer therapy following non-myeloablative but lymphodepleting chemotherapy for the treatment of patients with refractory metastatic melanoma. *J Clin Oncol.* 2005;23(10):2346–2357.

176. Boyiadzis MM, Dhodapkar MV, Brentjens RJ, et al. Chimeric antigen receptor (CAR) T therapies for the treatment of hematologic malignancies: clinical perspective and significance. *J Immunother Cancer.* 2018;6(1):137.

177. Heczey A, Louis CU, Savoldo B, et al. CAR T cells administered in combination with lymphodepletion and PD-1 inhibition to patients with neuroblastoma. *Mol Ther.* 2017;25(9):2214–2224.

178. Suryadevara CM, Desai R, Abel ML, et al. Temozolomide lymphodepletion enhances CAR abundance and correlates with antitumor efficacy against established glioblastoma. *OncoImmunology.* 2018;7(6):e1434464.

179. Klebanoff CA, Khong HT, Antony PA, Palmer DC, Restifo NP. Sinks, suppressors and antigen presenters: how lymphodepletion enhances T cell-mediated tumor immunotherapy. *Trends Immunol.* 2005;26(2):111–117.

180. Paulos CM, Wrzesinski C, Kaiser A, et al. Microbial translocation augments the function of adoptively transferred self/tumor-specific CD8+ T cells via TLR4 signaling. *J Clin Investig.* 2007;117(8):2197–2204.

181. Bettonville M, d'Aria S, Weatherly K, et al. Long-term antigen exposure irreversibly modifies metabolic requirements for T cell function. *Elife.* 2018;7.

182. Schietinger A, Philip M, Krisnawan VE, et al. Tumor-specific T cell dysfunction is a dynamic antigen-driven differentiation program initiated early during tumorigenesis. *Immunity.* 2016;45(2):389–401.

183. Philip M, Fairchild L, Sun L, et al. Chromatin states define tumour-specific T cell dysfunction and reprogramming. *Nature.* 2017;545(7655):452–456.

184. Mognol GP, Spreafico R, Wong V, et al. Exhaustion-associated regulatory regions in CD8(+) tumor-infiltrating T cells. *Proc Natl Acad Sci USA.* 2017;114(13). E2776-e85.

185. Rosenberg SA, Sherry RM, Morton KE, et al. Tumor progression can occur despite the induction of very high levels of self/tumor antigen-specific CD8+ T cells in patients with melanoma. *J Immunol.* 2005;175(9):6169–6176.

186. Singer M, Wang C, Cong L, et al. A distinct gene module for dysfunction uncoupled from activation in tumor-infiltrating T cells. *Cell.* 2016;166(6):1500–1511.e9.

187. Chihara N, Madi A, Kondo T, et al. Induction and transcriptional regulation of the co-inhibitory gene module in T cells. *Nature.* 2018;558(7710):454–459.

188. Pauken KE, Sammons MA, Odorizzi PM, et al. Epigenetic stability of exhausted T cells limits durability of reinvigoration by PD-1 blockade. *Science.* 2016;354(6316):1160–1165.

189. Hambardzumyan D, Gutmann DH, Kettenmann H. The role of microglia and macrophages in glioma maintenance and progression. *Nat Neurosci.* 2016;19(1):20–27.

190. Graeber MB, Scheithauer BW, Kreutzberg GW. Microglia in brain tumors. *Glia.* 2002;40(2):252–259.

191. Morantz RA, Wood GW, Foster M, Clark M, Gollahon K. Macrophages in experimental and human brain tumors. Part 2: studies of the macrophage content of human brain tumors. *J Neurosurg.* 1979;50(3):305–311.

192. Komohara Y, Ohnishi K, Kuratsu J, Takeya M. Possible involvement of the M2 anti-inflammatory macrophage phenotype in growth of human gliomas. *J Pathol.* 2008;216(1):15–24.

193. Wei J, Marisetty A, Schrand B, et al. Osteopontin mediates glioblastoma-associated macrophage infiltration and is a potential therapeutic target. *J Clin Investig.* 2019;129(1):137–149.

194. Chouaib S, Noman MZ, Kosmatopoulos K, Curran MA. Hypoxic stress: obstacles and opportunities for innovative immunotherapy of cancer. *Oncogene.* 2017;36(4):439–445.

195. Colegio OR, Chu NQ, Szabo AL, et al. Functional polarization of tumour-associated macrophages by tumour-derived lactic acid. *Nature.* 2014;513(7519):559–563.

196. Gray MJ, Poljakovic M, Kepka-Lenhart D, Morris Jr SM. Induction of arginase I transcription by IL-4 requires a

composite DNA response element for STAT6 and C/EBPbeta. *Gene*. 2005;353(1):98−106.

197. Pyonteck SM, Akkari L, Schuhmacher AJ, et al. CSF-1R inhibition alters macrophage polarization and blocks glioma progression. *Nat Med*. 2013;19(10):1264−1272.

198. Zhou W, Ke SQ, Huang Z, et al. Periostin secreted by glioblastoma stem cells recruits M2 tumour-associated macrophages and promotes malignant growth. *Nat Cell Biol*. 2015;17(2):170−182.

199. Margol AS, Robison NJ, Gnanachandran J, et al. Tumor-associated macrophages in SHH subgroup of medulloblastomas. *Clin Cancer Res*. 2015;21(6): 1457−1465.

200. Raychaudhuri B, Rayman P, Ireland J, et al. Myeloid-derived suppressor cell accumulation and function in patients with newly diagnosed glioblastoma. *Neuro Oncol*. 2011;13(6):591−599.

201. Raychaudhuri B, Rayman P, Huang P, et al. Myeloid derived suppressor cell infiltration of murine and human gliomas is associated with reduction of tumor infiltrating lymphocytes. *J Neuro Oncol*. 2015;122(2):293−301.

202. Hussain SF, Yang D, Suki D, Aldape K, Grimm E, Heimberger AB. The role of human glioma-infiltrating microglia/macrophages in mediating antitumor immune responses. *Neuro Oncol*. 2006;8(3):261−279.

203. Ugel S, De Sanctis F, Mandruzzato S, Bronte V. Tumor-induced myeloid deviation: when myeloid-derived suppressor cells meet tumor-associated macrophages. *J Clin Investig*. 2015;125(9):3365−3376.

204. Geiger R, Rieckmann JC, Wolf T, et al. L-arginine modulates T cell metabolism and enhances survival and antitumor activity. *Cell*. 2016;167(3):829−842.e13.

205. Ninomiya S, Narala N, Huye L, et al. Tumor indoleamine 2,3-dioxygenase (Ido) inhibits CD19-CAR T cells and is downregulated by lymphodepleting drugs. *Blood*. 2015; 125(25):3905−3916.

206. Zheng Y, Delgoffe GM, Meyer CF, Chan W, Powell JD. Anergic T cells are metabolically anergic. *J Immunol*. 2009;183(10):6095−6101.

207. Tang H, Liang Y, Anders RA, et al. PD-L1 on host cells is essential for PD-L1 blockade-mediated tumor regression. *J Clin Investig*. 2018;128(2):580−588.

208. Lin H, Wei S, Hurt EM, et al. Host expression of PD-L1 determines efficacy of PD-L1 pathway blockade-mediated tumor regression. *J Clin Investig*. 2018;128(2): 805−815.

209. Yamamoto TN, Lee PH, Vodnala SK, et al. T cells genetically engineered to overcome death signaling enhance adoptive cancer immunotherapy. *J Clin Investig*. 2019; 130.

210. Quail DF, Bowman RL, Akkari L, et al. The tumor microenvironment underlies acquired resistance to CSF-1R inhibition in gliomas. *Science*. 2016;352(6288):aad3018.

211. Butowski N, Colman H, De Groot JF, et al. Orally administered colony stimulating factor 1 receptor inhibitor PLX3397 in recurrent glioblastoma: an Ivy Foundation Early Phase Clinical Trials Consortium phase II study. *Neuro Oncol*. 2016;18(4):557−564.

212. Saha D, Martuza RL, Rabkin SD. Macrophage polarization contributes to glioblastoma eradication by combination immunovirotherapy and immune checkpoint blockade. *Cancer Cell*. 2017;32(2):253−267.e5.

213. Kamran N, Kadiyala P, Saxena M, et al. Immunosuppressive myeloid cells' blockade in the glioma microenvironment enhances the efficacy of immune-stimulatory gene therapy. *Mol Ther*. 2017;25(1):232−248.

214. Zhang F, Stephan SB, Ene CI, Smith TT, Holland EC, Stephan MT. Nanoparticles that reshape the tumor milieu create a therapeutic window for effective T-cell therapy in solid malignancies. *Cancer Res*. 2018;78(13): 3718−3730.

215. Long AH, Highfill SL, Cui Y, et al. Reduction of MDSCs with all-trans retinoic acid improves CAR therapy efficacy for sarcomas. *Cancer Immunol Res*. 2016;4(10):869−880.

216. Yeku OO, Purdon TJ, Koneru M, Spriggs D, Brentjens RJ. Armored CAR T cells enhance antitumor efficacy and overcome the tumor microenvironment. *Sci Rep*. 2017; 7(1):10541.

217. Heimberger AB, Abou-Ghazal M, Reina-Ortiz C, et al. Incidence and prognostic impact of FoxP3+ regulatory T cells in human gliomas. *Clin Cancer Res*. 2008;14(16): 5166−5172.

218. Gururangan S, Reap E, Schmittling R, et al. Regulatory T cell subsets in patients with medulloblastoma at diagnosis and during standard irradiation and chemotherapy (PBTC N-11). *Cancer Immunol Immunother*. 2017;66(12): 1589−1595.

219. Jacobs JF, Idema AJ, Bol KF, et al. Regulatory T cells and the PD-L1/PD-1 pathway mediate immune suppression in malignant human brain tumors. *Neuro Oncol*. 2009; 11(4):394−402.

220. El Andaloussi A, Lesniak MS. CD4+ CD25+ FoxP3+ T-cell infiltration and heme oxygenase-1 expression correlate with tumor grade in human gliomas. *J Neuro Oncol*. 2007;83(2):145−152.

221. Chang AL, Miska J, Wainwright DA, et al. CCL2 produced by the glioma microenvironment is essential for the recruitment of regulatory T cells and myeloid-derived suppressor cells. *Cancer Res*. 2016;76(19): 5671−5682.

222. Humphries W, Wei J, Sampson JH, Heimberger AB. The role of tregs in glioma-mediated immunosuppression: potential target for intervention. *Neurosurg Clin N Am*. 2010;21(1):125−137.

223. Wainwright DA, Balyasnikova IV, Chang AL, et al. Ido expression in brain tumors increases the recruitment of regulatory T cells and negatively impacts survival. *Clin Cancer Res*. 2012;18(22):6110−6121.

224. Vignali DA, Collison LW, Workman CJ. How regulatory T cells work. *Nat Rev Immunol*. 2008;8(7):523−532.

225. Liu C, Workman CJ, Vignali DA. Targeting regulatory T cells in tumors. *FEBS J*. 2016;283(14):2731−2748.

226. Beavis PA, Henderson MA, Giuffrida L, et al. Targeting the adenosine 2A receptor enhances chimeric antigen receptor T cell efficacy. *J Clin Investig*. 2017;127(3): 929−941.

227. Arce Vargas F, Furness AJS, Litchfield K, et al. Fc effector function contributes to the activity of human anti-CTLA-4 antibodies. *Cancer Cell.* 2018;33(4):649–663.e4.

228. Speiser DE, Ho PC, Verdeil G. Regulatory circuits of T cell function in cancer. *Nat Rev Immunol.* 2016;16(10):599–611.

229. Anderson KG, Stromnes IM, Greenberg PD. Obstacles posed by the tumor microenvironment to T cell activity: a case for synergistic therapies. *Cancer Cell.* 2017;31(3):311–325.

230. Chang CH, Curtis JD, Maggi Jr LB, et al. Posttranscriptional control of T cell effector function by aerobic glycolysis. *Cell.* 2013;153(6):1239–1251.

231. O'Sullivan D, van der Windt GJ, Huang SC, et al. Memory CD8(+) T cells use cell-intrinsic lipolysis to support the metabolic programming necessary for development. *Immunity.* 2014;41(1):75–88.

232. Bantug GR, Fischer M, Grahlert J, et al. Mitochondria-endoplasmic reticulum contact sites function as immunometabolic hubs that orchestrate the rapid recall response of memory CD8(+) T cells. *Immunity.* 2018;48(3):542–555.e6.

233. Gubser PM, Bantug GR, Razik L, et al. Rapid effector function of memory CD8+ T cells requires an immediate-early glycolytic switch. *Nat Immunol.* 2013;14(10):1064–1072.

234. van der Windt GJ, O'Sullivan D, Everts B, et al. CD8 memory T cells have a bioenergetic advantage that underlies their rapid recall ability. *Proc Natl Acad Sci USA.* 2013;110(35):14336–14341.

235. Delgoffe GM. Filling the tank: keeping antitumor T cells metabolically fit for the long haul. *Cancer Immunol Res.* 2016;4(12):1001–1006.

236. Liberti MV, Locasale JW. The Warburg effect: how does it benefit cancer cells? *Trends Biochem Sci.* 2016;41(3):211–218.

237. Strickland M, Stoll EA. Metabolic reprogramming in glioma. *Front Cell Dev Biol.* 2017;5:43.

238. Tanaka K, Sasayama T, Irino Y, et al. Compensatory glutamine metabolism promotes glioblastoma resistance to mTOR inhibitor treatment. *J Clin Investig.* 2015;125(4):1591–1602.

239. Bensaad K, Favaro E, Lewis CA, et al. Fatty acid uptake and lipid storage induced by HIF-1alpha contribute to cell growth and survival after hypoxia-reoxygenation. *Cell Rep.* 2014;9(1):349–365.

240. Agnihotri S, Zadeh G. Metabolic reprogramming in glioblastoma: the influence of cancer metabolism on epigenetics and unanswered questions. *Neuro Oncol.* 2016;18(2):160–172.

241. Bronte V, Zanovello P. Regulation of immune responses by L-arginine metabolism. *Nat Rev Immunol.* 2005;5(8):641–654.

242. Ho PC, Bihuniak JD, Macintyre AN, et al. Phosphoenolpyruvate is a metabolic checkpoint of anti-tumor T cell responses. *Cell.* 2015;162(6):1217–1228.

243. Rodriguez PC, Quiceno DG, Ochoa AC. L-arginine availability regulates T-lymphocyte cell-cycle progression. *Blood.* 2007;109(4):1568–1573.

244. Carr EL, Kelman A, Wu GS, et al. Glutamine uptake and metabolism are coordinately regulated by ERK/MAPK during T lymphocyte activation. *J Immunol.* 2010;185(2):1037–1044.

245. Ecker C, Guo L, Voicu S, et al. Differential reliance on lipid metabolism as a salvage pathway underlies functional differences of T cell subsets in poor nutrient environments. *Cell Rep.* 2018;23(3):741–755.

246. Scharping NE, Menk AV, Moreci RS, et al. The tumor microenvironment represses T cell mitochondrial biogenesis to drive intratumoral T cell metabolic insufficiency and dysfunction. *Immunity.* 2016;45(2):374–388.

247. Zhang L, Tschumi BO, Lopez-Mejia IC, et al. Mammalian target of rapamycin complex 2 controls CD8 T cell memory differentiation in a foxo1-dependent manner. *Cell Rep.* 2016;14(5):1206–1217.

248. Noman MZ, Desantis G, Janji B, et al. PD-L1 is a novel direct target of HIF-1alpha, and its blockade under hypoxia enhanced MDSC-mediated T cell activation. *J Exp Med.* 2014;211(5):781–790.

249. Barsoum IB, Smallwood CA, Siemens DR, Graham CH. A mechanism of hypoxia-mediated escape from adaptive immunity in cancer cells. *Cancer Res.* 2014;74(3):665–674.

250. Xu Y, Chaudhury A, Zhang M, et al. Glycolysis determines dichotomous regulation of T cell subsets in hypoxia. *J Clin Investig.* 2016;126(7):2678–2688.

251. Doedens AL, Phan AT, Stradner MH, et al. Hypoxia-inducible factors enhance the effector responses of CD8(+) T cells to persistent antigen. *Nat Immunol.* 2013;14(11):1173–1182.

252. Scharping NE, Menk AV, Whetstone RD, Zeng X, Delgoffe GM. Efficacy of PD-1 blockade is potentiated by metformin-induced reduction of tumor hypoxia. *Cancer Immunol Res.* 2017;5(1):9–16.

253. Jayaprakash P, Ai M, Liu A, et al. Targeted hypoxia reduction restores T cell infiltration and sensitizes prostate cancer to immunotherapy. *J Clin Investig.* 2018;128(11):5137–5149.

254. Brand A, Singer K, Koehl GE, et al. LDHA-associated lactic acid production blunts tumor immunosurveillance by T and NK cells. *Cell Metabol.* 2016;24(5):657–671.

255. Haas R, Smith J, Rocher-Ros V, et al. Lactate regulates metabolic and pro-inflammatory circuits in control of T cell migration and effector functions. *PLoS Biol.* 2015;13(7):e1002202.

256. Eil R, Vodnala SK, Clever D, et al. Ionic immune suppression within the tumour microenvironment limits T cell effector function. *Nature.* 2016;537(7621):539–543.

257. Chiang EY, Li T, Jeet S, et al. Potassium channels Kv1.3 and KCa3.1 cooperatively and compensatorily regulate antigen-specific memory T cell functions. *Nat Commun.* 2017;8:14644.

258. Allard B, Longhi MS, Robson SC, Stagg J. The ectonucleotidases CD39 and CD73: novel checkpoint inhibitor targets. *Immunol Rev.* 2017;276(1):121–144.

259. Xu S, Shao QQ, Sun JT, et al. Synergy between the ectoenzymes CD39 and CD73 contributes to adenosinergic immunosuppression in human malignant gliomas. *Neuro Oncol.* 2013;15(9):1160–1172.

260. Linden J, Cekic C. Regulation of lymphocyte function by adenosine. *Arterioscler Thromb Vasc Biol.* 2012;32(9):2097–2103.

261. Erdmann AA, Gao ZG, Jung U, et al. Activation of Th1 and Tc1 cell adenosine A2A receptors directly inhibits IL-2 secretion in vitro and IL-2-driven expansion in vivo. *Blood.* 2005;105(12):4707–4714.

262. Rodriguez G, Ross JA, Nagy ZS, Kirken RA. Forskolin-inducible cAMP pathway negatively regulates T-cell proliferation by uncoupling the interleukin-2 receptor complex. *J Biol Chem.* 2013;288(10):7137–7146.

263. Boussiotis VA, Freeman GJ, Taylor PA, et al. p27kip1 functions as an anergy factor inhibiting interleukin 2 transcription and clonal expansion of alloreactive human and mouse helper T lymphocytes. *Nat Med.* 2000;6(3):290–297.

264. Frumento G, Rotondo R, Tonetti M, Damonte G, Benatti U, Ferrara GB. Tryptophan-derived catabolites are responsible for inhibition of T and natural killer cell proliferation induced by indoleamine 2,3-dioxygenase. *J Exp Med.* 2002;196(4):459–468.

265. Zhai L, Ladomersky E, Lauing KL, et al. Infiltrating T cells increase Ido1 expression in glioblastoma and contribute to decreased patient survival. *Clin Cancer Res.* 2017;23(21):6650–6660.

266. Wainwright DA, Chang AL, Dey M, et al. Durable therapeutic efficacy utilizing combinatorial blockade against Ido, CTLA-4, and PD-L1 in mice with brain tumors. *Clin Cancer Res.* 2014;20(20):5290–5301.

267. Eshhar Z, Waks T, Gross G, Schindler DG. Specific activation and targeting of cytotoxic lymphocytes through chimeric single chains consisting of antibody-binding domains and the gamma or zeta subunits of the immunoglobulin and T-cell receptors. *Proc Natl Acad Sci USA.* 1993;90(2):720–724.

268. Maher J, Brentjens RJ, Gunset G, Riviere I, Sadelain M. Human T-lymphocyte cytotoxicity and proliferation directed by a single chimeric TCRzeta/CD28 receptor. *Nat Biotechnol.* 2002;20(1):70–75.

269. Ruella M, Maus MV. Catch me if you can: leukemia escape after CD19-directed T cell immunotherapies. *Comput Struct Biotechnol J.* 2016;14:357–362.

270. Nowak AK, Lake RA, Marzo AL, et al. Induction of tumor cell apoptosis in vivo increases tumor antigen cross-presentation, cross-priming rather than cross-tolerizing host tumor-specific CD8 T cells. *J Immunol.* 2003;170(10):4905–4913.

271. Bollard CM, Gottschalk S, Torrano V, et al. Sustained complete responses in patients with lymphoma receiving autologous cytotoxic T lymphocytes targeting Epstein-Barr virus latent membrane proteins. *J Clin Oncol.* 2014;32(8):798–808.

272. Hunder NN, Wallen H, Cao J, et al. Treatment of metastatic melanoma with autologous CD4+ T cells against NY-ESO-1. *N Engl J Med.* 2008;358(25):2698–2703.

273. Spitzer MH, Nolan GP. Mass cytometry: single cells, many features. *Cell.* 2016;165(4):780–791.

274. Angelo M, Bendall SC, Finck R, et al. Multiplexed ion beam imaging of human breast tumors. *Nat Med.* 2014;20(4):436–442.

275. Roybal KT, Rupp LJ, Morsut L, et al. Precision tumor recognition by T cells with combinatorial antigen-sensing circuits. *Cell.* 2016;164(4):770–779.

276. Kloss CC, Condomines M, Cartellieri M, Bachmann M, Sadelain M. Combinatorial antigen recognition with balanced signaling promotes selective tumor eradication by engineered T cells. *Nat Biotechnol.* 2013;31(1):71–75.

277. Fedorov VD, Themeli M, Sadelain M. PD-1- and CTLA-4-based inhibitory chimeric antigen receptors (iCARs) divert off-target immunotherapy responses. *Sci Transl Med.* 2013;5(215):215ra172.

278. Fousek K, Watanabe J, George A, et al. Targeting CD19-negative relapsed B-acute lymphoblastic leukemia using trivalent CAR T cells. *J Clin Oncol.* 2018;36(5 suppl):121.

279. Mukherjee M, Mace EM, Carisey AF, Ahmed N, Orange JS. Quantitative imaging approaches to study the CAR immunological synapse. *Mol Ther.* 2017;25(8):1757–1768.

280. Merouane A, Rey-Villamizar N, Lu Y, et al. Automated profiling of individual cell-cell interactions from high-throughput time-lapse imaging microscopy in nanowell grids (TIMING). *Bioinformatics.* 2015;31(19):3189–3197.

281. Turtle CJ, Hanafi LA, Berger C, et al. CD19 CAR-T cells of defined CD4+:CD8+ composition in adult B cell all patients. *J Clin Investig.* 2016;126(6):2123–2138.

282. Wong KM, Capasso A, Eckhardt SG. The changing landscape of phase I trials in oncology. *Nat Rev Clin Oncol.* 2016;13(2):106–117.

283. Onar A, Kocak M, Boyett JM. Continual reassessment method vs. traditional empirically based design: modifications motivated by Phase I trials in pediatric oncology by the Pediatric Brain Tumor Consortium. *J Biopharm Stat.* 2009;19(3):437–455.

284. Norelli M, Camisa B, Barbiera G, et al. Monocyte-derived IL-1 and IL-6 are differentially required for cytokine-release syndrome and neurotoxicity due to CAR T cells. *Nat Med.* 2018;24(6):739–748.

285. Giavridis T, van der Stegen SJC, Eyquem J, Hamieh M, Piersigilli A, Sadelain M. CAR T cell-induced cytokine release syndrome is mediated by macrophages and abated by IL-1 blockade. *Nat Med.* 2018;24(6):731–738.

286. Navai SA, Derenzo C, Joseph S, Sanber K., Byrd T, Zhang H, et al., editors. Administration of HER2-CAR T cells after lymphodepletion safely improves T cell expansion and induces clinical responses in patients with advanced sarcomas. AACR Annual Meeting; 2019; Atlanta, Georgia, United States.

287. Cheng Z, Wei R, Ma Q, et al. In vivo expansion and anti-tumor activity of coinfused CD28- and 4-1BB-engineered CAR-T cells in patients with B cell leukemia. *Mol Ther.* 2018;26(4):976–985.

288. Grossman SA, Ye X, Lesser G, et al. Immunosuppression in patients with high-grade gliomas treated with radiation and temozolomide. *Clin Cancer Res.* 2011;17(16): 5473–5480.

289. Alban TJ, Alvarado AG, Sorensen MD, et al. Global immune fingerprinting in glioblastoma patient peripheral blood reveals immune-suppression signatures associated with prognosis. *JCI Insight.* 2018;3(21).

290. Rajani KR, Carlstrom LP, Parney IF, Johnson AJ, Warrington AE, Burns TC. Harnessing radiation biology to augment immunotherapy for glioblastoma. *Front Oncol.* 2018;8:656.

291. Kim JE, Patel MA, Mangraviti A, et al. Combination therapy with anti-PD-1, anti-TIM-3, and focal radiation results in regression of murine gliomas. *Clin Cancer Res.* 2017;23(1):124–136.

292. Weiss T, Weller M, Guckenberger M, Sentman CL, Roth P. NKG2D-Based CAR T cells and radiotherapy exert synergistic efficacy in glioblastoma. *Cancer Res.* 2018;78(4): 1031–1043.

293. DeSelm C, Palomba ML, Yahalom J, et al. Low-dose radiation conditioning enables CAR T cells to mitigate antigen escape. *Mol Ther.* 2018;26(11):2542–2552.

294. Cao N, Li S, Wang Z, et al. NF-kappaB-mediated HER2 overexpression in radiation-adaptive resistance. *Radiat Res.* 2009;171(1):9–21.

295. Suarez ER, Chang de K, Sun J, et al. Chimeric antigen receptor T cells secreting anti-PD-L1 antibodies more effectively regress renal cell carcinoma in a humanized mouse model. *Oncotarget.* 2016;7(23):34341–34355.

296. Rupp LJ, Schumann K, Roybal KT, et al. CRISPR/Cas9-mediated PD-1 disruption enhances anti-tumor efficacy of human chimeric antigen receptor T cells. *Sci Rep.* 2017;7(1):737.

297. Nishio N, Diaconu I, Liu H, et al. Armed oncolytic virus enhances immune functions of chimeric antigen receptor-modified T cells in solid tumors. *Cancer Res.* 2014;74(18):5195–5205.

298. Tanoue K, Rosewell Shaw A, Watanabe N, et al. Armed oncolytic adenovirus-expressing PD-L1 mini-body enhances antitumor effects of chimeric antigen receptor T cells in solid tumors. *Cancer Res.* 2017;77(8): 2040–2051.

299. Pegram HJ, Lee JC, Hayman EG, et al. Tumor-targeted T cells modified to secrete IL-12 eradicate systemic tumors without need for prior conditioning. *Blood.* 2012; 119(18):4133–4141.

300. Chmielewski M, Kopecky C, Hombach AA, Abken H. IL-12 release by engineered T cells expressing chimeric antigen receptors can effectively Muster an antigen-independent macrophage response on tumor cells that have shut down tumor antigen expression. *Cancer Res.* 2011;71(17):5697–5706.

301. Riese MJ, Wang LC, Moon EK, et al. Enhanced effector responses in activated CD8+ T cells deficient in diacylglycerol kinases. *Cancer Res.* 2013;73(12):3566–3577.

CHAPTER 13

CAR 2.0: The Next Generation of Synthetic Receptor–Based Cellular Therapy for Cancer

ELAD JACOBY, MD • TERRY J. FRY, MD

INTRODUCTION

The growing clinical experience with chimeric antigen receptor (CAR) T-cells targeting CD19 has indicated that this therapy can induce remission in a high percentage of relapsed and refractory patients with B-cell precursor acute lymphoblastic leukemia (BCP-ALL) or B-cell non-Hodgkin's lymphoma (NHL) that is durable in some patients but has also highlighted a number of challenges. These include relapse of malignancy that retains expression of CD19 associated with lack of CAR persistence or the emergence of leukemia no longer expressing the target antigen. In addition, complex patterns of toxicities are being observed that, unlike cytokine release syndrome (CRS), can be unpredictable. These challenges have led to ongoing efforts to improve the CAR manufacturing platform and construct design. These improvements are also being developed to facilitate the expansion of this promising therapy to novel indications for other hematologic malignancies, solid tumors, and nonmalignant disorders. These challenges, along with potential solutions, are summarized in Table 13.1 and will be addressed throughout this chapter. The first three challenges have already been observed in patients treated with products targeting CD19 already approved by the Food and Drug Administration (FDA) and the European Medicines Agency (EMA), while the remaining represent gaps likely to emerge in the future design of CAR T-cells for hematologic and nonhematologic malignancies.

IMPROVING PERSISTENCE

The Advantage of Costimulation

The major design improvement leading to success of CAR T-cells in patients was the addition of a costimulatory domain to the CAR backbone,[1] providing a second signal in addition to that provided by the T-cell receptor signaling domain,[2] leading to enhanced T-cell engagement and persistence in preclinical models and clinical trials.[3,4] The two most common costimulatory domains included in the CAR construct are CD28 and 4-1BB (CD137) although others, such as OX40[5], have been tested in patients. Inherent differences between CD28 and 4-1BB in relation to T-cell activation via the endogenous T-cell receptor appear to have functional implications when implemented in the CAR design. CD28 is uniformly expressed on T-cells, is activated by binding to CD80 or CD86 on antigen-presenting cells, and leads to rapid activation of the T-cell with a skewing toward effector differentiation. 4-1BB, on the other hand, is expressed only on activated T-cells and, when engaged by its ligand (4-1BBL), leads to further stimulation of the T-cell but skewed toward a memory T-cell phenotype.[6] Consistent with this natural biology, preclinical work has shown that synthetic 4-1BB-containing CARs are less prone to T-cell exhaustion and lead to superior T-cell persistence in animal models.[7,8] Indeed, T-cell durability has been observed in many clinical trials using 4-1BB-based CARs and, although not directly compared, seems more prolonged than persistence of CD28-based CARs. Third-generation CARs, incorporating two costimulatory domains, introduce an additional layer of complexity and have shown superiority to second-generation CD28-based CARs in small series although results have been inconsistent.[9] Preclinical work incorporating ICOS in addition to 4-1BB has demonstrated superiority of these third-generation CARs in some studies[10] but have not been tested in patients. An alternative design was introduced, which uses the natural ligand for 4-1BB, 4-1BBL introduced into the T-cells with a CD28-based second generation CAR, and generates the complementary ligand activation by

Chimeric Antigen Receptor T-Cell Therapies for Cancer. https://doi.org/10.1016/B978-0-323-66181-2.00013-5

TABLE 13.1
Brief summary of challenges and potential solutions in CAR T-cell therapy.

Challenges	Potential Solutions
Loss of CAR T-cell persistence	• Improved costimulation to avoid exhaustion • PD-1 deletion in CAR product • Use of stem cell memory cells • Humanized scFv • Ensuring "physiologic" activation of CAR
Loss of target antigen on the malignant T-cells	• Combined targeting of several antigens
Short-term toxicity (CRS and ICANS)	• On/off switch • Suicide gene • CAR construct design (modifications to signaling domain or binding domain)
Specificity of targeting, preventing on-target, off-tumor effects	• Combined targeting and logic gating • Deletion of target from nonmalignant T-cells
Improved localization in the tumor microenvironment or CNS	• PD1-deleted T-cells as CAR backbone • Introduction of additional adhesion molecules or receptors (chemokines)
Using off-the-shelf platforms for cellular therapy	• Deletion of endogenous TCR • Use of NK cells as CAR platform

CAR, chimeric antigen receptor; *CNS*, central nervous system; *CRS*, cytokine release syndrome; *ICANS*, immune effector cell–associated neurotoxicity syndrome; *NK*, natural killer; *TCR*, T-cell receptor.

cis-signaling, leading to improved function and durability in preclinical models.[3] This approach, termed "armored CAR," is currently tested in a clinical trial (NCT03085173), with preliminary results demonstrating persistence in several patients.[11] Finally, targeted mutation-selective immune-receptor tyrosine-based activation motifs (ITAMs) in the CD3 zeta chain of CD28 containing CARs have also demonstrated improved persistence in preclinical studies, suggesting

that the alterations to the CAR design can modify in vivo behavior of CAR T-cells.[12]

TARGETING T-CELL INHIBITORY CHECKPOINTS

Exhaustion is a main contributor to loss of functionality and durability of T-cells stimulated through the endogenous T-cell receptor and is mediated by several receptors, including CTLA-4 and PD-1.[13] Administration of antibodies blocking these immune checkpoint pathways has led to long-term remissions in patients with solid tumors and Hodgkin's lymphoma, resulting in FDA and EMA approval. Theoretically, these agents could enhance activity and persistence of CAR T-cells, a question being studied in numerous clinical trials (for example, NCT03726515 and NCT03287817). As an engineering strategy, genetic deletion of PD-1 in T-cells prior to CAR transduction was performed and showed improved functionality in preclinical models.[14] This approach has not reached clinical trials yet.

Use of Memory-Driving Cytokines and T-Cell Subset Selection

Cytokines, mostly commonly interleukin-2 (IL-2),[15] have been used to support the expansion and persistence of transferred tumor-infiltrating nonengineered ex vivo expanded T-cells. The high levels of cytokines produced by activated CAR T-cells, demonstrated in both preclinical and clinical settings, have been sufficient to support expansion, persistence, and activity of CD19 CAR T-cells. However, the use of cytokines in the context of CAR T-cells has not been abandoned, as cytokines other than IL-2 are currently being used during the CAR T-cell production or to support T-cells in vivo to improved persistence.[16] Several groups are culturing T-cells with IL-7 and IL-15 with the intention of increasing central memory T-cell differentiation. Clinical grade IL-7 and IL-15 are available, and administration of these memory-driving gamma cytokines following CAR T-cell administration may be feasible, though this has yet to be tested. Use of stem cell memory T-cell subsets (T_{scm})[17] as the starting cellular product for CAR T manufacturing may lead to even better memory subsets and persistence.[18] Selective expansion of $CD8^+$ T_{scm} CAR T-cells may be facilitated by the addition of IL-7 and IL-21 in culture, potentially resulting in a superior product compared with nonselected CD28-based CAR T in preclinical models, but was dependent on cytokine support (due to lack of $CD4^+$ cells). Comparison of this approach to a "standard" 4-1BB-based CAR in humans has not been performed. To provide better cytokines without exogenous support, fourth-generation CARs have been generated using bicistronic vectors leading to continuous cytokine production along with CAR expression, resulting in reduced exhaustion and improved persistence.[19–21]

Anti—Chimeric Antigen Receptor Immune Response

T-cell exhaustion is not the sole reason for lack of persistence of CAR T-cells, as several groups have demonstrated an anti-CAR immune response, resulting in elimination of CAR T-cells.[22,23] CARs are composed of multiple foreign component that may be recognized by the immune system including the murine single-chain variable fraction (scFv) as well as several potential neoepitopes arising from nonphysiologic junctions, the C28-CD3zeta junction as an example. In the case of B-cell—targeting CARs, a humoral response is less likely because of B-cell aplasia as an expected side effect of CAR therapy, but a T-cell—mediated anti-CAR response has been demonstrated, resulting in loss of CAR+ T-cells and failure following reinfusion.[22,23] To overcome this, humanized scFvs have been incorporated into CAR design, leading to preclinical efficacy as well as early clinical success, even in patients failing a prior murine-scFv-based CD19 CAR[24,25] although it remains to be determined whether this approach will overcome poor responses to reinfusions. Abrogating potential immune response neoepitopes encoded by novel junction regions in the synthetic CAR will be more challenging.

PREVENTING LOSS OF TARGET ANTIGEN

Although CD19 was carefully chosen and is thought to be essential for BCP-ALL and NHL, loss of CD19 expression has been increasingly observed following targeted immunotherapy.[26] Indeed, two-thirds of patients with ALL relapsing after CD19 CAR T-cell products result from leukemic resistance mediated by loss of antigen. Antigen loss has been difficult to predict in patients prior to infusion of CAR T-cells and has been observed more commonly with long-persisting CAR T-cells, suggesting that strategies to sustain CAR T-cell persistence may increase this pattern of relapse.[27] The mechanisms of antigen loss are variable and include mutations affecting anchoring of CD19 to the membrane,[28] alternative splicing of exons 2, 4, 5, or 6 of CD19 affecting the extracellular domain,[29] trafficking defects, as well as more complex mechanism such as clonal evolution or lineage switch.[30–33] Since the 1960s, combination of cytotoxic agents targeting different pathways have been used successfully to induce durable remission in

patients with leukemia and other malignancies and have become the standard. Thus, combination targeting may be useful in preventing antigen loss as an escape mechanism from CAR T-cells.

Like CD19, CD22 is an alternative B-cell—restricted antigen expressed on the majority of BCP-ALL and NHL, although at lower antigen density than CD19.[34] CD22 has been successfully targeted by antibody conjugates, leading to clinical remissions in patients with ALL.[35,36] CD22 was also the second ALL antigen to be successfully targeted by CAR T-cells in clinical studies, but development of a clinically active CAR for CD22 entailed choosing a different scFv than that used for immunotoxins, targeting a more proximal epitope of CD22.[37] Embedding a 4-1BB costimulatory domain enhanced persistence and resulted in a 70% remission rate in the first clinical trial.[38] Despite persistence, the majority of patients relapsed after initial response, primarily due to antigen diminution/loss, again demonstrating the challenges in single antigen targeting. Importantly, the disadvantage of single-antigen targeting is not unique to hematologic malignancies. One of the first reports of success following intraventricular administration of an IL13-receptor α2 (IL13Rα2) CAR for a patient with glioblastoma, a deep and prolonged remission was followed by recurrence of a lesion, lacking IL13Rα2[39] and a similar pattern of antigen loss has been observed in multiple patients receiving an EGFRvIII targeted CAR.[40]

The availability of two clinically validated CAR constructs expressed on the same malignancy has enabled the testing of the logical hypothesis that combined targeting of two or more antigens expressed on the malignant cell, which may reduce antigen loss and lead to superior outcome. This may be achieved through several methods as depicted in Fig. 13.1:

1. Coinfusion of two different CAR T-cell products manufactured separately.
2. Cotransduction of two CARs into the same T-cell using separate viral vectors, resulting in the possibility of both single-CAR-expressing T-cells and double-CAR-expressing T-cells.
3. Uniform introduction of two CARs using the same viral vector (using a bicistronic vector) resulting in a single dual-targeted CAR T-cell population.
4. Transduction with a single CAR construct endowed with bispecificity using via two separate antigen-binding domains (tandem or bivalent CARs).

All of the above methods have been used in preclinical studies, and some are already in clinical trials.

B-cell NHL, arising from mature B-cells, expresses both CD19 and CD20, and CD20-based antibodies

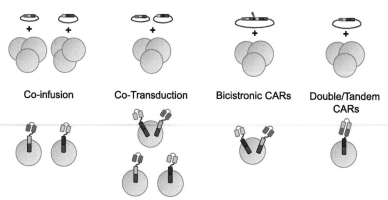

FIG. 13.1 Models of dual chimeric antigen receptor (CAR) targeting. Four models of targeting two antigens to prevent antigen negative relapse: (1) coinfusion of two separately transduced T-cells, resulting in two different CAR T-cell populations. (2) Cotransduction of the same bulk of cells with two different CARs, resulting in two single-transduced populations and one double-transduced population. (3) Cotransduction of T-cells with a single vector encoding for two different CARs, which will be expressed in a 1:1 ratio on the same cell. (4) Transduction of a single double-targeting CAR, with two single chain variable fractions against both antigens, with the same signaling domains. In all cotransduction options (1—3), the costimulatory domain and primary signaling chain can be different in each CAR, while in the double or tandem CAR, this is the same predefined unit.

are given as standard of care for these patients. Thus, a combined CD19-CD20 tandem CAR was designed and has demonstrated efficacy against the CD19-CD20 double-positive Burkitt lymphoma cell line Raji.[41] Dual CD19 and CD22 CAR targeting has been shown to be effective in preclinical models of ALL.[38,42] Importantly, the CD22 moiety has shown clinical efficacy in eradicating leukemic cells not expressing CD19, and the tandem CAR construct was superior to sequential coinfusion and to cotransduction of both CD19 and CD22 CARs.[42] Other bispecific CARs showing preclinical efficacy are, for example, the bicistronic CD19-CD123 CAR, adding the targeting of CD123, the receptor for IL3, known to be expressed on acute myeloid leukemia (AML) and have retained expression on B-ALL despite loss of CD19,[43] and a tandem CD19-CD37 CAR, targeting B-cell and, potentially, T-cell malignancies.[44] In solid tumors, a tandem CAR targeting IL13Rα2 and HER2 resulted in improved outcome of mice with orthotopically implanted glioblastoma compared with single targeting or other forms of pooled combined targeting or cotransduction of cells.[45] Currently, several clinical trials are evaluating combined targeting of CD19 and CD22 for ALL and NHL, CD19 and CD20 for NHL, BCMA and CD19 for myeloma as well as other combinations, with preliminary data showing efficacy of the approach, but true

value in terms of improved durability of remissions awaiting long-term results.

REDUCING SHORT-TERM TOXICITY

Robust activation of immune effector cells via the CAR has led to severe toxicities, termed CRS and immune effector cell—associated neurotoxicity syndrome (ICANS). Detailed clinical, pathophysiological, and management aspects of these syndromes are covered in another chapters of this book. Here, we will discuss several methods of receptor and cellular design that aim to abrogate or control these adverse events. Most have been only tested in preclinical models, and given the complexity of modeling CRS and ICANS, effectiveness in reducing toxicity will require human trials.

Genetic engineering of T-cells with constructs that, if expressed and activated, will lead to apoptosis, termed "suicide gene," has been used in the setting of allogeneic donor lymphocyte infusion for more than two decades. The most extensively tested suicide gene is the inducible caspase 9 (iCasp9), which initiates the intrinsic pathway of apoptosis but is resistant to physiologic signals of the apoptosome, and can only dimerize and signal when binding to the synthetic dimerizing drug rimiducid.[46,47] Use of rimiducid following iCasp9-engineered haploidentical lymphocyte infusion leads to rapid resolution of graft-versus-host disease (GVHD),[48] demonstrating safety and feasibility of this approach. Several groups have included an iCasp9 in the vector encoding for the CAR, but no clinical use in this context has been reported thus far. In vivo deletion of CAR T-cells may be also achieved via antibodies targeting a nonsignaling protein expressed along with the CAR, such as truncated EGFR (tEGFR). Coexpression of a CAR with tEGRF is used in clinical trials,[49] and CAR T-cell elimination by cetuximab was achieved in murine models, reverting B-cell aplasia and hypogammaglobulinemia.[50]

Short-term CAR expression may also be achieved by nonintegrating methods of CAR transduction, such as mRNA electroporation. In the first clinical trial reported using this method, four patients with Hodgkin's lymphoma received several infusions of CD19-CAR-T-cells, resulting in transient CAR persistence (days) and limited remissions in these patients, with no immune-based toxicity.[51]

Given the importance of CAR T-cell persistence for some forms of malignancy, a more balanced control switch may be desired, in which the CAR activation may be switched on or off according to a pharmacological signal. One nonengineered controlled that has been reported preclinically is dasatinib, a tyrosine-kinase inhibitor known to target Src, Abl1, Fyn, and Lck, thus inhibiting the downstream CAR signaling, with full recovery of CAR T-cell function once drug is stopped.[52,53] Since myeloid cells are essential for CAR-mediated toxicity, GM-CSF neutralization, achieved by either inhibitory antibodies or genetic knockout from the CAR T-cells, resulted in reduction of CRS and CNS inflammation in murine models, without impacting the CAR efficacy.[54]

On/off switches of CAR expression can be achieved also through synthetic-Notch receptor system. Here, T-cells are transduced to express two different receptors, in which the antigen recognition of one (signal A) will trigger the expression of the other CAR, resulting in an AND logic gate.[55] Absence of signal A will stop transcription, and CAR expression will be limited by its natural turnover.[55,56]

Last, minor changes in nonsignaling areas may have vast impact on CAR efficacy and outcome. Changes in several amino acids around the transmembrane hinge of CD19-4-1BB-based CARs led to limited but controlled cytokine activations in vitro and to clinical remissions in vivo with 14 of 15 reported patients having no CRS and 1 having grade 1 CRS.[57]

IMPROVING TUMOR SPECIFICITY

The main barrier in expanding the success of CD19 CAR T-cells to other malignancies is the concern for on-target, off-tumor toxicities, given lack of tumor specificity of many antigens selected as CAR targets. This effect was initially seen when using T-cell receptor (TCR)—based immunotherapy, where T-cells aiming at targeting MAGE-A3 restricted via HLA-A:01 or HLA-A:02 recognized titin or MAGE-A12, leading to fatal cardiac[58] and neurologic[59] toxicity, respectively. In B-cell malignancies, an on-target, off-tumor effect is almost unanimously seen, resulting in B-cell aplasia following CAR T-cell activation, but this lacks significant morbidity since patients can receive supplementation of immunoglobulin. While choosing different targets that may be expressed on normal cells, this effect may have devastating results. Rarely, a cell-surface expressed antigen can be found to be restricted to malignant cells, necessitating rigorous efforts to discover off-tumor expression even at low levels to prevent severe on-target, off-tumor toxicity, including the use of normal tissue microarray and induced pluripotent stem cell—based assays.[60]

We previously described combined signaling for multi-targeting aiming to prevent antigen loss, and for controlled expression to prevent toxicity. Similarly, multi-targeting using a combinatorial approach may lead to better targeting despite shared antigens between tumor and normal tissue. One approach is to abandon highly functional second-generation CARs and to split the signal with two scFvs, one providing signal 1 and the other providing signal 2 (Fig. 13.2A). Only through combined interactions will the CAR provide a sustained signaling and thus may spare normal cells. Another approach is using a second-generation CAR combined with an inhibitory CAR, incorporating a PD-1 signal, leading to SHP2 activation and subsequent inhibition of CD28-based and ZAP70 signaling, for example (Fig. 13.2B). In this case, the negative signal provides protection for normal cells expressing the targeted antigen. This approach is being explored in AML, which expresses many targetable antigens with some overlap with normal hematopoietic progenitor and stem cells, and through proteomic studies, targets may be identified and combinations provided.[61]

Another approach for prevention of on-target, off-tumor effects is removing the target from normal tissues. This is applied in T-cell malignancies, since the T-cell leukemia/lymphoma expression repertoire is similar to those on normal T-cells, and transduction with CARs may lead to fratricide. Several options have emerged for targeting T-ALL, either through targeting T-cell leukemia/lymphoma-specific antigens not expressed on normal T-cells (such as CD37),[44] through selection of a portion of the T-cells to target via selective TCR expression,[62] via natural selection in the culture of

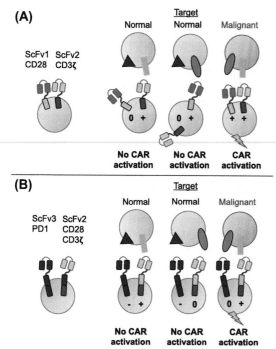

(A)

(B)

FIG. 13.2 Methods of cotargeting to prevent on-target, off-tumor toxicity. The chimeric antigen receptor (CAR) T-cells are depicted in the left side. Normal cells (gray) express not only some of the targets but also nontumor antigens, while the malignant T-cells have two predefined targets and lack one normal antigen. In example A (top), upon recognition of antigen, CAR1 will provide costimulation via CD28, and CAR2 will provide primary CD3-zeta signaling. Only if both antigens are on the same cell, will the CAR T-cell achieve sufficient stimuli to activate. In example B (bottom), the T-cell is transduced with a second-generation CAR targeting one antigen that is shared between normal and malignant tissue. The T-cells also express a negative CAR (via ScFv3) that has an inhibitory signaling domain such as the PD1 intracellular ITIMs. Thus, CAR T-cells will activate only in the presence of the targeted antigen (by ScFv2) and in the absence of the negative ligand for scFv3.

CD5-low T-cells using a CD5 CAR,[63] or following knockout of CD3 by TALEN-mediated disruption or CD7 by CRISPR/Cas9 mechanisms, followed by transduction of CD3 or CD7 CARs, respectively.[64–66] Some of these approaches are entering the clinical arena (e.g., NCT03690011). Removing the normal target from nonmalignant cells, as performed with CD7-CARs, has been also conceptualized in preclinical work in AML, where rhesus macaques received CD33-deleted hematopoietic stem cells, which were resistant to CD33-directed CARs given as treatment for AML.[67] Despite potential of such knockouts in hematopoietic

tissues, this will be difficult when dealing with antigens expressed in solid organs. Thus, for solid malignancies, addressing off-tumor targeting is to be performed by limitation of CAR expansion and achieved by either cotransduction of suicide genes, on/off switches or repeated infusion of very-short persisting RNA-based CARs, as described in a previous section.

IMPROVING TUMOR LOCALIZATION

A major barrier of advancing CAR T-cells into solid tumors is not just antigen specificity but also the suppressive microenvironment surrounding the malignant cells, creating a barrier for T-cell infiltration. The minimal manipulation of the microenvironment carried by the lymphodepleting conditioning, as performed routinely prior to CAR T-cells administered for hematologic malignancies, may not be sufficient for solid tumors.

A simple case of targeting the microenvironment is by disrupting the PD1-PDL1-mediated immune suppression in PDL1+-expressing tumors, as was shown in a model of genetic disruption of PD1 on the T-cells prior to CAR transduction.[14] The use of cytokine-augmented CARs, as discussed before, may improve localization and trafficking in the suppressive tumor microenvironment. IL-18 and IL-21 were found to increase effector functions of anti-CEA CAR T-cells, inducing regression of large established pancreatic tumors in murine models and altering the microenvironment by reducing myeloid-derived suppressor cells and regulatory T-cells.[68]

More complex challenges present when targeting tumors in the central nervous system (CNS), which are considered incurable, and lay in a restricted immune tissue. CARs targeting HER2 and IL13Rα2 have been designed for glioblastoma, the most aggressive CNS tumor, and have shown preclinical success in orthotopically injected xenograft models.[69,70] However, when administered intravenously, poor trafficking of T-cells was observed into tumor lesions in the CNS.[40] Improved response was seen with direct intraventricular injection, leading to remissions and limited only by loss of antigen expression,[39] but this injection mechanism is complex and may not be feasible in many institutions. Interestingly, CD19-CAR-T-cells have been shown to penetrate the CNS and eliminate residual leukemic cells,[22] eluding to differences between solid tumors and leukemia in this compartment.

USING OFF-THE-SHELF PLATFORMS FOR CELLULAR THERAPY

Availability of CAR T-cells as an off-the-shelf product will further revolutionize the field of adoptive T-cell therapy. Currently, in academic center–based clinical trials, the waiting time from apheresis to cell administration ranges between 7 and 14 days on average. In FDA- and EMA-approved products, this is currently longer (average ~ 1 month), leading to a significant dropout of 5%–30% between patients infused and those actually receiving therapy.[71–73] Generation of cellular products ready-to-use from third-party donors requires eliminating the risks of GVHD driven by the effector cells and of rejection of the foreign cells by the host immune system. To use T-cells for this cause, use of nonallogeneic TCR or its deletion by TALEN[74] or CRISPR/Cas9[75] may abrogate GVHD but will not ensure engraftment and persistence of delivered cells. The use of viral-specific T-cells, which have been used in third parties and are controlled for a viral-specific nonallogeneic TCR, has been successful against viral infections[76] but has shown limited efficacy as a platform for CARs.[77,78] TCR-deleted third-party cells have been administered to patients, following extensive manipulation of the cells, including CD19 CAR transduction, TALEN mRNA electroporation aiming to delete *TRAC* and *CD52*, followed by a final step of αβ-TCR depletion using immunomagnetic beads on a cliniMACS system.[79] Thus, cells were absent of potential GVHD (via TCR deletion) and were resistant to alemtuzumab, an anti-CD52 monoclonal antibody, that was given for conditioning of the patient, resulting in broad deletion of CD52 expressing B, T, and NK cells capable of rejection of third-party cells. This approach led to clinical remission in two initial reported patients but, despite deletion of the TCR from third-party cells, resulted in brief GVHD episodes controlled with medical therapy. Also, prolonged alemtuzumab-induced immune suppression necessitated a consolidative hematopoietic stem cell transplantation.[79] As mentioned before, using a CRISPR/Cas9 system for gene editing not only may result in avoidance of GVHD due to the absence of the native TCR but may also lead to more physiologic expression of the CAR, if it "highjacks" the normal regulatory elements for the T-cells.[66,75] Several concerns regarding off-target gene editing have been raised using CRISPR technologies, leading to undesired genomic insertions and deletions,[80] and screening for such should be standardized when clinical-grade products are generated. Nevertheless, despite lacking GVHD potential, these cells are likely to be rejected by the host, given different MHC expression or its lack-of.

An alternative solution relies on abandoning the regular T-cells as effectors, and using other lymphocyte effectors, such as natural killer (NK) lymphocytes, known to be able to mediate effector functions across HLA barriers, or γδT-cells, with similar safety profiles across HLA mismatches. Limitations of using NK cells as CAR platforms are mainly caused by limited in vivo expansion and persistence, even if CAR signaling is designed specifically for NKs.[81,82] A potential solution was recently described using cord blood–derived NK cells, which are naïve but, via IL-21 and 41BBL stimulation (bound to feeder K562 cells), lead to appropriate expansion and successful transduction in vitro. The transduced cells expressed, along with a CD19 CAR, an iCasp9 safety switch, and interleukin-15 (IL15), an important cytokine for NK cell proliferation and T-cell memory.[83] These NK cells have a median expansion of over 2000-fold, with a potential of 100 products made from 1 cord blood. Preliminary data show durable remissions accompanied by a very low toxicity profile, making this a promising approach with relatively minimal intervention for off-the-shelf cells.

SUMMARY

CAR T-cells are one of the first genetically modified cells produced to be approved for commercial use by several regulatory agencies. Technological advances in genome editing are likely to change the landscape of CAR T-cells in the future, addressing many of the challenges seen today using these cells. Multiple targeting, crossing immune-restricted barriers, controlled durability, and even immediate availability of off-the-shelf CARs are possibilities that once seemed remote are currently within our reach.

REFERENCES

1. Gross G, Waks T, Eshhar Z. Expression of immunoglobulin-T-cell receptor chimeric molecules as functional receptors with antibody-type specificity. *Proc Natl Acad Sci.* 1989;86(24):10024–10028. https://doi.org/10.1073/pnas.86.24.10024.
2. Sadelain M. CAR therapy: the CD19 paradigm. *J Clin Invest.* 2015;125(9):3392–3400. https://doi.org/10.1172/JCI80010.
3. Zhao Z, Condomines M, van der Stegen SJC, et al. Structural design of engineered costimulation determines tumor rejection kinetics and persistence of CAR T cells. *Cancer Cell.* 2015;28(4):415–428. https://doi.org/10.1016/j.ccell.2015.09.004.
4. Savoldo B, Ramos CA, Liu E, et al. CD28 costimulation improves expansion and persistence of chimeric antigen receptor-modified T cells in lymphoma patients. *J Clin Invest.* 2011;121(5):1822–1826. https://doi.org/10.1172/JCI46110.
5. Pulè MA, Straathof KC, Dotti G, Heslop HE, Rooney CM, Brenner MK. A chimeric T cell antigen receptor that

augments cytokine release and supports clonal expansion of primary human T cells. *Mol Ther.* 2005;12(5):933–941.

6. Chester C, Sanmamed MF, Wang J, Melero I. Immunotherapy targeting 4-1BB: mechanistic rationale, clinical results, and future strategies. *Blood.* 2018;131(1):49–57. https://doi.org/10.1182/blood-2017-06-741041.

7. Long AH, Haso WM, Shern JF, et al. 4-1BB costimulation ameliorates T cell exhaustion induced by tonic signaling of chimeric antigen receptors. *Nat Med.* 2015;21(6): 581–590. https://doi.org/10.1038/nm.3838.

8. Kawalekar OU, O'Connor RS, Fraietta JA, et al. Distinct signaling of coreceptors regulates specific metabolism pathways and impacts memory development in CAR T cells. *Immunity.* 2016;44(2):380–390. https://doi.org/10.1016/j.immuni.2016.01.021.

9. Ramos CA, Rouce R, Robertson CS, et al. In vivo fate and activity of second- versus third-generation CD19-specific CAR-T cells in B cell non-Hodgkin's lymphomas. *Mol Ther.* September 2018. https://doi.org/10.1016/J.YMTHE.2018.09.009.

10. Guedan S, Posey AD, Shaw C, et al. Enhancing CAR T cell persistence through ICOS and 4-1BB costimulation. *JCI Insight.* 2018;3(1):1–17. https://doi.org/10.1172/jci.insight.96976.

11. Park JH, Palomba ML, Batlevi CL, et al. A phase I first-in-human clinical trial of CD19-targeted 19-28z/4-1BBL "armored" CAR T cells in patients with relapsed or refractory NHL and CLL including Richter's transformation. *Blood.* 2018;132:224. https://doi.org/10.1182/blood-2018-99-117737.

12. Feucht J, Sun J, Eyquem J, et al. Calibration of CAR activation potential directs alternative T cell fates and therapeutic potency. *Nat Med.* 2019;25:82–88. https://doi.org/10.1038/s41591-018-0290-5.

13. Wherry EJ. T cell exhaustion. *Nat Immunol.* 2011;12(6): 492–499. https://doi.org/10.1038/ni.2035.

14. Rupp LJ, Schumann K, Roybal KT, et al. CRISPR/Cas9-mediated PD-1 disruption enhances anti-tumor efficacy of human chimeric antigen receptor T cells. *Sci Rep.* 2017; 7(1):737. https://doi.org/10.1038/s41598-017-00462-8.

15. Rosenberg SA, Packard B, Aebersold PM, et al. Use of tumor-infiltrating lymphocytes and interleukin-2 in the immunotherapy of patients with metastatic melanoma. *N Engl J Med.* 1988;319(25):1676–1680.

16. Dwyer CJ, Knochelmann HM, Smith AS, et al. Fueling cancer immunotherapy with common gamma chain cytokines. *Front Immunol.* 2019;10:263. https://doi.org/10.3389/fimmu.2019.00263.

17. Gattinoni L, Zhong X-S, Palmer DC, et al. Wnt signaling arrests effector T cell differentiation and generates CD8+ memory stem cells. *Nat Med.* 2009;15:808.

18. Sabatino M, Hu J, Sommariva M, et al. Generation of clinical-grade CD19-specific CAR-modified CD8+ memory stem cells for the treatment of human B-cell malignancies. *Blood.* 2016;128(4):519–529. https://doi.org/10.1182/blood-2015-11-683847.

19. Hoyos V, Savoldo B, Quintarelli C, et al. Engineering CD19-specific T lymphocytes with interleukin-15 and a suicide gene to enhance their anti-lymphoma/leukemia effects and safety. *Leukemia.* 2010;24(6):1160–1170. https://doi.org/10.1038/leu.2010.75.

20. Chmielewski M, Abken H. TRUCKs: the fourth generation of CARs. *Expert Opin Biol Ther.* 2015;15(8):1145–1154. https://doi.org/10.1517/14712598.2015.1046430.

21. Hu B, Ren J, Luo Y, et al. Augmentation of antitumor immunity by human and mouse CAR T cells secreting IL-18. *Cell Rep.* 2017;20(13):3025–3033. https://doi.org/10.1101/111260.

22. Lee DW, Kochenderfer JN, Stetler-Stevenson M, et al. T cells expressing CD19 chimeric antigen receptors for acute lymphoblastic leukaemia in children and young adults: a phase 1 dose-escalation trial. *Lancet.* 2015; 385(9967):517–528. https://doi.org/10.1016/S0140-6736(14)61403-3.

23. Turtle CJ, Riddell SR, Maloney DG, et al. CD19 CAR–T-cells of defined CD4+:CD8+ composition in adult B cell ALL patients. *J Clin Invest.* 2016;126(6):2123–2138. https://doi.org/10.1172/JCI85309DS1.

24. Sommermeyer D, Hill T, Shamah SM, et al. Fully human CD19-specific chimeric antigen receptors for T-cell therapy. *Leukemia.* 2017;31(10):2191–2199. https://doi.org/10.1038/leu.2017.57.

25. Maude SL, Barrett DM, Rheingold SR, et al. Efficacy of humanized CD19-targeted chimeric antigen receptor (CAR)-Modified T cells in children and young adults with relapsed/refractory acute lymphoblastic leukemia. *Blood.* 2016;128(217).

26. Mejstríková E, Hrusak O, Borowitz MJ, et al. CD19-negative relapse of pediatric B-cell precursor acute lymphoblastic leukemia following blinatumomab treatment. *Blood Cancer J.* 2017;7(12):659. https://doi.org/10.1038/s41408-017-0023-x.

27. Hay KA, Gauthier J, Hirayama AV, et al. Factors associated with durable EFS in adult B-cell ALL patients achieving MRD-negative CR after CD19 CAR-T cells. *Blood.* 2019; 133(15). https://doi.org/10.1182/blood-2018-11-883710.

28. Orlando EJ, Han X, Tribouley C, et al. Genetic mechanisms of target antigen loss in CAR19 therapy of acute lymphoblastic leukemia. *Nat Med.* 2018;1. https://doi.org/10.1038/s41591-018-0146-z.

29. Sotillo E, Barrett DMDM, Black KLKL, et al. Convergence of acquired mutations and alternative splicing of CD19 enables resistance to CART-19 immunotherapy. *Cancer Discov.* 2015;5(12):1282–1295. https://doi.org/10.1158/2159-8290.CD-15-1020.

30. Evans AG, Rothberg PG, Burack WR, et al. Evolution to plasmablastic lymphoma evades CD19-directed chimeric antigen receptor T cells. *Br J Haematol.* 2015;171(2): 205–209. https://doi.org/10.1111/bjh.13562.

31. Jacoby E, Nguyen SM, Fountaine TJ, et al. CD19 CAR immune pressure induces B-precursor acute lymphoblastic leukaemia lineage switch exposing inherent leukaemic plasticity. *Nat Commun.* 2016;7(May):12320. https://doi.org/10.1038/ncomms12320.

32. Gardner R, Wu D, Cherian S, et al. Acquisition of a CD19 negative myeloid phenotype allows immune escape of

MLL-rearranged B-ALL from CD19 CAR-T cell therapy. *Blood*. 2016. https://doi.org/10.1182/blood-2015-08-665547.

33. Oberley MJ, Gaynon PS, Bhojwani D, et al. Myeloid lineage switch following chimeric antigen receptor T-cell therapy in a patient with TCF3-ZNF384 fusion-positive B-lymphoblastic leukemia. *Pediatr Blood Cancer*. 2018; 65(9):e27265. https://doi.org/10.1002/pbc.27265.

34. Shah NN, Stetler-Stevenson M, Yuan CM, et al. Characterization of CD22 expression in acute lymphoblastic leukemia. *Pediatr Blood Cancer*. 2015;62(6):964−969. https://doi.org/10.1002/pbc.

35. Wayne AS, Shah NN, Bhojwani D, et al. Phase I Study of the anti-CD22 immunotoxin moxetumomab pasudotox for childhood acute lymphoblastic leukemia. *Blood*. 2017;130(14):5−9. https://doi.org/10.1182/blood-2017-02-749101.

36. Kantarjian HM, DeAngelo DJ, Stelljes M, et al. Inotuzumab ozogamicin versus standard therapy for acute lymphoblastic leukemia. *N Engl J Med*. 2016;375(8):740−753. https://doi.org/10.1056/NEJMoa1509277.

37. Haso W, Lee DW, Shah NN, et al. Anti-CD22-chimeric antigen receptors targeting B-cell precursor acute lymphoblastic leukemia. *Blood*. 2013;121(7):1165−1174. https://doi.org/10.1182/blood-2012-06-438002.

38. Fry TJ, Shah NN, Orentas RJ, et al. CD22-targeted CAR T cells induce remission in B-ALL that is naive or resistant to CD19-targeted CAR immunotherapy. *Nat Med*. 2018; 24(1):20−28. https://doi.org/10.1038/nm.4441.

39. Brown CE, Alizadeh D, Starr R, et al. Regression of glioblastoma after chimeric antigen receptor T-cell therapy. *N Engl J Med*. 2016;375(26):2561−2569. https://doi.org/10.1056/NEJMoa1610497.

40. O'Rourke DM, Nasrallah MP, Desai A, et al. A single dose of peripherally infused EGFRvIII-directed CAR T cells mediates antigen loss and induces adaptive resistance in patients with recurrent glioblastoma. *Sci Transl Med*. 2017; 0984(July).

41. Schneider D, Xiong Y, Wu D, et al. A tandem CD19/CD20 CAR lentiviral vector drives on-target and off-target antigen modulation in leukemia cell lines. *J Immunother Cancer*. 2017;5(1):1−17. https://doi.org/10.1186/s40425-017-0246-1.

42. Qin H, Ramakrishna S, Nguyen S, et al. Preclinical development of bivalent chimeric antigen receptors targeting both CD19 and CD22. *Mol Ther Oncolytics*. 2018; 11(December):127−137. https://doi.org/10.1016/j.omto.2018.10.006.

43. Ruella M, Barrett DM, Kenderian SS, et al. Dual CD19 and CD123 targeting prevents antigen-loss relapses after CD19-directed immunotherapies. *J Clin Invest*. 2016; 126(10):3814−3826. https://doi.org/10.1172/JCI87366.

44. Scarfò I, Ormhøj M, Frigault MJ, et al. Anti-CD37 chimeric antigen receptor T cells are active against B- and T-cell lymphomas. *Blood*. 2018;132(14):1495−1506. https://doi.org/10.1182/blood-2018-04-842708.

45. Hegde M, Mukherjee M, Grada Z, et al. Tandem CAR T cells targeting HER2 and IL13R α 2 Mitigate tumor antigen

46. Straathof KC, Pulè MA, Yotnda P, et al. An inducible caspase 9 safety switch for T-cell therapy. *Blood*. 2005;105(11): 4247−4254. https://doi.org/10.1182/blood-2004-11-4564.

47. Zhou X, Brenner MK. Improving the safety of T-Cell therapies using an inducible caspase-9 gene. *Exp Hematol*. 2016; 44(11):1013−1019. https://doi.org/10.1016/j.exphem.2016.07.011.

48. Di Stasi A, Tey S-KK, Dotti G, et al. Inducible apoptosis as a safety switch for adoptive cell therapy. *N Engl J Med*. 2011; 365(18):1673−1683. https://doi.org/10.1056/NEJMoa1106152.

49. Gardner RA, Finney O, Annesley C, et al. Intent to treat leukemia remission by CD19 CAR T cells of defined formulation and dose in children and young adults. *Blood*. 2017; 129(25):3322−3331. https://doi.org/10.1182/blood-2017-02-769208.

50. Paszkiewicz PJ, Fräßle SP, Srivastava S, et al. Targeted antibody-mediated depletion of CD19 CAR-T cells permanently reverses B cell aplasia. *J Clin Invest*. 2016. https://doi.org/10.1172/JCI84813.

51. Svoboda J, Rheingold SR, Gill SI, et al. Non-viral RNA chimeric antigen receptor modified T cells in patients with Hodgkin lymphoma. *Blood*. 2018;132(10). https://doi.org/10.1182/blood-2018-03-837609.

52. Weber EW, Lynn RC, Sotillo E, Lattin J, Xu P, Mackall CL. Pharmacologic control of CAR-T cell function using dasatinib. 2018;3(5):711−717. https://doi.org/10.1182/bloodadvances.2018028720.

53. Mestermann K, Giavridis T, Weber J, et al. The tyrosine kinase inhibitor dasatinib acts as a pharmacologic on/off switch for CAR T cells. *Sci Transl Med*. 2019;11(499): eaau5907. https://doi.org/10.1126/scitranslmed.aau5907.

54. Sterner RM, Sakemura R, Cox MJ, et al. GM-CSF inhibition reduces cytokine release syndrome and neuroinflammation but enhances CAR-T cell function in xenografts. *Blood*. 2018;133(7):697−709. https://doi.org/10.1182/blood-2018-10-881722.

55. Roybal KT, Rupp LJ, Morsut L, et al. Precision tumor recognition by T cells with combinatorial antigen-sensing circuits. *Cell*. 2016;164(4):770−779. https://doi.org/10.1016/j.cell.2016.01.011.

56. Srivastava S, Salter AI, Liggitt D, et al. Logic-gated ROR1 chimeric antigen receptor expression rescues T cell-mediated toxicity to normal tissues and enables selective tumor targeting. *Cancer Cell*. 2019;35(3):489−503.e8. https://doi.org/10.1016/j.ccell.2019.02.003.

57. Ying Z, Huang XF, Xiang X, et al. A safe and potent anti-CD19 CAR T cell therapy. *Nat Med*. 2019:86. https://doi.org/10.1038/s41591-019-0421-7.

58. Linette GP, Stadtmauer EA, Maus MV, et al. Cardiovascular toxicity and titin cross-reactivity of affinity-enhanced T cells in myeloma and melanoma. *Blood*. 2013;122(6): 863−872. https://doi.org/10.1182/blood-2013-03-490565.

59. Morgan RA, Chinnasamy N, Abate-daga DD, et al. Cancer regression and neurologic toxicity following anti-MAGE-

A3 TCR gene therapy. *J Immunother.* 2014;36(2):133−151. https://doi.org/10.1097/CJI.0b013e3182829903.Cancer.

60. Qin H, Cho M, Haso W, et al. Eradication of B-ALL using chimeric antigen receptor-expressing T cells targeting the TSLPR oncoprotein. *Blood.* 2015;126(5):629−639. https://doi.org/10.1182/blood-2014-11-612903.

61. Perna F, Berman SH, Soni RK, Hendrickson RC, Brennan CW, Sadelain M. Integrating proteomics and transcriptomics for systematic combinatorial chimeric antigen receptor therapy of AML article integrating proteomics and transcriptomics for systematic combinatorial chimeric antigen receptor therapy of AML. *Cancer Cell.* 2017;32(4): 506−519.e5. https://doi.org/10.1016/j.ccell.2017.09.004.

62. Maciocia PM, Wawrzyniecka PA, Philip B, et al. Targeting the T cell receptor β-chain constant region for immunotherapy of T cell malignancies. *Nat Med.* 2017;(October). https://doi.org/10.1038/nm.4444.

63. Mamonkin M, Rouce RH, Tashiro H, Brenner MK. A T-cell − directed chimeric antigen receptor for the selective treatment of T-cell malignancies. *Blood.* 2015;126(8):983−993. https://doi.org/10.1182/blood-2015-02-629527.

64. Gomes-Silva D, Srinivasan M, Sharma S, et al. CD7-edited T cells expressing a CD7-specific CAR for the therapy of T-cell malignancies. *Blood.* 2017. https://doi.org/10.1182/blood-2017-01-761320.

65. Rasaiyaah J, Georgiadis C, Preece R, Mock U, Qasim W. TCR ab/CD3 disruption enables CD3-specific antileukemic T cell immunotherapy Find the latest version: TCR αβ/CD3 disruption enables CD3-specific antileukemic T cell immunotherapy. *JCI Insight.* 2018;3(13): e99442. https://doi.org/10.1172/jci.insight.99442.

66. Cooper ML, Choi J, Staser K, et al. An "off-the-shelf" fratricide-resistant CAR-T for the treatment of T cell hematologic malignancies. *Leukemia.* 2018;32(9):1970−1983. https://doi.org/10.1038/s41375-018-0065-5.

67. Kim MY, Yu KR, Kenderian SS, et al. Genetic inactivation of CD33 in hematopoietic stem cells to enable CAR T cell immunotherapy for acute myeloid leukemia. *Cell.* 2018; 173(6):1439−1453.e19. https://doi.org/10.1016/j.cell.2018.05.013.

68. Chmielewski M, Abken H, CAR T. Cells releasing IL-18 convert to T-Bethigh FoxO1low effectors that exhibit augmented activity against advanced solid tumors. *Cell Rep.* 2017;21(11):3205−3219. https://doi.org/10.1016/j.celrep.2017.11.063.

69. Ahmed N, Ratnayake M, Savoldo B, et al. Regression of experimental medulloblastoma following transfer of HER2-specific T cells. *Cancer Res.* 2007;67(12):5957−5964. https://doi.org/10.1158/0008-5472.CAN-06-4309.

70. Ahmed N, Salsman VS, Kew Y, et al. HER2-specific T cells target primary glioblastoma stem cells and induce regression of autologous experimental tumors. *Clin Cancer Res.* 2010;16(2):474−485. https://doi.org/10.1158/1078-0432.CCR-09-1322.

71. Maude SL, Latesch T, Buechner J, et al. Tisagenlecleucel in children and young adults with B-cell lymphoblastic leukemia. *N Engl J Med.* 2018;378(5):439−448. https://doi.org/10.1056/NEJMoa1709866.

72. Neelapu SS, Locke FL, Bartlett NL, et al. Axicabtagene ciloleucel CAR T-cell therapy in refractory large B-cell lymphoma. *N Engl J Med.* 2017;377(26). https://doi.org/10.1056/NEJMoa1707447.

73. Schuster SJ, Bishop MR, Tam CS, et al. Tisagenlecleucel in adult relapsed or refractory diffuse large B-cell lymphoma. *N Engl J Med.* 2019;380(1):45−56. https://doi.org/10.1056/NEJMoa1804980.

74. Poirot L, Philip B, Schiffer-Mannioui C, et al. Multiplex genome edited T-cell manufacturing platform for "off-the-shelf" adoptive T-cell immunotherapies. *Cancer Res.* 2015;75(18):3853−3864. https://doi.org/10.1158/0008-5472.CAN-14-3321.

75. Eyquem J, Mansilla-Soto J, Giavridis T, et al. Targeting a CAR to the TRAC locus with CRISPR/Cas9 enhances tumour rejection. *Nature.* 2017:1−19. https://doi.org/10.1038/nature21405.

76. Leen AM, Bollard CM, Mendizabal AM, et al. Multicenter study of banked third-party virus-specific T cells to treat severe viral infections after hematopoietic stem cell transplantation. *Blood.* 2013;121(26):5113−5123. https://doi.org/10.1182/blood-2013-02-486324.

77. Cruz CRY, Micklethwaite KP, Savoldo B, et al. Infusion of donor-derived CD19-redirected virus-specific T cells for B-cell malignancies relapsed after allogeneic stem cell transplant: a phase 1 study. *Blood.* 2013;122(17):2965−2973. https://doi.org/10.1182/blood-2013-06-506741.

78. Rossig C, Pule M, Altvater B, et al. Vaccination to improve the persistence of CD19CAR gene-modified T cells in relapsed pediatric acute lymphoblastic leukemia. *Leukemia.* 2017;31(5):1087−1095. https://doi.org/10.1038/leu.2017.39.

79. Qasim W, Zhan H, Samarasinghe S, et al. Molecular remission of infant B-ALL after infusion of universal TALEN gene-edited CAR T cells. *Sci Transl Med.* 2017;2013(January):1−9. https://doi.org/10.1126/scitranslmed.aaj2013.

80. Cullot G, Boutin J, Toutain J, et al. CRISPR-Cas9 genome editing induces megabase-scale chromosomal truncations. *Nat Commun.* 2019;10(1):1136. https://doi.org/10.1038/s41467-019-09006-2.

81. Töpfer K, Cartellieri M, Michen S, et al. DAP12-Based activating chimeric antigen receptor for NK cell tumor immunotherapy. *J Immunol.* 2015;194(7):3201−3212. https://doi.org/10.4049/jimmunol.1400330.

82. Li Y, Hermanson DL, Moriarity BS, et al. Human iPSC-derived natural killer cells engineered with chimeric antigen receptors enhance anti- tumor activity article human iPSC-derived natural killer cells engineered with chimeric antigen receptors enhance anti-tumor activity. *Cell Stem Cell.* 2018;23:181−192. https://doi.org/10.1016/j.stem.2018.06.002.

83. Liu E, Tong Y, Dotti G, et al. Cord blood NK cells engineered to express IL-15 and a CD19-targeted CAR show long-term persistence and potent antitumor activity. *Leukemia.* 2018;32(2):520−531. https://doi.org/10.1038/leu.2017.226.

CHAPTER 14

Regulatory Issues in Gene-Modified Immune Effector Cell Therapy

KENNETH CORNETTA, MD • KRISHNA V. KOMANDURI, MD

REGULATORY ISSUES IN GENE-ENGINEERED T-CELLS

Cancer immunotherapy using T-cells engineered to expressed T-cell receptors (TCR) or chimeric antigen receptors (CAR) has moved from investigational agents into approved treatments.[1,2] Approval by the US Food and Drug Administration (FDA) requires licensed products to be both safe and efficacious. Engineered cell products transduced with integrating vectors (gammaretroviral and HIV-1-based lentiviral vectors, referred to here as retroviral and lentiviral vectors, respectively) present unique safety concerns related to the infusion of cell products and the potential adverse events associated with gene therapy. To determine the risk associated with engineered T-cells, regulators have required a challenging array of testing requirements that include analysis of the vector product, the transduced cell product, and postinfusion monitoring of patients for up to 15 years. In this chapter, we will focus on these safety issues and discuss current and proposed changes to FDA requirements related to the use of engineered T-cells.

GENERATING AND TESTING VECTOR PRODUCTS

TCR- and CAR T-cell products are typically generated by ex vivo transduction of T-cells with a retroviral or lentiviral vector. Regulators consider the transduced cell product the investigational agent, but the unique safety concerns related to gene therapy vectors has resulted in a series of regulatory guidance documents that affect those who manufacture vector and those who utilize the vector products to modify T-cells (Table 14.1).

Retroviral and lentiviral vectors are membrane-bound RNA viruses, and while HIV-1 is considerably more complex, retroviral and lentiviral vectors are similar in overall design (Fig. 14.1A and B). One major difference is that many retroviral vectors retain the native viral long terminal repeats (LTRs) which are required for integration and also contain the promoter and enhancer sequences used to drive transgene expression.[3] Lentiviral vectors use self-inactivating LTRs requiring an internal promoter to drive transgene expression.[4] As discussed below, retention of the gammaretroviral LTR has significant safety implications.

Vector products can be manufactured by two different methods (Fig. 14.1C and D). Traditionally, clinical retroviral vectors were generated in packaging cell lines which contained three integrated plasmids.[5] Since the vector genome has been stripped of key viral genes required for viral replication, a plasmid expressing the *gag*/pol sequences is needed to package the vector RNA into viral particles. A third plasmid encoding an envelope glycoprotein plasmid is also stably introduced into the cell line. The envelope is expressed on the virion surface and directs the particles to specific receptors on a target cell. Human cells lack the receptor for many gammaretroviruses, so alternative envelopes (such as the Gibbon Ape Leukemia Virus envelope) are used to "pseudotype" the vector particles. Packaging cells can generate vectors over many days and can be used to generate Master Cell Banks (MCBs) of the cell line, thereby providing a consistent product as the vector moves from Phase I through licensure.

The other method commonly used, particularly for lentiviral vectors, has been transient transfection (Fig. 14.1D).[6] In this method the plasmids are transfected into cell lines and the vector harvested over 1–2 days. Pseudotyping is also used for most lentiviral vectors as the native HIV-1 envelope glycoprotein would limit infection to CD4+ cells. Many lentiviral vectors contain the vesicular stomatitis virus G glycoprotein (VSV-G) which provides high level of gene transfer into most mammalian cell types. An advantage of transient transfection is it bypasses the prolonged period of clone selection and MCB generation associated with packaging

Chimeric Antigen Receptor T-Cell Therapies for Cancer. https://doi.org/10.1016/B978-0-323-66181-2.00014-7

TABLE 14.1
Current and Draft Guidance Documents Outlining Testing Requirements for Gene Therapy Product Testing.

Current Guidance Documents	Draft Documents
Points to Consider in the Characterization of Cell Lines Used to Produce Biologicals (July 12, 1993)	Chemistry, Manufacturing, and Control (CMC) Information for Human Gene Therapy Investigational New Drug Applications (INDs); Draft Guidance for Industry
Guidance for Industry: Guidance for Human Somatic Cell Therapy and Gene Therapy (March 30, 1998)	Long-Term Follow-up After Administration of Human Gene Therapy Products; Draft Guidance for Industry
Guidance for Industry: Gene Therapy Clinical Trials—Observing Subjects for Delayed Adverse Events (November 2006)	Testing of Retroviral Vector-Based Human Gene Therapy Products for Replication Competent Retrovirus During Product Manufacture and Patient Follow-up; Draft Guidance for Industry
Guidance for Industry: Supplemental Guidance on Testing for Replication Competent Retrovirus in Retroviral Vector Based Gene Therapy Products and During Follow-up of Patients in Clinical Trials Using Retroviral Vectors (November 2006)	Human Gene Therapy for Hemophilia; Draft Guidance for Industry
Guidance for Industry: Preclinical Assessment of Investigational Cellular and Gene Therapy Products (November 2013)	Human Gene Therapy for Rare Diseases; Draft Guidance for Industry
Guidance for Industry: Determining the Need for and Content of Environmental Assessments for Gene Therapies, Vectored Vaccines, and Related Recombinant Viral or Microbial Products (March 2015)	Human Gene Therapy for Retinal Disorders; Draft Guidance for Industry
Considerations for the Design of Early-Phase Clinical Trials of Cellular and Gene Therapy Products; Guidance for Industry (June 2015)	
Recommendations for Microbial Vectors Used for Gene Therapy; Guidance for Industry (September 2016)	

cell lines making it the quickest path to a Phase I trial. A possible downside is lot to lot variability of the transient method which could be an issue for later phase trials. There are now lentiviral packaging cell lines in development, and some retroviral vectors used clinically have been generated by transient transfection. The science of vector production is rapidly developing, particularly as industry seeks to meet the consistency challenges around manufacturing licensed products.

The FDA guidance documents listed in Table 14.1 provide testing requirements for cell lines used in vector manufacture along with the tests required on the vector product (see Table 14.2). The majority of assays listed in Table 14.2 are not unique to vector production and are required for generating any biologic product. Requirements are tailored to the cell line species of origin. If cell lines of more than one species are utilized (ex. using the "ping-pong" method to obtain high-titer packaging

cell line clones[7]), expanded testing is required to cover pathogens from the relevant species. As shown in Table 14.2, excluding virus contamination is a major focus of release testing for the cell line and the vector product. Since the cells used in manufacture are in fact generating viral particles, excluding replication competent retroviruses within the large number of vector particles has proven to be a major challenge for product development (discussed in detail below).

The FDA does require some specific tests when HEK293 and HEK293T-cell lines are used in vector manufacturing. Both lines contain genetic material from the adenovirus E1A region, and HEK293T-cells also contain sequences from the SV40 large T antigen. FDA requires vectors generated in these cell lines to be tested to ensure there is no passage of these viral sequences to transduced cells. Since some cellular DNA frequently contaminates vector products, evaluating

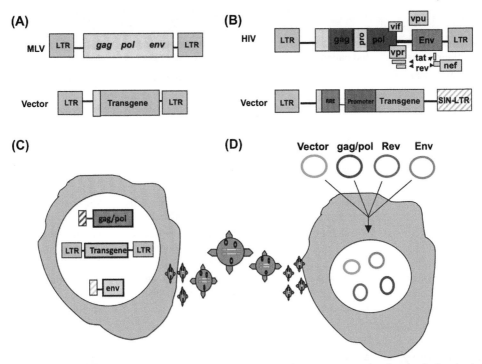

FIG. 14.1 Retroviral and lentiviral vectors. The basic genome of a gamma retrovirus (murine leukemia virus, MLV) and a lentivirus (human immunodeficiency virus 1, HIV) are depicted in **(A)** and **(B)**, respectively. **(C)** The diagram illustrates a retroviral packaging cell that has three plasmids integrated into the cell genome expressing retroviral *gag/pol*, an envelope glycoprotein that will be expressed on the surface of the vector particle (env), and a plasmid containing the vector sequence with the transgene of interest flanked by retroviral long terminal repeats (LTR). **(D)** Representation of the transient transfection method for lentiviral vector production where four plasmids are transfected into a cell such as HEK293T. The plasmids include HIV *gag/pol*, an env plasmid (typically the vesicular stomatitis virus G glycoprotein), the vector plasmid, and HIV-1 Rev gene.

transduced cells shortly after transduction will generally be positive by qPCR and other methods. Indiana University has utilized a 21-day assay, testing cells within the culture at approximately 5, 11, and 21 days. E1A or SV40 sequences in the culture decrease over time and most are negative by day 11.

Testing will also be required to show transduced cell products contain intact vector sequences. Retroviral and lentiviral vectors are prone to alternate splicing. In some cases, vectors may be generated that contain the full-length vector and an additional truncated transcript. The ratio can vary. If sequencing alone is used to analyze packaging cell lines and vector products, care must be taken to assure significant truncated transcripts can be detected. In addition to sequencing, Southern blots may be useful in documenting intact vector sequences in transduced cells. The US FDA has also required testing for residual total DNA or residual plasmid DNA, depending on the manufacturing method. Other product-specific testing may be required, such as residual benzonase in products where benzonase is used to reduce residual plasmid after transient transection. Specific limits for DNA and benzonase have not be published, and the requirement is generally to "report results" on the product Certificate of Analysis. Acceptable limits will likely be required as products move from Phase I to licensure.

RISK OF RCR AND RCL AND TESTING OF VECTOR PRODUCTS

As mentioned above, excluding replication competent retroviruses or lentivirus (RCR and RCL, respectively) has been a major concern of regulators. The design of early retroviral packaging cell lines contained significant homology between the vector and packaging sequences and RCR development during vector production was well documented.[8] Gammaretroviruses are slowly

TABLE 14.2
Testing Requirements for Retroviral and Lentiviral Vector Products.

Master Cell Bank Tests	Indication	Vector Supernate Test	Indication
Sterility with bacteriostasis/fungistasis	All cell lines	Sterility with bacteriostasis/fungistasis	All products
Mycoplasma with mycoplasmastasis	All cell lines	Mycoplasma with mycoplasmastasis	All products
In vivo virus assay	All cell lines	In vitro virus assay for adventitious agents	All products
In vitro virus assay for adventitious agents	All cell lines	Endotoxin	All products
Bovine virus assay	All cell lines	RCR assay—ecotropic virus (medium and EOP cells)	Murine packaging cell lines
Porcine virus assay	All cell lines	RCR assay—amphotropic/xenotropic viruses (medium and EOP cells)	All retroviral products
Mouse antibody production/LCM virus assay	All cell lines	RCL assay—Lentiviruses (medium and EOP cells)	All lentiviral products
Transmission electron microscopy	All cell lines	Vector titer	All products
Cell Identity assay	All cell lines	Vector function	All products
qPCR virus panel (HIV 1/2, HTLVI/II, hepatitis B and C, HHV 6 and 8, EBV, CMV, B19)	All cell lines	Bovine virus assay	All products (unless serum and reagents shown to be bovine virus free)
Vector insert stability (Southern Blot or other method)	Producer cell lines	Porcine virus assay	All products (unless trypsin and reagents shown to be porcine virus free)
RCR assay—ecotropic virus (medium and EOP cells)	Murine packaging cell lines	Passage of E1A DNA	If HEK293 or HEK293T-cells used
RCR assay—amphotropic/xenotropic viruses (medium and EOP cells)	All cell lines	Passage of SV40 large T antigen DNA	If HEK293 T-cells used
		Residual DNA	All products
		Vector sequence and/or vector insert stability	All products
		Residual benzonase	All products

transforming retroviruses and the Moloney murine leukemia virus (MLV), frequently used as the backbone for retroviral vectors, is known to cause lymphoma in mice. The LTR enhancer is felt to be an important factor in determining the predilection for causing lymphoma in mice, and its insertion is frequently found near the *pim-1* gene.[9] Additional mutagenic effects are required as *pim-1* transgenics do not have an increased risk of malignancy, but exposure of these mice to RCR lead rapidly to lymphoma with virus insertions near *c-myc*

and *n-myc*.[10] The potential risk for humans was noted in a variety of early safety studies. Mice injected with an RCR that arose from the PA12 packaging cell line led to lymphoma that appeared similar to that caused by the parent MLV.[11] While a large volume of RCR infused into immunocompetent, nonhuman primates did not appear to cause disease,[12] inadvertent exposure of an immunosuppressed rhesus monkey during a bone marrow transplant experiment led to T-cell lymphoma.[13]

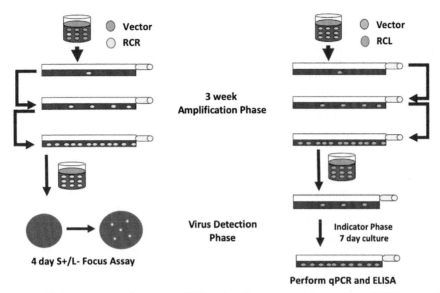

FIG. 14.2 Replication competent retrovirus (RCR) and replication competent lentivirus (RCL) testing. Current methods used in the National Gene Vector Biorepository at Indiana University are illustrated. The left figure depicts testing for RCR with RCL testing shown on the right. The 3 week amplification is mandated by the US FDA to allow slow growing recombinant viruses to expand to a detectable level. The PG4 sarcoma+/leukemia− (S+/L−) cell line is used to detect RCR. Gamma retroviruses transform S+/L− cell lines and foci of transformed cells indicate the presence of an RCR. For RCL detection, the combination of an ELISA method for detecting HIV capsid (p24), and a quantitative PCR (qPCR) based method for detecting reverse transcriptase (product-enhanced reverse transcriptase, PERT), are used.

Having identified malignancy as a potential risk from RCR exposure, the FDA developed a specific guidance for clinical trials using retroviral vectors entitled "Supplemental Guidance on Testing for Replication Competent Retrovirus in Retroviral Vector Based Gene Therapy Products and During Follow-up of Patients in Clinical Trials Using Retroviral Vectors."[14] Testing was required on 5% of the vector product and 1% of the end-of-production (EOP) cells (up to a maximum of 10^8 cells). If vector is generated in a packaging cell, cell line testing is also required. The method of testing is suggested in the FDA guidance. For testing RCR in vector products, molecular assays are not sufficiently sensitive and likely to yield false-positive results due to carryover of packaging cell line DNA. Cell-based assays have been recommended and the material must be passaged on a cell line that is highly infectable and capable of expanding RCR to high titer. Since retroviral vectors have been pseudotyped with a variety of viral envelopes, a validated RCR detection method specific for the envelope must be used.[11,15−17]

The other challenge in detecting an RCR is understanding the potential RCR genome. Most recombinant viruses arising from packaging cell lines contain sequences from the vector and packaging plasmids, but not in all cases. In mice, gammaretroviruses can recombine in vivo to form novel viruses with increased pathogenicity (reviewed in Cornetta et al.[18]). RCR have also been reported to contain genomic sequences from the packaging cell line used in early gene transfer experiments.[19,20]

A variety of cell-based assays have been reported for the testing of retroviral and lentiviral vectors.[3,21−28] These cell-based assays, commonly used to screen vector and cell products, are similar and the basics are depicted in Fig. 14.2. Vector supernatant or end-of-production (EOP) cells are cultured with a cell line that is used to amplify virus to high titer. Since the assay must be capable of detecting a recombinant virus whose growth kinetics is unknown, regulators have required the extended passage (approximately 3 weeks of culture) to detect a slow-growing virus. Since the large number of vector particles could inhibit infection of the amplification cells (receptor interference), a large number of cells are required in the assay. Commercially available RCR and RCL testing can cost between $8000 and $18,000 per sample.

There is currently no public repository of testing results for retroviral products used in clinical trials. If a patient had been exposed in the United States, it would have been public knowledge based on the past reporting requirements to the US National Institute of Health Recombinant DNA Advisory Committee. To date, no such disclosure has been reported for RCR or RCL. This is likely due, in part, to improved vector and packaging cell line design.[29,30–33]

While the FDA guidance around RCR was developed prior to the use of lentiviral vector products, regulators have applied the same requirements. Lentiviral vectors by their design with self-inactivating long terminal repeats removing HIV-1 enhancers and promoters, removal of the HIV-1 accessory proteins and sequences such as Tat, frequent use of transient vector production methods, and the lack of direct malignant transformation by HIV-1 insertions predict an even safer profile for this vector class.[34] While there is less experience with lentiviral vector products, reports have also supported the generation of RCL-free vector material using current production methods for clinical products.[21,33,35]

CELL PRODUCT ISSUES

RCR and RCL Screening in T-Cell Products

Concerned that the stringent testing requirement for vector product would still miss an RCR, the FDA had required testing of ex vivo treated cells (1% of the transduced cells up to 10^8 cells). Given the concerns about sensitivity and the potential false-positive results (due to carryover of packaging cell line DNA or plasmid DNA), a cell-based assay has generally been required. The NIH-sponsored National Gene Vector Biorepository (NGVB) at Indiana University screened 282 cell products from 14 clinical trials for RCR; all were negative for RCR by a cell-based assay. Moreover, blood collected at > 30 days post infusion was also negative for RCR using qPCR or ELISA methods.[32] The NGVB also performed screening for RCL on 460 CAR T-cell products from 375 patients participating in 26 clinical trials. All were negative for RCL, as were blood samples from 296 patients screened for viral envelope (collected > 30 days post infusion).[35] Additional reports have now been published providing further support for decreasing the RCR/RCL testing requirement for T-cell products.[31,33] The FDA is currently finalizing a new Guidance for Industry "Testing of Retroviral Vector-Based Human Gene Therapy Products for Replication Competent Retrovirus During Product Manufacture and Patient Follow-up; Draft Guidance for Industry" that is expected to greatly decrease or eliminate RCR/RCL testing of T-cell products. One potential alternative may be to utilize qPCR to identify

sequences that would be present in an RCR/RCL but not in the vector genome (for example the viral envelope DNA). Samples taken shortly after transduction would be expected to be positive due to carryover of cell line or plasmid DNA, but a decline in copy number over time would be inconsistent with an RCR/RCL. Given the extended culture period for the cell-based RCR/RCL testing, the FDA has generally required these assays be performed retrospectively. If the qPCR assay is required, it may be required for product release.

Posttrial Monitoring for RCR/RCL

The existing Guidance for Industry on RCR/RCL testing requires posttrial monitoring for RCR and RCL at multiple time points after infusion of gene-transduced cells. Testing is to be performed on a pretreatment sample then 3, 6, and 12 months post treatment and then yearly up to 15 years (or as long as vector is detected in the patient). A commentary from multiple centers performing gene transfer found no evidence of RCR in 29 clinical trials performed in five centers in the United States.[31] The NIH-funded NGVB program also assists with posttrial monitoring and has tested 1745 samples for RCR (GALV or RD114 envelope) and 461 for RCL (VSV-G), representing material from 64 retroviral and 12 lentiviral clinical trials. All have been negative. The University of Pennsylvania also presented data on the safety of T-cell products from retroviral and lentiviral trials.[33] The negative data have led to calls for revisions to the current US FDA guidelines,[31] and as noted above for testing T-cell products, a draft Guidance document is being finalized. The new Guidance is expected to decrease posttrial monitoring sample testing after sufficient (as yet to be determined) safety data have been accrued for the clinical product.[36] Novel vector systems will likely still require extensive evaluation for replication competent virus.

Monitoring for Insertional Mutagenesis

It was hoped that RCR-free vector preparations would eliminate the risk of malignancy in clinical gene therapy applications, but that has proven not to be the case. The gene therapy field was challenged by the development of T-cell leukemia in children treated with retroviral vectors that conferred the *IL2RG* gene as a treatment for X-linked severe combined immunodeficiency. Shortly after this report, children treated with retroviral vectors for Wiskott–Aldrich syndrome and chronic granulomatous disease also developed malignancies. The mechanism by which disease developed is complex, and just like murine malignancies, the LTR enhancer and promotor appear to be key factors in the transformation. LMO-2 was a common gene associated with the site of vector integration but not in all cases.[37,38] It is of interest that children treated in a similar manner for another SCID, adenosine deaminase deficiency (ADA), have not developed leukemia. Reasons for the different outcomes may be related to differences in the LTR promoter and enhancers, the cell pool at risk for mutagenesis, and the difference between a gene involved with growth regulation (*IL2RG*) and a housekeeping gene (ADA) (see review by Niehnhuis et al.[39]). While a gamma retroviral vector has been approved for use in Europe for the treatment of ADA deficiency, the field has generally moved to lentiviral vectors when the target is hematopoietic stem cells (HSCs). Regulators have also been concerned that the number of vector insertions per cell could increase the risk of malignancy. Therefore, preclinical development must include transduction protocols that minimize the number of vector insertions per cell while still correcting the cell phenotype. Regulators often require monitoring transduced cell products for insertion site frequency (i.e., vector copy number per cell) in infused populations.

Despite the reports of leukemia, many TCR- and CAR T-cell applications still use retroviral vectors. Arguments put forth to support the continued use of retroviral vectors include a lack of malignancy in retroviral TCR- and CAR T-cell therapy trials and the potential decreased risk of leukemia development in differentiated T-cells as compared to undifferentiated HSC cells.

To date, there are no documented malignancies associated with lentiviral vectors, but two studies document the potential for growth dysregulation related to lentiviral insertion. In an HSC trial in which a β-globin lentiviral vector was utilized as a treatment for thalassemia, a clonal population of red cell precursors expanded. The patient required phlebotomy due to elevated red cell number. Evaluation of the clonal population documented insertion of the vector into the HMGA2 gene, and the integration site generated a truncated RNA that was insensitive to let-7 mircoRNA regulation. More recently, a lentiviral vector used in a CAR T-cell patient was found to disrupt the methylcytosine dioxygenase TET2 gene.[40] In this circumstance, there was a concurrent hypomorphic mutation in the second TET2 allele. Therapeutic outcome was obtained in both instances, and progression to malignancy has not been reported. Nevertheless, these findings support continued monitoring for clonal populations in both lentiviral and retroviral clinical trials. Monitoring guidelines are often negotiated with the FDA based on the vector type, cell target, transgene, and disease being treated.

Monitoring for insertional events that alter cell growth can involve two steps. The first is determining if there is clonal expansion. For example, hematopoietic stem cell correction of a genetic disease is expected to provide long-term persistence of gene-corrected cells which make up the majority of blood cells in circulation. In this case, monitoring for clonal dominance will be required. If the population is heterogeneous, detailed insertion site analysis may not be required. If there is a predominant clone, further studies may be required to determine if the expansion is due to altered cell growth related to vector integration. For CAR- or TCR-expressing T-cells, there may be evidence of dominant clones initially that typically decrease over the first year post treatment. Insertion site analysis is generally required in cases where there is exceedingly high levels of gene-marked cells or the cells become detectable after a period of undetectability. The methods for insertion site analysis are evolving and require a team experienced in complex PCR methodology, high-throughput sequencing, and bioinformatic analysis.[41] Regulators have not set specific testing methodology for insertion site analysis.

Macroscopic Regulation of Immune Effector Cell Therapies

The remainder of this chapter will discuss the regulation of immune effector cell therapies, including CAR T and other adoptive T-cell therapies, at the level of the laboratory and clinical cellular therapy program, rather than at the level of an individual therapeutic agent (e.g., a gene-modified T-cell product for a specific indication). While the frameworks for clinical deployment of adoptive cellular immunotherapies outside of the investigational setting are nascent and continue to evolve rapidly, we will present a current overview and also discuss likely future determinants of regulation at the immunotherapy center level.

FDA Standards for Tiered Regulation of Cellular Therapies

In 2005, the FDA outlined a tiered approach to the overall regulation of what they categorized as "Human Cells, Tissues, and Cellular and Tissue-Based Products (HCT/Ps)" encompassing a variety of cellular products that could potentially be used to treat human diseases. Prior to this reassessment, routinely employed clinical cellular therapies (beyond the routine use of transfusions of peripheral blood components) consisted primarily of therapies using bone marrow— and/or peripheral blood—derived hematopoietic cell transplantation (HCT) products.

While the era of HCT began in 1957 with the initial (noncurative) use of allogeneic marrow transplantation, clinical application expanded significantly in the late 1960s, following the first successful applications of HCT to treat both nonmalignant diseases (e.g., immunodeficiency states) and diseases including acute myeloid leukemia. In the intervening decades, HCT has expanded to a broad range of centers, with over 175 centers performing allogeneic transplants in the Be The Match network operated by the National Marrow Donor Program (NMDP) at the time of this writing.[42]

The increasing emergence of a broad range of cellular therapies (e.g., mesenchymal stromal cells and putative stem cells derived from a variety of placental, umbilical cord, and adult tissues) prompted an FDA reassessment of the need for more strict regulatory requirements. This included the definition of a "minimally manipulated" product, defined by two criteria: (1) For structural tissue, processing that does not alter the original relevant characteristics of the tissue relating to the tissue's utility for reconstruction, repair, or replacement and (2) For cells or nonstructural tissues, processing that does not alter the relevant biological characteristics of cells or tissues.[43] Products that fit these two criteria included autologous and hematopoietic progenitor cell products used for hematopoietic reconstitution or nonmalignant and malignant diseases treatable by autologous and allogeneic HCT, as well as donor lymphocyte products obtained from allogeneic donors intended to achieve donor-derived host chimerism or to treat relapse following allogeneic HCT. The practical result is that therapies using minimally manipulated products may be conducted, as reaffirmed by the FDA in 2005, without the need for an investigational new drug (IND) authorization.

While minimally manipulated HCT/Ps including autologous and allogeneic HCT products and donor lymphocyte infusions are less regulated than engineered T-cell therapies, their use is still associated with significant clinical risks. These include risks of infusion reactions, potential marrow aplasia related to primary or secondary graft failure, and, for allogeneic products, the morbidity and mortality associated with graft-versus-host disease (GVHD). While mortality within 100 days of autologous HCT is now less than 1%–2% in most centers, 100-day mortality after allogeneic HCT may be 10% or higher depending on patient risk and graft source.

Despite these clear risks, one reason for the lack of tighter FDA regulation of autologous and allogeneic HCT is a largely voluntary system of accreditation,

registry reporting, and, more recently, the establishment of a federally supported outcomes registry, the stem cell therapeutic outcomes database (SCTOD). In aggregate, these systems have driven consistent improvements in the quality of cellular therapy programs, created an unprecedented transparency of individual center outcomes, and provided a strong safety net for patients seeking both established and experimental therapies. Additionally, private payers have created networks of centers of excellence (COEs) with defined criteria for volume and quality. Since it is highly likely that these systems will be used to similarly drive quality and ensure safety in engineered T-cell therapies, key elements that may be applied to these emerging therapies will be discussed in the next sections.

Accreditation of HCT and Immune Effector Cell Therapies by FACT

The American Society for Transplantation and Cellular Therapy (ASTCT, previously known as the American Society for Blood and Marrow Transplantation—ASBMT) and the International Society for Cellular Therapy (ISCT) have independently and jointly provided crucial support and advocacy for the needs of cellular therapy patients, researchers, and clinicians. In 1996, the ASTCT and ISCT worked together to form the Foundation for Accreditation of Cellular Therapy (FACT), a nonprofit corporation founded to provide a peer network of experts committed to improving practices in stem cell transplantation and other cellular therapies. FACT established guidelines and processes for voluntary accreditation based on robust standard operating procedures (SOPs) governing the collection, cryopreservation, and infusion of cellular products that creates a framework of safe and effective clinical practices that ensures safety in care and drives continuous process improvement. FACT standards for HCT govern three broad areas: (1) clinical programs, (2) collection of cellular products, and (3) cellular processing. Standards for hematopoietic cellular therapy, now jointly published with the Joint Accreditation Committee ISCT-Europe and EBMT (JACIE) are updated every few years to ensure their relevance to evolving practices and are now in their seventh edition. FACT provides training, educational activities, written guidelines and accreditation, which is maintained through formal independent review of standards and practices, and site inspection, which must be performed at least every 3 years. It is estimated that more than 90% of eligible HCT programs in the United States and their associated collection and cell processing facilities maintain voluntary accreditation, in part due to the requirement for FACT accreditation to qualify for inclusion into the COE networks of major private insurance payers.

Recognizing the value of FACT standards for clinical programs, cell therapy laboratories, and collection facilities supporting non-HCT cellular therapies (e.g., experimental therapies in the field of regenerative medicine), FACT developed a set of "Common Standards" that could be applied to centers involved in cellular therapies but that do not perform HCT. Recognizing the likelihood of impending approvals for CAR T-cell therapies targeting CD19-positive malignancies, FACT leadership (consisting of appointed members representing both ASTCT and ISCT) established an immune effector cell (IEC) task force that also included representatives from the American Society for Gene and Cellular Therapy (ASGCT) and the Society for Immunotherapy of Cancer (SITC).[44] These efforts led to the development of the first-edition standards and an accreditation program that were first published in 2017, prior to the approval later that year of the CAR T-cell therapies tisagenlecleucel and axicabtagene ciloleucel. As with HCT accreditation, programs are responsible for accreditation related to the services they provide (e.g., clinical management, collection, cell processing) in the continuum of care of patients receiving IEC therapies, defined as including T-cell and NK therapies, including both gene-modified and ex vivo–expanded cell products.

Registry Reporting of Outcomes of HCT and Engineered T-Cell Therapies

Early in the HCT era, a prescient group of leaders including Mortimer M. Bortin at the Medical College of Wisconsin (MCW) recognized the value of a data repository for the nascent field of hematopoietic transplantation. At that time, there were fewer than 12 centers in the United States actively performing HCT, and no more than 50 transplants performed nationwide. In 1986, the United States Navy established a registry of donors, and a separate data repository was created to track outcomes of HCTs performed using unrelated registry donors, with these collective efforts known as the National Marrow Donor Program (NMDP), also now known colloquially as Be The Match.

In 2004, these two registry efforts merged into what is now known as the Center for International Blood and Marrow Transplant Research, a remarkable registry that now collates data from virtually all of the allogeneic HCTs and a significant majority of the autologous HCTs performed in the United States. The CIBMTR now collects data not only from the United States but from almost 50 countries worldwide, and the registry now contains outcomes data from more than 425,000

HCT procedures. Furthermore, donor and recipient research samples have been collected for a majority of transplanted patients, serving as a significant repository enabling translational research. The CIBMTR performs several critical functions, including: (1) enabling research that has significantly advanced clinical and basic understanding of determinants of HCT outcomes, with significant support from funding agencies including the NIH and yielding over 1000 publications in peer-reviewed journals since 1972; (2) supporting quality improvement, with CIBMTR data audits used by programs and also by FACT as a measure of data quality and integrity; (3) facilitating risk-adjusted outcomes reporting valuable to programs, potential patients, governmental agencies providing oversight of HCT and for third-party payers.

STEM CELL THERAPEUTICS OUTCOMES DATABASE

Recognizing the importance of transparency in outcomes reporting to assuring patient safety, the US Congress advanced legislation that created a national risk-adjusted outcomes Stem Cell Therapeutics Outcomes Database (SCTOD). The SCTOD was first established as part of the C.W. Bill Young Cell Transplantation Program, authorized by the Stem Cell Therapeutic and Research Act of 2005 (Public Law 109−129)[45] and reauthorized by the Stem Cell Therapeutic and Research Reauthorization Act of 2010 (Public Law 111−264),[46] and the Stem Cell Therapeutic and Research Reauthorization Act of 2015 (Public Law 114−104).[47]

As the contract holder, the CIBMTR, utilizing principal resources at both MCW and the NMDP, was charged with collecting data on all allogeneic (related and unrelated) HCTs performed in the United States, and on all HCTs done with products procured through the NMDP but performed outside of the United States. The SCTOD database allows analysis of NMDP registry utilization, center-specific outcomes, assessment of the size of donor registry and cord blood inventory, and the facilitation of studies related to patient access and availability of HCT.

SCTOD BUILDS ON THE FOUNDATION OF THE CIBMTR

As discussed above, motivated by a desire to advance research using aggregated data and to drive quality improvement, transplant physicians and researchers early on established a national data registry with enormous reach and impact. The establishment of the

SCTOD builds upon this infrastructure and expertise involving data collection, management, and analysis supporting both quality management and research publications. As noted previously, SCTOD data represent a subset of CIBMTR data, which in addition to mandatory data submission for all allogeneic HCTs performed in the United States, include voluntarily submitted autologous transplantation data from domestic CIBMTR centers and autologous and allogeneic transplantation data from international CIBMTR centers.

In managing the SCTOD, the CIBMTR collaborates with transplant centers to:

- Develop data reporting requirements for allogeneic transplants in the United States
- Manage a related donor–recipient research sample repository
- Design and maintain systems to collect data and make it publicly available
- Study center-specific outcomes
- Collect data on novel therapeutic uses of hematopoietic stem cells

EXTENSION OF CIBMTR EFFORTS TO COLLECT IMMUNE EFFECTOR CELL OUTCOMES DATA

As of this writing, there are no impending national governmental mandates to require analogous reporting of engineered T-cell therapy data, as for allogeneic HCT data. However, given similar collective benefits in the field of cellular immunotherapy (e.g., facilitation of research, value of outcomes data for quality improvement, potential for creation of risk-adjusted measures of center performance visible to patients or payers), leaders within the CIBMTR worked with representatives of the NMDP, ASTCT, FACT, and other key stakeholders (e.g., FDA, Centers for Medicare and Medicaid Services, CMMS) to develop a framework for immune effector cell outcomes data. Substantial progress has been made, including the development of forms-based reporting of key clinical data, including indications, comorbidities, toxicities, and ultimate outcomes of engineered T-cell therapies.

Recognizing the rapid evolution of the field, especially following the 2017 approval of the first two CAR T-cell therapies, the CIBMTR has reacted rapidly to developments in the cellular therapy community. For example, the ASTCT united experts in a June 2018 consensus conference to harmonize the grading and reporting of CAR T-cell toxicities.[48] In October 2018, a draft set of guidelines was presented at the CIBMTR data summit on engineered T-cell therapies, and discussed with key stakeholders (including representatives from FDA, CMMS, payers, developers, and key affiliated organizations, including ASTCT and FACT). Within months, CIBMTR draft forms had been revised to incorporate the newly published consensus criteria.[48] It has been proposed, but not yet resolved, that a robust reporting system (either voluntary or mandatory) might best facilitate achievement of both academic and regulatory goals. For example, the ASTCT consensus statement suggested the elimination of redundant reporting through the CIBMTR registry and to the FDA for required risk evaluation and management strategies (REMS) for events arising following CAR T therapies.

CENTERS OF EXCELLENCE AND THEIR ROLE IN PROGRAM REGULATION AND QUALITY IMPROVEMENT
Payer-based COE Networks

There are over 150 centers in the United States performing allogeneic HCT (i.e., HCT using a donor, who may be a family member or a registry-derived volunteer unrelated donor) and an even greater number of centers where autologous HCT (i.e., using stem cells harvested from the patient, as with CAR T-cells) is performed.[49] Many large payers have developed HCT COE plan language restricting or encouraging referrals to a subset of these HCT centers. Criteria for inclusion in a plan or network COE program typically include sufficient volume to demonstrate experience of a multidisciplinary clinical team, a requirement for accreditation, and achievement of quantitative metrics of quality which may include risk-adjusted rates of survival (either absolute or relative to peer institutions providing similar services).[49] Additional criteria may include geographical distribution (to increase patient access and/or limit travel which may be costly and which can impair caregiver access and familial support). Finally, there is usually a commitment to contracted care rates that promote an incentive on value-based care.[49]

Manufacturer-Based "COE-like" Cellular Therapy Networks

The pivotal trials performed to date by individual manufacturers of CAR T-cell products typically utilized a relatively small (e.g., <30) group of cellular therapy centers. As with payer-defined criteria, manufacturers identified institutions that were skilled in clinical care of cellular therapy patients and also in clinical research for the disease (acute lymphoblastic leukemia or non-Hodgkin lymphoma to date) targeted in initial trials. Because manufacturers desired to keep complication rates low for both ethical reasons and to yield superior survival outcomes needed for approval, most centers included were already those in traditional allogeneic HCT COE networks. With approval, manufacturers have an incentive to increase the number of sites where therapies are available, while ensuring that complication rates remain low, particularly as outcomes data are being closely compared across sites and competing products. For example, as of the time of this writing, there are 71 centers authorized by Kite/Gilead to deliver axicabtagene ciloleucel for lymphoma and 95 centers authorized by Novartis to deliver tisagenlecleucel for leukemia in children and lymphoma in adults. While criteria for inclusion into manufacturer networks are proprietary, the limitation of approved cellular immunotherapies to a subset of potential sites serves as a de facto regulation based on quality, volume, and economic factors.

Unique aspects of payer COE selection criteria and other issues relevant to immune effector cell therapies for cancer are:

Volume: Rather than using minimal volumes as an entry hurdle for determining COE status, payers may develop measures of total experience with novel therapies and participation in clinical trials as surrogates for volume. As the number of available therapies increases, experienced centers are likely to develop platforms that improve outcome across diseases and unique cell therapy types.[49]

Potential conflicts between manufacturer and payer networks: Initially, payers will likely have to accept de facto COEs created by manufacturers of cell therapy products and established in the process of pivotal trials leading to approvals. However, because payer and manufacturer standards and goals in COE creation may at times differ (e.g., with respect to emphasis on value vs. scientific expertise), patient access may be impaired as those seeking therapies will need to find overlap between the requirements of their payer and their clinical and geographic needs. Over time, payers may appropriately exert pressure on manufacturers to include centers that fit their needs for regional clinical access and (likely) value-based needs, although all parties have an inherent interest in maintaining quality standards and outcomes. Earlier-stage therapies will likely continue to be provided through a more limited network of experienced clinical trial sites, while more mature and lower-risk therapies are more likely to find their way to community-based providers with broader geographic access.

Outcomes: As noted above for HCT programs, governmental regulations require transparency and standardized reporting of risk-adjusted survival outcomes, accomplished via the SCTOD and facilitated by the CIBMTR and NMDP. Specialty societies including the ASTCT and informed payers are looking beyond simple outcomes such as mortality at defined posttreatment periods to include metrics of timely evaluation and treatment and other factors including quality of life. These may come to play a more important role with respect to high-cost durable therapies.

Quality standards and accreditation: For COE inclusion, virtually all payers require FACT accreditation of all aspects of the program relevant to the delivery of HCT (e.g., clinical program, collection, cell processing). Already, some payers are already requesting evidence of compliance with the first edition (2017) FACT standards for immune effector cell therapies for inclusion in nascent immunotherapy COE networks.

IMPACTS OF HIGH COSTS AND STILL UNCERTAIN VALUE OF CURRENT T-CELL THERAPIES

Unlike organ acquisition costs in solid organ transplant, and stem cell acquisition costs in autologous and allogeneic HCT, the product cost for current CAR T-cell therapies is high, often many times higher than the typical costs for the clinical care services alone, even in patients without serious adverse effects. For example, initial retail prices for both axicabtagene ciloleucel and tisagenlecleucel were set at $373,000, which includes manufacturing and product procurement, but excludes the significant costs of associated care, which may be substantial especially when toxicities develop. This results in a much higher ratio of product costs to other care costs. In contrast to autologous and allogeneic HCT, the engineered product is often the primary driver of total cost, lessening the ability to create incentives for center efficiency that help to maintain cost containment.

While a discussion of costs and value is beyond the scope of this chapter, frameworks assessing cost per quality-adjusted life years (QALY) gained, an accepted metric of value, have recently been developed, albeit with limited real-world data available to date detailing costs for the entire cycle of patient care. With these caveats, assessments including the initial value assessment of the first two approved CAR T-cell therapies published by the Institute for Clinical and Economic Review (ICER) in 2018 have established a process for ongoing iterative review of the therapeutic value.[50] As expected, given the earlier intervention and greater potential years of life saved for pediatric leukemia patients relative to older adults with lymphoma, value assessments have been more favorable for similar products when applied to pediatric CD19+ ALL[51] versus adults with relapsed and refractory CD19+ lymphomas.[52] The reason for the discussion of costs here is that the high costs (and still relatively uncertain value) of these developing therapies will likely be a strong driver of patient selection, COE network inclusion, and decisions by both private and public payers to cover one or more therapies for a specific indication. Therefore, it is very possible that despite the FDA approval of multiple products for each indication, individual patients may find themselves restricted by these considerations not historically limiting access to other approved therapies.

SUMMARY OF REGULATORY ISSUES AT THE PROGRAM LEVEL

As discussed, the regulation of novel cellular therapies extends beyond the considerable regulatory issues that are already covered by existing and evolving standards designed to limit the risks of novel human gene therapies. These include the use of retroviral and lentiviral transduction approaches to engineer cancer-specific T-cells that are typically expanded ex vivo for therapeutic use and have demonstrated remarkable efficacy in the setting of otherwise refractory malignancies. As noted, the more gradual evolution of the field of hematopoietic cell transplantation has provided context for the societal and regulatory landscape into which these novel therapies have emerged. Already, the FDA has taken a relatively removed stance with respect to HCT therapies, arguably due to the incredible efforts of the HCT community to develop voluntary but highly demanding systems that include SOP-driven clinical care, quality improvement, third-party inspection, and accreditation. Additionally, a highly evolved registry has made remarkable contributions to patient safety, clinical research, and risk-adjusted outcomes reporting that have been endorsed and adopted by federal regulators seeking to improve access to curative cellular therapies while ensuring transparency of outcomes data and patient safety. Finally, the unique economic issues and need for specialized expertise have driven both governmental and private payers to develop de facto standards to limit care to centers likely to maximize access, while optimizing safety. The increasing and remarkable costs of novel therapies will for the foreseeable future maintain consolidation of these therapies within relatively limited networks of centers, compared to other complex therapies not requiring cellular therapy. Increasingly, it is likely that payer frameworks will evolve further to include milestone-based or value-based payment

systems that will better assure a favorable balance of cost to quality. These novel financial models will be needed to ensure that therapies are applied in a cost-effective manner and to encourage development of the most effective and least toxic therapies that may achieve clinical and societal benefit.

ACKNOWLEDGMENTS

Dr. Cornetta's effort was supported, in part, with Federal funds from the National Heart, Lung, and Blood Institute, National Institutes of Health, Department of Health and Human Services, under Contract No. 75N92019D00018 for the National Gene Vector Biorepository Program. Dr. Komanduri acknowledges Stephanie Farnia (BCBS), Patricia Martin (Anthem), and Ronald Potts (INTERLINK and Kaiser Permanente) and members of the Massachusetts Institute of Technology Project on Financing of Curative Therapies in the United States (MIT FoCUS) for helpful discussions related to centers of excellence networks.

COI disclosures: Dr. Cornetta has no disclosures. Dr. Komanduri has provided ad hoc consulting to Kite/Gilead, Novartis, Celgene/Juno, Autolus, Atara, Kiadis, and Takeda. He has no equity positions and no licensed intellectual property.

REFERENCES

1. U.S. Food and Drug Administration. *FDA Approves CAR-T Cell Therapy to Treat Adults with Certain Types of Large B-Cell Lymphoma*. 2017.
2. U.S. Food and Drug Administration. KYMRIAH (tisagenlecleucel). 2018, 05/07/18, July 31, 2018; Available from: https://www.fda.gov/BiologicsBloodVaccines/ CellularGeneTherapyProducts/ApprovedProducts/ ucm573706.htm.
3. Cornetta K, Wilson CA. Safety of retroviral vectors: regulatory and technical considerations. In: Dropulic BACB, ed. *Concepts in Genetic Medicine*. John Wiley & Sons, Inc.; 2008:277–288.
4. Schambach A, Zychlinski D, Ehrnstroem B, Baum C. Biosafety features of lentiviral vectors. *Hum Gene Ther*. 2013;24(2):132–142.
5. Miller AD. Retrovirus packaging cells. *Hum Gene Ther*. 1990;1(1):5–14.
6. Merten O, Charrier S, Laroudie N, et al. Large scale manufacture and characterisation of a lentiviral vector produced for clinical ex vivo gene therapy application. *Hum Gene Ther*. 2011;22:343–356.
7. Kozak SL, Kabat D. Ping-pong amplification of a retroviral vector acheives high-level gene expression: human growth hormone production. *J Virol*. 1990;64:3500–3508.
8. Muenchau DD, Freeman SM, Cornetta K, Zwiebel JA, Anderson WF. Analysis of retroviral packaging lines for

generation of replication-competent virus. *Virology*. 1990; 176:262−265.

9. Cuypers HT, et al. Murine leukemia virus-induced T-cell lymphomagenesis: integration of proviruses in a distinct chromosomal region. *Cell*. 1984;37(1):141−150.

10. van Lohuizen M, Verbeek S, Krimpenfort P, et al. Predisposition to lymphomagenesis in pim-1 transgenic mice: cooperation with c-myc and N-myc in murine leukemia virus-induced tumors. *Cell*. 1989;56(4):673−682.

11. Cornetta K, Nguyen N, Morgan RA, Muenchau DD, Hartley J, Anderson WF. Infection of human cells with murine amphotropic replication-competent retroviruses. *Hum Gene Ther*. 1993;4:579−588.

12. Cornetta K, Moen RC, Culver K, et al. Amphotropic murine leukemia retrovirus is not an acute pathogen for primates. *Hum Gene Ther*. 1990;1:13−26.

13. Donahue RE, Kessler SW, Bodine D, et al. Helper virus induction T cell lymphoma in nonhuman primates after retroviral mediated gene transfer. *J Exp Med*. 1992;176: 1125−1135.

14. U.S. Food and Drug Administration, Guidance for industry − supplemental guidance on testing for replication competent retrovirus in retroviral vector based gene therapy products and during follow-up of patients in clinical trials using retroviral vectors. U.S. Food and Drug Adminstration. November 2006.

15. Chen J, Reeves L, Cornetta K. Safety testing for replication-competent retrovirus (RCR) associated with Gibbon Ape Leukemia Virus pseudotyped retroviral vectors. *Hum Gene Ther*. 2001;12:61−70.

16. Reeves L, Duffy L, Koop S, Fyffe J, Cornetta K. Detection of ecotropic replication-competent retroviruses: comparison of S+/L- and marker rescue assays. *Hum Gene Ther*. 2002; 13:1783−1790.

17. Duffy L, Koop S, Fyffe J, Cornetta K. *Extended S+/L− Assay for Detecting Replication Competent Retroviruses (RCR) Pseudotyped with the RD114 Viral Envelope*. Preclinica; 2003 May/June:53−59.

18. Cornetta K, Morgan RA, Anderson WF. Safety issues related to retroviral-mediated gene transfer in humans. *Hum Gene Ther*. 1991;2(1):5−14.

19. Chong H, Starkey W, Vile RG. A replication-competent retrovirus arising from a split-function packaging cell line was generated by recombination events between the vector, one of the packaging constructs, and endogenous retroviral sequences. *J Virol*. 1998;72:2663−2670.

20. Garrett E, Miller AR, Goldman J, Apperley JF, Melo JV. Characterization of recombinant events leading to the production of an ecotropic replication-competent retrovirus in a GP+envAM12-derived producer cell line. *Virology*. 2000;266:170−179.

21. Cornetta K, Yao J, Jasti A, et al. Replication competent lentivirus analysis of clinical grade vector products. *Mol Ther*. 2011;19:557−566.

22. Sastry L, Cornetta K. Detection of replication competent retrovirus and lentivirus. *Methods Mol Biol*. 2009;506: 243−263.

23. Escarpe P, Zayek N, Chin P, et al. Development of a sensitive assay for detection of replication-competent recombinant lentivirus in large-scale HIV-based vector preparations. *Mol Ther*. 2003;8:332−341.

24. Corre G, Dessainte M, Marteau JB, et al. "RCL-Pooling assay": a simplified method for the detection of replication-competent Lentiviruses in vector Batches using sequential pooling. *Hum Gene Ther*. 2016;27(2):202−210.

25. Farley DC, McCloskey L, Thorne BA, et al. Development of a replication-competent lentivirus assay for dendritic cell-targeting lentiviral vectors. *Mol Ther Methods Clin Dev*. 2015;2:15017.

26. Forestell SP, Dando JS, Bohnlein E, Rigg RJ. Improved detection of replication-competent retrovirus. *J Virol Methods*. 1996;60:171−178.

27. Miskin J, Chipchase D, Rohll J, et al. A replication competent lentivirus (RCL) assay for equine infectious anaemia virus (EIAV)-based lentiviral vectors. *Gene Ther*. 2006;13: 196−205.

28. Wilson CA, Ng T, Miller AE. Evaluation of recommendations for replication-competent retrovirus testing associated with use of retroviral vectors. *Hum Gene Ther*. 1997; 8:869−874.

29. Miller AD, Buttimore C. Redesign of retrovirus packaging cell lines to avoid recombination leading to helper virus production. *Mol Cell Biol*. 1986;6:2895−2902.

30. Miller AD, Garcia JV, Von Suhr N, Lynch CM, Wilson C, Eiden MV. Construction and properties of retrovirus packaging cells based on gibbon ape leukemia virus. *J Virol*. 1991;65:2220−2224.

31. Bear AS, Morgan RA, Cornetta K, et al. Replication-competent retroviruses in gene-modified T cells used in clinical trials: is it time to revise the testing requirements? *Mol Ther*. 2012;20(2):246−249.

32. Cornetta K, Duffy L, Feldman SA, et al. Screening clinical cell products for replication competent retrovirus: the national gene vector biorepository experience. *Mol Ther Methods Clin Dev*. 2018;10:371−378.

33. Marcucci KT, Jadlowsky JK, Hwang WT, et al. Retroviral and lentiviral safety analysis of gene-modified T cell products and infused HIV and oncology patients. *Mol Ther*. 2018;26(1):269−279.

34. Modlich U, Navarro S, Zychlinski D, et al. Insertional transformation of hematopietic cells by self-inactiving lentiviral and gammaretroviral vectors. *Mol Ther*. 2009;17: 1919−1928.

35. Cornetta K, Duffy L, Turtle CJ, et al. Absence of replication-competent lentivirus in the clinic: analysis of infused T cell products. *Mol Ther*. 2018;28:280−288.

36. U.S. Food and Drug Administration, ed. *Testing of Retroviral Vector-Based Human Gene Therapy Products for Replication Competent Retrovirus during Product Manufacture and Patient Follow-Up Draft Guidance of Industry*. Center for Biologics Evaluation and Research; 2018.

37. Braun CJ, Boztug K, Paruzynski A, et al. Gene therapy for Wiskott-Aldrich syndrome—long-term efficacy and genotoxicity. *Sci Transl Med*. 2014;6(227):227ra33.

38. Stein S, Ott MG, Schultze-Strasser S, et al. Genomic instability and myelodysplasia with monosomy 7 consequent to EVI1 activation after gene therapy for chronic granulomatous disease. *Nat Med.* 2010;16:198−204.

39. Nienhuis AW, Dunbar CE, Sorrentino BP. Genotoxicity of retroviral integration in hematopoietic cells. *Mol Ther.* 2006;13:1031−1049.

40. Fraietta JA, Nobles CL, Sammons MA, et al. Disruption of TET2 promotes the therapeutic efficacy of CD19-targeted T cells. *Nature.* 2018;558(7709):307−312.

41. Biasco L, Rothe M, Buning H, Schambach A. Analyzing the genotoxicity of retroviral vectors in hematopoietic cell gene therapy. *Mol Ther Methods Clin Dev.* 2018;8:21−30.

42. NMDP Transplant Center Listing. Available from: https://bethematch.org/tcdirectory/search/.

43. U.S. Food and Drug Administration. *Regulatory Considerations for Human Cells, Tissues, and Cellular and Tissue-Based Products: Minimal Manipulation and Homologous Use.* Guidance for Industry and Food and Drug Administration Staff; 2017.

44. Maus MV, Nikiforow S. The why, what, and how of the new FACT standards for immune effector cells. *J Immunother Cancer.* 2017;5(1):36.

45. Stem Cell Therapeutic and Research Act. 2005. Available from: https://www.govinfo.gov/content/pkg/STATUTE-119/pdf/STATUTE-119-Pg2550.pdf.

46. Stem Cell Therapeutic and Research Reauthorization Act. 2010. Available from: https://www.congress.gov/111/plaws/publ264/PLAW-111publ264.pdf.

47. Stem Cell Therapeutic and Research Reauthorization Act. 2015. Available from: https://www.govinfo.gov/content/pkg/PLAW-114publ104/pdf/PLAW-114publ104.pdf.

48. Lee DW, Santomasso BD, Locke FL, et al. ASTCT consensus grading for cytokine release syndrome and neurologic toxicity associated with immune effector cells. *Biol Blood Marrow Transplant.* 2019;25(4):625−638.

49. Komanduri KV, Potts R, Martin P. Role of Centers of Excellence (COE) Networks in the Delivery of Curative Cellular Therapies in Oncology. MIT NEWDIGS Research Brief 2018F209-v026-COE. 2018. Available from: https://newdigs.mit.edu/sites/default/files/FoCUS%20Research%20Brief%202018F209v026_0.pdf.

50. ICER. *Chimeric Antigen Receptor TCell Therapy for B-Cell Cancers: Effectiveness and Value;* 2018 [cited Jun 9 2018; Available from: https://icer-review.org/wp-content/uploads/2017/07/ICER_CAR_T_Final_Evidence_Report_032318.pdf.

51. Lin JK, Lerman BJ, Barnes JI, et al. Cost effectiveness of chimeric antigen receptor Tcell therapy in relapsed or refractory pediatric B-cell acute lymphoblastic leukemia. *J Clin Oncol.* 2018. JCO2018790642.

52. Lin JK, Muffly LS, Spinner MA, et al. Cost effectiveness of chimeric antigen receptor Tcell therapy in multiply relapsed or refractory adult large Bcell lymphoma. *J Clin Oncol.* 2019. JCO1802079.

Index

Note: Page numbers followed by "f" indicate figures, "t" indicates tables.

Printed and bound by CPI Group (UK) Ltd, Croydon, CR0 4YY

03/10/2024

01040349-0001